"It is to the political credit of psychoanalysis', wrote Michel Foucault in the *History of Sexuality*, that in contrast to psychiatry and the German psychotherapy of the Nazi years, the 'Freudian endeavour' remained 'in theoretical and practical opposition to fascism'. In this magisterial historical work, Laura Sokolowsky details how the Berlin Psychoanalytic Institute resisted attempts to replace psychoanalysis with therapies based on identification and suggestion, practices more conducive to totalitarianism. In so doing she draws some significant lessons about the current travails of psychoanalysis in the context of contemporary politics and the prevailing state of the discourse of the master."

– Scott Wilson, Professor of Media and Communication, Kingston School of Art, London

"Laura Sokolowsky has given us that precious thing – a history which illuminates the urgent stakes of our present. Detailing the socially engaged innovations that marked the Berlin Psychoanalytic Institute's first flowering during the Weimar years, but also tracking its painful compromises with a Nazi regime that burned Freud's books, this lucid work provides us with a reminder: to remain subversive, psychoanalysis must be guided not by state power but by the desire of Freud and Lacan. In an era of the neoliberalisation of health, Laura Sokolowsky's brilliantly evoked history could not be more timely."

– Colin Wright, Associate Professor of Critical Theory, University of Nottingham

Psychoanalysis Under Nazi Occupation

Laura Sokolowsky's survey of psychoanalysis under Weimar and Nazism explores how the paradigm of a 'psychoanalysis for all' became untenable as the Nazis rose to power.

Mainly discussing the evolution of the Berlin Institute during the period between Freud's creation of free psychoanalytic centres after the founding of the Weimar Republic and the Nazi seizure of power in 1933, the book explores the ideal of making psychoanalysis available to the population of a shattered country after World War I, and charts how the Institute later came under Nazi control following the segregation and dismissal of Jewish colleagues in the late 1930s. The book shows how Freudian standards resisted the medicalisation of psychoanalysis for purposes of adaptation and normalisation, but also follows Freud's distinction between sacrifice (where you know what you have given up) and concession (an abandonment of position through compromise) to demonstrate how German psychoanalysts put themselves at the service of the fascist master, in the hope of obtaining official recognition and material rewards.

Discussing the relations of psychoanalysis with politics and ethics, as well as the origin of the Lacanian movement as a response to the institutionalisation of psychoanalysis during the Nazi occupation, this book is fascinating reading for scholars and practitioners of psychoanalysis working today.

Laura Sokolowsky is a psychoanalyst and member of the École de la Cause Freudienne and the World Association of Psychoanalysis. She is the current director of the psychoanalytical journal *La Cause du désir*.

The Lines of the Symbolic in Psychoanalysis Series

Series Editor:
Ian Parker, *Manchester Psychoanalytic Matrix*

Psychoanalytic clinical and theoretical work is always embedded in specific linguistic and cultural contexts and carries their traces, traces which this series attends to in its focus on multiple contradictory and antagonistic 'lines of the Symbolic'. This series takes its cue from Lacan's psychoanalytic work on three registers of human experience, the Symbolic, the Imaginary and the Real, and employs this distinctive understanding of cultural, communication and embodiment to link with other traditions of cultural, clinical and theoretical practice beyond the Lacanian symbolic universe. The Lines of the Symbolic in Psychoanalysis Series provides a reflexive reworking of theoretical and practical issues, translating psychoanalytic writing from different contexts, grounding that work in the specific histories and politics that provide the conditions of possibility for its descriptions and interventions to function. The series makes connections between different cultural and disciplinary sites in which psychoanalysis operates, questioning the idea that there could be one single correct reading and application of Lacan. Its authors trace their own path, their own line through the Symbolic, situating psychoanalysis in relation to debates which intersect with Lacanian work, explicating it, extending it and challenging it.

Schizostructuralism
Divisions in Structure, Surface, Temporality, Class
Daniel Bristow

Obscenity, Psychoanalysis and Literature
Lawrence and Joyce on Trial
William Simms

Lacan, Mortality, Life and Language
Clinical and Cultural Explorations
Berjanet Jazani

Psychoanalysis Under Nazi Occupation
The Origins, Impact and Influence of the Berlin Institute
Laura Sokolowsky

Psychoanalysis Under Nazi Occupation

The Origins, Impact and Influence of the Berlin Institute

Laura Sokolowsky

Translated by
Janet Haney and John Haney

Routledge
Taylor & Francis Group
LONDON AND NEW YORK

First published 2022
by Routledge
2 Park Square, Milton Park, Abingdon, Oxon OX14 4RN

and by Routledge
605 Third Avenue, New York, NY 10158

Routledge is an imprint of the Taylor & Francis Group, an informa business

British Library Cataloguing-in-Publication Data
A catalogue record for this book is available from the British Library

Library of Congress Cataloging-in-Publication Data
A catalog record has been requested for this book

ISBN: 978-1-032-10518-5 (hbk)
ISBN: 978-1-032-10519-2 (pbk)
ISBN: 978-1-003-21568-4 (ebk)

DOI: 10.4324/9781003215684

Typeset in Times New Roman
by Taylor & Francis Books

Contents

Tables

Acknowledgements

I would like to thank my colleagues at the École de la Cause Freudienne for their questions and comments. In particular I would like to thank Marie-Hélène Brousse, Jean-Claude Maleval and Laurent Ottavi for reading the manuscript so attentively. I would also like to thank Pierre Naveau for his listening, as well as my friend Marina Lusa for her indefatigable support.

I greatly appreciate the assistance provided by the Freud Archives at the Library of Congress in Washington, D.C., and especially Leonard Bruno. I am also grateful to the library of the London Institute of Psychoanalysis for having allowed me to consult many unpublished documents.

Finally, without the love and patience of my companion Jean-Michel and my two children, Louise and Corentin, I would not have been able to bring this book to completion. I thank them with all my heart.

Series preface

Each and every history is a 'history of the present', something that psychoanalysts know well, whether they are listening to the patching together of a life narrative in the clinic or piecing together the cultural-political conditions for the development of psychoanalysis as such. At stake in this compelling and necessary exploration of the life and times of the 'Berlin Institute' is the way that the attempt to formalise training of psychoanalysts between the First and Second World Wars, and then as the Nazis held central Europe in their grip, resonates with and informs present-day debates over the nature of our practice, how we learn it and how it is validated.

Laura Sokolowsky builds up a case – through careful examination of archival materials and analytic conceptual reflection on existing histories of 'Freud's Free Clinics' in Budapest, Vienna and Berlin – that we should attend to what she calls 'the crucial signifier' of adaptation. Adaptation as key signifier of the attempts by Freud and his colleagues to address the threat of medicalisation, reframing of psychoanalytic clinic work as a therapeutic endeavour and the rise of fascism, cues us into a series of errors and traps.

The errors are, Sokolowsky shows us in this indispensable and properly psychoanalytic study of the attempt to make psychoanalysis both 'accessible' and 'respectable', a function of the symbolic structuring of the clinic and then the increasing popularity of psychoanalysis in Germany between the wars. In this sense, the errors were unavoidable, and the configuring of psychoanalysis as a social intervention carried in its wake fear of how it might escape into the wild – 'wild analysis' in popular culture and in the hands of the lay analysts, particularly those who were not medically trained, was viewed as a threat. Such fear determined, appeared to logically and inevitably lead to the application of rules governing training and application of psychoanalysis, what today would be called 'good governance' by those who profoundly misunderstand what psychoanalysis is really about.

The traps comprise the different responses to these fears, responses which bind the psychoanalysts all the more into the very forms of conformism and surveillance that Freud himself warned against. Would that we could take heed of the sharp choice that Freud posed between what must be sacrificed to protect the integrity of psychoanalytic theory and practice or what concessions many of his colleagues, unwittingly or deliberately, were willing to make to the enemy.

This book traces the symbolic context in which psychoanalysis became sedimented as a cultural form, crystallised as an institution, bureaucratised, and we are thereby able to notice the imaginary effects of that, in justification for bad choices and bad faith on the part of some involved, as the institutions of psychoanalysis – here the Berlin Institute – encountered the real; deadly forking paths led away from psychoanalysis as such, paths back into medicine and into therapy.

Psychoanalytic clinical and theoretical work circulates through multiple intersecting antagonistic symbolic universes. This series opens connections between different cultural sites in which Lacanian work has developed in distinctive ways, in forms of work that question the idea that there could be single correct reading and application. The Lines of the Symbolic in Psychoanalysis series provides a reflexive reworking of psychoanalysis that transmits Lacanian writing from around the world, steering a course between the temptations of a metalanguage and imaginary reduction, between the claim to provide a god's eye view of psychoanalysis and the idea that psychoanalysis must everywhere be the same. And the elaboration of psychoanalysis in the symbolic here grounds its theory and practice in the history and politics of the work in a variety of interventions that touch the real.

Ian Parker
Manchester Psychoanalytic Matrix

List of acronyms used

BPV	Berliner Psychoanalytische Vereinigung (Berlin Psychoanalytic Association, 1910–1926)
DPG	Deutsche Psychoanalytische Gesellschaft (German Psychoanalytic Society, 1926–1936)
DAÄGP	Deutsche Allgemeine Ärtzliche Gesellschaft für Psychotherapie (German General Medical Society for Psychotherapy)
IPA	International Psychoanalytical Association
KPD	Kommunistische Partei Deutschlands (Communist Party of Germany)
NSDAP	Nationalsozialistische Deutsche Arbeiterpartei (National Socialist German Workers' Party, aka Nazi Party)
SPD	Sozialdemokratische Partei Deutschlands (Social Democratic Party of Germany)
WPV	Wiener Psychoanalytische Vereinigung (Vienna Psychoanalytic Association)

Introduction

Freud's warning regarding therapy

Throughout the 1920s, Sigmund Freud led a battle against the psychoanalytic association that he had founded in 1910. His defence of lay psychoanalysis pitted him against those colleagues who wanted to turn his discovery into a credible and respectable practice that would be useful to society and on a par with medicine. This tendency to medicalise psychoanalysis was fiercely contested by Freud, to the point where he envisaged resigning from the International Psychoanalytical Association (IPA) should it maintain its position in relation to the rejection of non-doctors. Where had this medicalising tendency come from? Did it come about because some practitioners wanted to assure their academic or professional reputations? Was it because psychiatrists who had trained as psychoanalysts wanted to preserve their prerogatives at a moment when psychoanalysis was becoming fashionable and attracting other professions – teachers, educators and psychologists? Was medicalisation linked to historical circumstances or to ideological choices?

What Freud saw was the danger of transforming psychoanalysis into a healing technique, of adapting it to social norms. The insertion of a chapter on Freudian theory into a psychiatric manual was hardly, he felt, a good omen. It didn't represent progress or recognition. It signalled an assimilation of psychoanalysis by the current discourse and provided proof that his own discourse was about to lose its subversive element. It implied that the best way of resisting psychoanalysis was to turn it into psychotherapy. Some eighty years later, French psychoanalysts refused the enactment of a regulatory amendment stipulating that only doctors and certified psychologists would be authorised to practise any kind of psychotherapy. Presented as a precautionary measure meant to protect patients from charlatans who would set themselves up as psychotherapists without having received adequate training, this amendment gave doctors privileges as exorbitant as they were unjustified: hence, doctors become psychotherapists without having to prove themselves through any kind of training in the matter; they could then go on to prescribe therapies using their established diagnostic protocols and could even choose – and evaluate – different treatments. The

DOI: 10.4324/9781003215684-1

supremacy accorded to psychiatrists by this legislative mechanism triggered a protest by psychoanalysts of different schools. Many of them denounced the ambiguity of the term 'psychotherapy' employed at the time. And so, some years later and in different places, we find psychotherapy striving to absorb psychoanalysis. This had already happened in Freud's time. The events that took place in France at the beginning of the twenty-first century – in the country where psychoanalysis resists diverse attempts intended to weaken and discredit it – show that the battle is far from over.

Freud, originally a doctor, began by treating hysterics' symptoms by means of hypnosis. However, it was by renouncing the powers that medicine had conferred on him that he invented a singular technique based on the speech of the patient: one speaks, the other listens and interprets what is said in a manner that is punctuated and rather rare. The analyst is responsible for the unfolding of the analysis, but he does not direct his patient. Psychoanalysis is born of the refusal to make suggestions; it is distinguished in that regard from psychotherapy. Ultimately, the only power of psychoanalysis is the power of speech, not the power of the psychoanalyst. Psychoanalysis certainly has therapeutic effects, but it does not proceed from the desire to cure; it does not aim at the relief of psychic suffering, at access to greater liberty or at the strengthening of individual autonomy. The psychoanalyst does not dispense advice on getting better; he does not invite anyone to free themselves from a behaviour that doesn't fit in. The analyst has a certain knowledge, but he or she does not know in advance what the patient is suffering from or how to remedy it. The knowledge of the psychoanalyst comes from his or her own analysis; it results from an extraction of unconscious knowledge – from a knowledge unknown to the subject. Pursuant to this decipherment, the unbearable sadness of existence is transformed into a function supporting a new desire. The desire of the analyst stems from a journey – sometimes a long one – which is not that of a cure in the classical sense of the term. The journey is not a return to the state that preceded the illness. Analysis does not cure, it transforms – it modifies the relation to the symptom. One doesn't succeed in changing oneself totally: the constant revealed by the symptom is the repetition of a mode of drive jouissance. What one does succeed in modifying is the way of making do with this symptomatic repetition insofar as it leaves in the body a trace of a singular event – the contingent encounter with jouissance. What Freud distinguished as trauma, Jacques Lacan defined as a traumatism of language to the extent that the symbolic is marked by a lack. There is something that is impossible to say, to symbolise, to signify. The rapport between the sexes is marked by this impossible, which Lacan called the nonexistence of the sexual rapport. This relation between man and woman cannot be written, and from that there is hardly any remedy. That is the reason why love is a substitute for this non-rapport; it is a creation, a symptomatic invention proper to each. Psychoanalysis does not aim at a cure because nothing is capable of curing speaking beings of this flaw, this non-rapport. On the contrary, acknowledging the weight of speech once heard, forgotten, but foundational – made with a drive jouissance resulting from a traumatic encounter whose effects have not ceased to create one's destiny – has nothing to do with psychotherapy understood as a corrective adaptation of the individual to his environment. Psychoanalysis does not aim at the eradication of the symptom considered in isolation. The essential question for psychoanalysis is the status of the symptom. Throughout the history of the analytic movement, the training of psychoanalysts examines this non-therapeutic dimension. Freud's battle against the medicalisation of psychoanalysis is still with us today. It turns out that psychoanalysts themselves can sometimes forget to take care of the future of 'their science'. It is nevertheless customary to establish a distinction between the therapeutic application of psychoanalysis and the formation of analysts. Pure psychoanalysis, or didactic analysis, would not be a therapeutic technique. It's just that one can ask oneself if the destiny of psychoanalysis isn't at stake, structurally, on this score: when it identifies with therapeutics, psychoanalysis is threatened. It no longer unsettles – it adapts and assimilates. Freud did not think otherwise. His astounding formula, according to which therapeutics could kill science, had the sense of a warning. And yet the inventor of psychoanalysis never ceased to work on the development of his discovery. How can we assure the diffusion of psychoanalysis in society? How should we transmit it to future generations?

On the treatment of neuroses in free clinics

The future of psychoanalysis was evoked differently by Freud at different times. The first scansion of his reflection accompanied the creation of the IPA in 1910. The second was enunciated shortly before the end of World War I, in September 1918. Two years later, in the autumn of 1920, Freud was called as an expert witness to testify in front of a parliamentary commission tasked with ascertaining whether or not military doctors had abused their duty of care in relation to soldiers who had been traumatised by war. On that occasion, Freud recalled that psychoanalysis had been applied on a large scale during the last months of the conflict. He reiterated what he had said two years earlier, during the IPA's Fifth Congress, on the subject of the application of psychoanalysis to the masses. The creation of the Berlin Psychoanalytic Polyclinic for the Treatment of Nervous Diseases, which was inaugurated in the spring of 1920, inscribed itself in a series of developments in analytic therapeutics.

At the moment of the creation of the IPA, at a congress in Nuremberg in 1910, Freud had already put the emphasis on therapeutics. He had indicated that civilised sexual morality imposed limits on drive satisfactions. Without this barrier to jouissance, there would be no civilisation. Faced with the conflicts resulting from the necessity of repressing the drive, many human beings took refuge in illness. The psychoanalyst does not have the right to approach life as a fanatic for hygiene or therapy, said Freud, who pointed out that a 'good number of those who now take flight into illness would not [be able to] support the conflict'.[1] They would succumb or would cause much worse problems. Because neuroses offer protection against harm, Freud believed that they have a biological function of protection. Leading on from that, they also have a social justification. Symptoms have a reason for being – there is always an intention in illness. To deny that would be to believe that neuroses have nothing of the real about them, Freud said.

Since repression is a balancing factor on the collective scale, it would be nonsensical to want to cure all neuroses. They have a social utility – their secondary benefit is not purely subjective. If symptoms have a regulatory function, it would be necessary to take some precautions before doing without them. We know that psychoanalysis does not have an ambition to cure at any price, and we also know that the disappearance of the symptom is not the end in itself of a psychoanalytic cure. The therapeutic effect is certainly not the last word of an analysis, and the disappearance of the symptom is not equivalent to the resolution of the neurosis. What is expressed via the mask of the symptom is a desire that one does not want and that one represses. Freud said that the prophylactic action of psychoanalysis would be determinant for its future. The fact that it's not necessary to cure every neurosis must not put obstacles in the way of the duty to elucidate that is incumbent on psychoanalysts. Regrouping in the form of an international association, he said, would allow analysts to combat ignorance and to enlighten the masses because the energy wasted in the production of symptoms would be made available for the transformation of civilisation. The diffusion of psychoanalytic concepts would produce an authentic enlightenment of the masses because guarding against the neuroses would be linked to the introduction of a new knowledge into civilisation. It would be necessary not to recoil from the risk of revealing the secret of the neuroses while overturning the social order.

Freud did not pretend that it would be possible to eradicate neurosis from civilisation. He was, however, betting on the dissemination of psychoanalytic concepts as a prophylactic action. To convince people that his arguments were well-founded, he borrowed an example from the domain of belief. It had become rare for women to have apparitions of the Virgin Mary once the church began to ask doctors to examine these visionaries, he said. If the call to medical knowledge had had immediate repercussions in the sense of a scarcity of visionary phenomena, it was no less certain that psychoanalytical revelations would have an effect on those who found refuge in neurosis. The diffusion of psychoanalytic knowledge would produce a therapeutic action and would do so, moreover, on a collective scale.

In his 1910 speech, Freud addressed the diffusion of psychoanalytic concepts – which is to say, knowledge in the public domain and not unconscious knowledge, which is deciphered in the cure. Lacan, for his part, was to state – in 1971 – that psychoanalysis does not add knowledge to the body of knowledge already in existence. The Freudian discovery introduced a subversion into the structure of knowledge itself. It's a question of an articulated knowledge that has nothing to do with the ego: it is a knowledge that doesn't know itself. This new status of knowledge is bound up with a new discourse, named by Lacan as the discourse of the psychoanalyst, 'one that is not easy to maintain and which, up to a certain point, has yet to be begun'.[2] One's resistance to psychoanalysis comes from the misunderstanding (indeed, the rejection) of the ex-centricity of knowledge in its unconscious form in relation to the ego and its mastery. In other words, the discourse of the psychoanalyst sustains itself in a relation to knowledge which is not that of the subject of knowledge. Consequently, reproaching psychoanalysts for wanting to escape from the protocols of scientific experimentation misses the point. It's not a question of will, or of a refusal, but of a difference regarding the structure of the knowledge in play. If analysis demonstrates the existence of an unknown knowledge, what is this knowledge that does not know itself? This is the fundamental problem of psychoanalysis. From a purely therapeutic perspective, such an orientation can seem unsettling. Psychoanalysis has therapeutic effects, but it is not a therapy as such. The reason is simple: the symptom as defined by psychoanalysis is not conceived of as an abnormal phenomenon that disturbs good cognitive functioning and the individual's adaptation to his or her environment. Besides, the Freudian thesis concerning the function of the symptom insofar as it cannot be healed prefigures the thesis that Lacan developed many years later. For Lacan, there is a coherence between the unconscious and the symptom: the symptom is defined by the way in which each of us enjoys the unconscious insofar as the unconscious determines us.[3] There can be no drive without a symptom. In his last teaching, Lacan further radicalises the function of the symptom. It becomes the sinthome – it knots the real, the symbolic and the imaginary. The fourth ring has a function that situates it beyond decipherment and meaning.

Freud delivered his other great discourse on the future of psychoanalysis at the end of September 1918. Since the creation of the IPA eight years earlier, the world had changed. By the autumn of 1918, the war was already lost for the German and Austro-Hungarian coalition. This conferred a particular significance on Freud's comments on the discipline's future prospects, delivered a few weeks before the Armistice, which came into effect in November 1918. Confronted by the extent of the traumas of World War I, as well as by the immense disarray and dilapidated state structures of the former Central European powers, Freud explained that it was no longer necessary to focus solely on the effects of the dissemination of psychoanalytic knowledge. Psychoanalysts were going to have to engage in the reconstruction of a civilisation marked by catastrophe. He proceeded to a rigorous revision of the therapeutic data then available and indicated new lines of advance in psychoanalysis. He suggested, in particular, that it would be necessary to create free psychoanalytic centres to treat people who had been most severely affected by the ravages of war. He expressed himself as follows:

> Now let us assume that by some kind of organization we succeeded in increasing our numbers to an extent sufficient for treating a considerable mass of the population. On the other hand, it is possible to foresee that at some time or other the conscience of society will awake and remind it that the poor man should have just as much right to assistance for his mind as he now has to the life-saving help offered by surgery; and that the neuroses threaten public health no less than tuberculosis, and can be left as little as the latter to the impotent care of individual members of the community. When this happens, institutions or out-patient clinics will be started, to which analytically-trained physicians will be appointed, so that men who would otherwise give way to drink, women who have nearly succumbed under their burden of privations, children for whom there is no choice but between running wild or neurosis, may be made capable, by analysis, of resistance and of efficient work. Such treatments will be free. It may be a long time before the State comes to see these duties as urgent. Present conditions may delay its arrival even longer. Probably these institutions will first be started by private charity. Some time or other, however, it must come to this.[4]

Six weeks before the end of the war, representatives of the governments of the Central Powers (Austria-Hungary and Germany) attended the IPA's Fifth Congress, which took place at the Hungarian Academy of Sciences in Budapest. The Royal and Imperial Ministry of War in Vienna sent medical staff: two majors, a general and a commander. The German government sent two majors. The psychoanalysts were welcomed by the mayor of the city, and a boat was on hand to take them on a trip down the Danube. Therapy for war neurosis was on the programme. A discussion on the theme took place, with contributions from Freud, Karl Abraham, Sándor Ferenczi, Ernst Simmel and Ernest Jones. According to Jones, it was Simmel's published work on war neuroses that had first caught the interest of the governmental, medical and military authorities.[5] It's important to remember that it was in front of an assembly composed of psychoanalysts and military doctors that Freud suggested creating psychoanalytic centres in the army. This mixed audience must be remembered in order to avoid misinterpretation. Without due care, one risks transforming the inventor of psychoanalysis into an idealistic therapist or a humanist do-gooder. Freud was neither one nor the other.

The incidence of war neuroses

Therapy for war neuroses was a major bet for the psychoanalytic movement during this period. It now became possible to contemplate obtaining official recognition of psychoanalysis. Medical doctors hostile to such a development would have found it more difficult to discredit a practice recognised by the authorities. But what explains these government representatives' interest in psychoanalysis? By the winter of 1917–1918, the interminable and murderous war on the Western and Eastern fronts had severely impacted the morale of soldiers and civilians alike. Wounded soldiers continued to flood the health services. Furthermore, the increase in war neuroses was also linked to the decline of patriotic ideals, to a collapse in morale as much as to the next defeat. Discouragement and exhaustion progressively took hold of the civilian populations, which were facing mounting economic difficulties. They also affected the fighting spirit, that part of the personality described by Freud as a kind of identification that leads the combatant to despise danger and to think himself immortal. The growth in the number of war neuroses was also linked to this decline of heroic and patriotic ideals. Military psychiatrists found themselves in difficulties when faced with the failure of the electric-shock treatments they were administering to multitudes of traumatised soldiers. In September 1918, psychoanalysis – or, rather, a mixed and derivative version of psychoanalysis – came just in time to prove its worth. Those of Freud's students who had been called to the colours had obtained considerable therapeutic success in the treatment of war neuroses. The comprehensive presentation that Ferenczi made at the Budapest congress demonstrated how the psychic source of neuroses was a factor in this. The collective experience of war had produced a considerable number of serious neuroses from which all mechanical and organic effect was excluded. The neurologists had to admit that they had not taken sufficient account of the psychic nature of these symptoms.[6]

Ferenczi recalled that people suffering from war neuroses were often considered by psychiatrists to be malingerers and were treated by electric shocks with results that were mixed, not to say tragic. These electrical treatments were based on terror. The expected result was the replacement of one aversion by another, with the traumatised soldier ending up being more terrorised by the electric shocks than by the prospect of returning to combat. The problem was that it was always necessary to increase the force of the electric current, and some soldiers had not survived this treatment. For their part, the analytically trained psychiatric doctors like Simmel and Max Eitingon had obtained good results by using a cathartic process. The method employed by Simmel at one military hospital consisted of a combination of cathartic hypnosis and dream interpretation, both in a waking state and under hypnosis. Simmel claimed to have made the symptoms disappear after an average of two or three sessions. This combined and shortened method did not aim at the analytic healing of the entire personality. That was not the aim of this brief application of analytic therapy in time of war. Further clinical examination would be indispensable before one could be in a position to claim long-term therapeutic effects.

This use of psychoanalysis clearly had a humanitarian aim. With the soldiers suffering from traumatic neuroses being perceived as malingerers by the military authorities, the treatment they received essentially punished them for their so-called cowardice by means of repeated sessions of excruciatingly painful electrotherapy. In Austria, Dr Michal Kozlowski, an assistant of the celebrated Dr Julius Wagner-Jauregg, was in charge of the electrical treatments at Wagner-Jauregg's clinic. This disquieting personage allowed his sadistic tendencies to express themselves with impunity in applying the electrical brushes to the chests and testicles of terrified soldiers. 'My cures are incisive,' he sarcastically declared.[7] This truly nightmarish figure, seemingly straight out of a Nazi concentration camp, was also called before the Austrian Parliamentary Commission in October 1920. The commission had been tasked with investigating abuses committed by military psychiatrists accused of having subjected traumatised soldiers to excessive electric shocks. In front of a public audience, Freud delivered an expert report that contradicted, on a certain number of points, the arguments put forward by the representatives of official psychiatry. On this occasion, Freud emphasised that, before the end of the war, the psychoanalytic method had given very convincing results in the treatment of revolving-door cases of war neuroses: 'There was a psychoanalytic congress in Budapest and the Austrian government sent a senior doctor to find out what was going on because it wanted to set up psychoanalytic services for the treatment of these illnesses,' said Freud.

Psychoanalysis presented itself as an alternative to the violence of a method that demonstrated technology's grip on humanity, which the war had accelerated. Based on an electrical apparatus that permitted the production-line treatment of individuals in specialised service centres, the faradisation sessions could last half an hour or even longer. They generally took place before a team that was as terrified as the patient himself. It was also about provoking fear in those who were going to be subjected to the same treatment. The unfortunate soldier was held down and given shocks up to the point where he emitted terrifying cries. Others were subjected to gymnastic exercises up to the point of complete exhaustion. Some soldiers were placed in isolation cells for several weeks. All these violent measures were supported by the psychiatrists of the period, who claimed to have been put under pressure by the military authorities, who were demanding results. One argument in their defence was that electroshock therapy was used on hysterical patients in peacetime. In reality, the technique had been taken up because it was quick and cheap, and was then adapted to the treatment of the masses. The treatments adopted in military hospitals by Freud's students clearly ran contrary to these cruel and, it seems, less effective methods. The mixed method set up by Simmel was presented as an alternative to the violence of electroshock treatment. Moreover, it allowed a response to the argument that the psychoanalytic method was of no use in large-scale treatments. When Freud specified that one had to mix the pure gold of analysis with the copper of suggestion in psychoanalytic centres, he had in mind the practice inaugurated by his colleagues and students during the war.

The volume bringing together the contributions on the therapy of war neuroses presented at the Budapest congress was published the following year, with an introduction by Freud. He referred to the presence of government representatives and to the hopes raised by the analytic treatment of these ailments. He also recalled the engagement to establish psychoanalytic centres where doctors with analytic training would work. The Minister for War was thanked for his participation in the congress by Ferenczi in his capacity as president of the IPA.

Beyond the project of creating free treatment centres, taking psychoanalysis to a whole new level was the key issue. Freud imagined the social mission of psychoanalysis in a world overturned by war, stressing the necessity of rebuilding a civilisation that had been devastated by the death drive. But had he foreseen that an increase in the authority of psychoanalysis could result in recognition by the state? Probably not – Freud's correspondence hardly goes in this direction. It seems, rather, that he was surprised by the sudden interest of the military authorities, coming as it did at a time when fatigue and desire to see an end to the war were prevalent. Freud's attention to the therapy of war neuroses responded first of all to an opportunity that was not calculated. It was about not losing an opportunity to present the theory of neuroses in front of representatives of medicine and official psychiatry. From a scientific point of view, on the other hand, Freud didn't believe that the battle concerning war neuroses had been won. This had served to convince the medical corps of the importance of the psychogenesis of neurotic troubles, and he had put the emphasis on the gain of the illness, on the flight into illness. But even though Freud had taken this position a little late, the fact remained that no one had been able to carry out a deep analysis of a case of war neurosis. One could not, said Freud, draw valid conclusions. The analytic therapy of war neuroses was above all conceived as a way of popularising the practice in the medical corps. It was going to be up to Freud to draw decisive conclusions from certain facts that had still not been clarified, such as the repetition of unpleasure in the dreams of those traumatised by war. The question of repetition in traumatic dreaming was developed during the period 1919–1920 and appears in the second part of *Beyond the Pleasure Principle.*

The turning point of Budapest

In the wake of the Fifth Congress, Budapest seemed to offer the most favourable conditions for the creation of a first psychoanalytic institution. On 9 October 1918, a decree from the Austro-Hungarian Ministry of War entitled 'Further Implementation of Neurological Services for the Treatment of War Neuroses' referred explicitly to the methods employed by psychoanalysts in military hospitals. Freud noted, however, the lack of discernible financial support. During the same period, Ferenczi was contacted by the head of health services in the Budapest military command. In the report that he delivered to the Ministry of War, Ferenczi recommended that a psychoanalytic outpost be created in the capital. He thought it preferable to begin with a small establishment that would receive about thirty patients. He was hoping to get Max Eitingon or István Hollós to assist him.

In March 1919, the communist politician and activist Béla Kun established the Hungarian Soviet Republic, which, during the 103 days of its existence, offered the hope that Hungary would be the first country where psychoanalysis would enjoy official recognition. An unprecedented enthusiasm for psychoanalysis was apparent there, in large part due to the personality of Ferenczi, who was both a physician and a psychoanalyst. The health insurance system would, it was hoped, open a psychoanalytic dispensary for workers as well as a psychoanalytic clinic for which Ferenczi would be responsible. In the same vein, medical students wanted to establish a student psychoanalytic association which would be placed under his stewardship. Was the influence of the Russian Revolution going to play a role in the institutional development of psychoanalysis? The conspicuously optimistic Ferenczi wanted to believe it. He wrote to Freud that psychoanalysis was being courted from all sides and that private practice would be totally suppressed. From then on, psychoanalysts would work in hospitals. One can also date from this period the insertion of psychoanalysis into the university discourse, since Ferenczi was to be named holder of the first chair in psychoanalysis at Budapest University. In the face of these encouraging prospects, Freud's more prudent nature led him to demonstrate a certain reserve. For Freud, psychoanalysis had to protect its independence at all costs. Besides, he had no faith in Kun's regime. It was not so much the prospect of official recognition that disturbed him – it was the development of a psychoanalysis cut off from all private practice, as suggested by Ferenczi.

It quickly became necessary to recognise the fact that events were not going to turn out the way Ferenczi had hoped. Beginning in August 1919, an unprecedented wave of reactionary and anti-Semitic terror unfolded in Hungary when Rear-Admiral Miklós Horthy seized power. Many Hungarian analysts had to emigrate. Some, including Sándor Radó and Jenö Harnick, decided to rejoin the group of analysts who were working with Karl Abraham in Berlin. The death of Dr Anton von Freund in January 1920 completely put an end to the hope of opening a psychoanalytic clinic in Budapest. Von Freund, who came from a family of brewers and had a doctorate in law, was extremely wealthy. He had dreamed of devoting himself to teaching, but he went into his father's business, where he had great success as a manufacturer and administrator. This professional success did nothing, however, to satisfy his true interests – social work and scientific activity. What truly motivated von Freund was the ideal of social justice. It was Freud – who had cured von Freund of a serious neurosis – who put him in touch with Ferenczi. Von Freund had been General Secretary of the IPA since the Budapest congress. Knowing himself to be seriously ill, he wished to place his fortune at the service of the analytic cause. He actually had a fund drawn from the immense profits realised by his industrial enterprises during the war. A significant amount of money was transferred to Freud with the agreement of the mayor of Budapest. This donation served to finance the Internationaler Psychoanalytischer Verlag, the psychoanalytic publishing house, in 1918. At the same time, von Freund wanted to create a centre for analytical teaching and theory. This project failed due to the political upheavals that intervened shortly after the premature death of this great defender of analysis in January 1920. At the time of von Freund's passing, Freud spoke of the circumstances that had necessitated the move to Berlin. He recalled that von Freund had wanted to help the masses by means of psychoanalysis. The social necessity of alleviating the neurotic misery of the poor had led him to the project of opening a psychoanalytic institute where analysis would be cultivated, taught and made accessible to the people. There was a plan to train psychoanalysts there, many of them doctors. The establishment would pay their fees for the clinical treatment of the poor. The Budapest institute would have become a centre for further scientific research in analysis.[8] Ferenczi would have been its scientific director and von Freund would have been in charge of running it. Von Freund's death put an end to the philanthropic project, and the Horthy regime had no time for psychoanalysis. Freud emphasised that the first psychoanalytic polyclinic had been opened in Berlin by Eitingon just a few weeks after the death of von Freund. Eitingon took the place of von Freund on Freud's 'secret committee'. (This was the designation given to the IPA's informal directorate, which was established in 1912–1913, at the time of Freud's conflict with Jung and Alfred Adler.)

What happened in Hungary demonstrates that the creation of a psychoanalytic institution depends on a variety of factors. Firstly, the insertion of such an institution into society can suffer directly from a deficit of democratic functioning. Authoritarian forms of government never favour the development of psychoanalysis. Indeed, this confirms the opinion of Freud, who held that psychoanalysis lends support to society's resistances. Nevertheless, this movement can also be understood in the opposite sense: psychoanalysis has no chance of blossoming under totalitarian regimes when watchwords and the depersonalising slogans of propaganda come to suture the flaw inherent in the subject of the unconscious. This flaw, which takes us back to the gap between signified and signifier, can permit a space vis-à-vis the most alienating master signifiers. As a result, the possibility of setting up a psychoanalytic institution cannot be abstracted from the political context and the prevailing state of the discourse of the master. The Hungarian interlude clearly demonstrates this. In Europe, the extension of psychoanalysis applied to therapy in its institutional form happened in an atmosphere where freedom of expression and artistic and political renewal carried it for a time through the most destructive manifestations of identification with a leader. This brief interlude lasted fifteen years, when there was a democratic regime in Germany. In a totalitarian regime, therapies based on identification and suggestion both threaten and replace psychoanalysis. The history of the Berlin Psychoanalytic Institute throws light on this process in an exemplary manner.

Secondly, it is also a matter of personalities and contingency. At the beginning of the 1920s, the first generation of psychoanalysts were seized by the urgency of working towards the 'propagation of the psychoanalytic species'.[9] Also, a veritable gale of panic swept over the analytic community at the moment when they believed that Sigmund Freud's days were numbered. This led to the accelerated establishment of new modalities of analytic formation. From this perspective, it was essential to arrange sufficiently important clinical material. Without the presence of analysts capable of ensuring teaching, without the existence of a psychoanalytical society sufficiently organised to welcome and to offer sufficient guarantees to psychoanalysts in formation as well as to patients received for consultation and without the appropriate financial means, the Berlin Institute would never have seen the light of day.

Notes

1 Sigmund Freud, 'The Future Prospects of Psychoanalytic Therapy' (1910), in *The Standard Edition of the Complete Psychological Works of Sigmund Freud*, trans. James Strachey, Alix Strachey and Alan Tyson, vol. 11 (London: Vintage, 2001), p. 150.
2 Jacques Lacan, *Talking to Brick Walls: A Series of Presentations in the Chapel at Sainte-Anne Hospital*, trans. A. R. Price (Cambridge: Polity, 2017), p. 18.
3 Jacques Lacan, 'Le séminaire de Jacques Lacan' (1975), *Ornicar?*, no. 4 (1975), 106.
4 Sigmund Freud, 'Lines of Advance in Psychoanalytic Therapy' (1919), *Standard Edition*, vol. 17, p. 167.
5 Ernst Simmel, *Kriegs-Neurosen und psychisches Trauma* (Munich and Leipzig: Otto Nemnich, 1918). See also Ernest Jones (ed.), *Psychoanalysis and the War Neuroses* (London: International Psychoanalytical Press, 1921), vol. 2, pp. 30–43.
6 Sándor Ferenczi, 'Psychoanalysis of War Neurosis', given at the Symposium on Psychoanalysis and the War Neuroses held at the Fifth International Psychoanalytical Congress, Budapest, September 1918. Published in a collection with Karl Abraham, Ernst Simmel, Ernest Jones and Sigmund Freud, *The International Psychoanalytical Library*, vol. 2 (1921), pp. 5–21.
7 Kurt R. Eissler, *Freud as an Expert Witness: The Discussion of War Neuroses Between Freud and Wagner-Jauregg* (Madison, CT: International Universities Press, 1986).
8 Sigmund Freud, 'Dr. Anton von Freund' (1920), *Standard Edition*, vol. 18, pp. 267–268.
9 Max Eitingon, 'Report on the Berlin Psychoanalytic Polyclinic (March 1920–June 1922)', *Bulletin of the International Psychoanalytical Association*, no. 4 (1923), 265.

Part I

Berlin at the centre of the psychoanalytic movement

Chapter 1

The golden age of the Berlin Institute

Weimar: a democratic interval for psychoanalysis

The Berlin Institute and the Berlin Polyclinic prospered under the Weimar Republic, which was established following the abdication of Kaiser Wilhelm II – on 9 November 1918 – after four years of a ruthless war in which 1.8 million Germans soldiers had died and more than 4 million had been wounded. Some weeks after the signing of the Armistice, workers' uprisings took place in Berlin and Munich. An attempted revolution by the Spartacists was brutally repressed by the Reichswehr (the successor to the German imperial army) at the beginning of 1919. Throughout the thirteen years that followed, the Social Democrats remained in power despite constant governmental reshuffles and a catastrophic social and economic situation. It was during this time that the first psychoanalytic institute was developed and became a pole of attraction comparable to Vienna. From its opening, the influx of patients far exceeded its capacity. In its first decade, analysts undertook 1,955 consultations, and 363 analyses were completed. Hundreds of patients – adults, adolescents and children – were treated in the polyclinic founded by Karl Abraham, Max Eitingon and Ernst Simmel in February 1920.

This boom in applied psychoanalysis also served to form a new generation of analysts, after that of Freud and his students. A training institution was attached to the polyclinic, which is why the social extension of psychoanalysis was intrinsically linked to the politics of the IPA's development. From the moment of its creation in 1910, the IPA realised that the admission of new members would oblige it to guarantee their competence by assuming social responsibility for their practice. The period in which it sufficed to be recognised as an analyst by Freud, and to study the works of psychoanalysis while analysing your own dreams with your colleagues, was over. The institutionalisation of didactic analysis, put in place for the first time in Berlin by Max Eitingon, profoundly modified the existing relationship between analysis and the analyst. One passed imperceptibly from the question of the formation of the analyst to the problem of selecting candidates. The generalisation of didactic psychoanalysis obliged the subject to rethink and reformulate the question of the end

DOI: 10.4324/9781003215684-3

of analysis to the point where 'the usually sufficient mark, that of a lasting distancing from symptoms'[1] was no longer sufficient.

The training dispensed by the Berlin Institute rested on three fundamental aspects of the curriculum: didactic analysis, theoretical training and practical formation. Cycles of introductory courses on psychoanalysis were proposed for social workers, teachers, lawyers and psychologists. A particular cycle of studies was aimed more specifically at those people – generally doctors – who wished to become analysts. In 1923, this training was placed under the guardianship of a teaching commission that elaborated directives for teaching activity and for training. These directives were reformulated in 1929 in order to render them more adequate for the orientation of training at an international level. In the first phase, the duration of the training was from one to one and a half years. The obligatory didactic analysis lasted about six months. Theoretical teaching was dispensed in the form of an obligatory course that lasted two semesters. Once judged capable, candidates undertook a practical stage in the polyclinic by taking patients into treatment. Up until 1922, Eitingon selected all the patients who applied to the polyclinic and also supervised the treatments undertaken by new analysts. The regulation of the training, which was progressively put in place at the Berlin Institute, served as the model for the institutes in Vienna, Budapest, London and New York that IPA members went on to create. Without the existence of a polyclinic that made psychoanalysis accessible to a great number of patients, this training policy would hardly have been conceivable.

At the beginning of the 1930s, the Berlin group was quite proud of the work it had done in diffusing the practice invented by Freud throughout the wider culture. At that time, who could have foreseen the persecution and extermination of Europe's Jews that would soon be wiping analysis off the map in Germany? The Weimar democratic interval ended abruptly when Adolf Hitler was designated Chancellor of the Reich by President Paul von Hindenburg on 30 January 1933. The director of the Berlin Institute emigrated to Palestine, and the Nazis took over the institute's premises in order to install a centre of Aryan psychotherapy directed by Matthias Göring, a cousin of Hermann Göring, Hitler's Minister of the Interior and a future Reichsmarschall. Some German psychoanalysts trained by the old institute agreed to work there. In 1945, Allied bombing destroyed the premises, which had been fitted out by Freud's son Ernst. The transition from the old institution, directed by Jews, to the new one, placed under Hermann Göring's guardianship, has been the subject of several carefully documented studies. The pitiful attempt to safeguard German psychoanalysis led by Ernest Jones, president of the IPA since 1932, has been well known for a long time. Analysts Carl Müller-Braunschweig and Felix Boehm worked with the Nazi administration in order to integrate the German Psychoanalytic Society (Deutsche Psychoanalytische Gesellschaft, or DPG) and the Berlin Institute into the National Socialist state. (This took place shortly after the public burning of Freud's books.) Boehm entered into correspondence with Jones; he wrote precise reports regarding the manner in which he had gone about convincing the Nazi administration that it was in the interests of the new regime to preserve psychoanalysis.[2] The full extent of the shameless collaboration of certain psychoanalysts with the Hitler regime, along with the painful evidence of the fact that the IPA had not punished them as it should have, only came to light in the decades after the war. The weight accorded to these pathetic events, which took place after 1933, has focused attention on the darkest period of German psychoanalysis. As a consequence of this, questions relating to the Berlin Polyclinic during its thirteen years of effective operation were sidelined.

The history of this institution, from its creation to its confiscation by the Nazis, has largely been viewed as the internal business of the IPA. Only a few authors – such as Moustapha Safouan – have been interested in the origins of didactic analysis and have used the institute's training data. In general, the Berlin Polyclinic has been of little interest to analytic movements outside the IPA's sphere of influence.[3] The interest that has been taken relates to the training curriculum invented in Berlin. Little interest has been taken in the clinical practice.

The American sociologist Elizabeth Ann Danto, whose *Freud's Free Clinics* was published in 2005, has focused on the first IPA institutions, Alfred Adler's centres for child rearing and Wilhelm Reich's Sex-Pol project. But psychoanalysis itself and the discourse that it supports are missing. In Danto's work, this demanding and complex discipline appears frozen in a portrait marked by nostalgia for a bygone epoch. In her vision, the world's first psychoanalytic institution was directed by enthusiastic souls carried away by the whirlwind that was Berlin during the Roaring Twenties. The analysts, she says, didn't worry about their time – they strove to give free care, and they were all militant socialists. Concern for the general wellbeing was stronger than egotistical sentiments. Everything was placed under the benediction of a highly optimistic Freud immersed in the effervescence of Red Vienna. This heroic portrait of a community of analysts seduced by progressive ideals remains intriguing. Even if it's true that some analysts who worked in Berlin – such as Otto Fenichel, Ernst Simmel and Siegfried Bernfeld – were socialists, and if others, like Wilhelm Reich, were convinced communists, to argue that a single momentum swept the analytical community along in a desire for social transformation remains a wild generalisation. After the tragic events of 1933, the secret community of leftist Freudians in exile on American soil were unable to stop the transformation of American psychoanalysis into a medical speciality. But who would say that they failed in the USA, having once succeeded in Europe? Truly, tensions did exist in the Berlin group for the simple reason that these psychoanalysts were not all politically engaged in the exact same way. The vision proposed by Danto tends to separate the Berlin experiment from its historical, political and clinical roots even though she believes that she is putting those factors in the foreground. All the spiritual and social complexity of Germany, as well as that of Central Europe, disappears in Danto's fusion of behaviours, along with the tensions, violence, paradoxes and extraordinary creativity that were in evidence before the disaster that befell Germany in 1933. For Danto, all good intentions will triumph in a happy ending as long as men are able to help one another. Even though she tells us how many chairs there were in the waiting room of the polyclinic, we end up wondering where analysis itself may have gone.

Ultimately, Danto's version of psychoanalysis at the beginning of the 1920s is simply a critique of the contemporary healthcare system in North America. It is a denunciation of managed care, in which only the rich can access proper care. This is undoubtedly the reason why she describes the emphasis on the provision of free care by the Freudian institutes in Berlin as the ne plus ultra of psychoanalysis. But this does not correspond to the state of mind of the analysts of the era, who adapted themselves as best they could to the economic conditions of an epoch characterised by a general impoverishment of the population. To pretend otherwise would be to pass a bit too quickly over some interesting questions. The founders of the Berlin Institute specifically refused to offer totally free treatments – which, of course, ran counter to the vision put forward by Freud in Budapest. To ask the patient himself to assess the price that he thought he could pay for his treatment at the polyclinic effectively adapted the analytic tool to the economic conditions of this period of crisis but did not give up on the principle of a clinical and subjective reference point. One must also keep in mind the fact that the first of the free clinics rejected the possibility of free analysis for all. For clinical and diagnostic reasons it was not made into a universal principle. Free psychoanalysis was not an end in itself. If one wanted psychoanalysis to last, if one hoped to form psychoanalysts, it was necessary to make sacrifices, and the founders of the Berlin Polyclinic were in agreement on this pragmatic point of view. It was a necessity, not an ideal.

Made in Berlin

The Berlin-style training had been developed so that it could be exported elsewhere, and principles had been challenged – a radically different conception had come to the fore, one that diverged from the idea of analysts being produced on the basis of their own analysis. This is incontestable. However, it's also safe to say that a decisive step was taken when a handful of analysts began to receive patients at the Berlin Institute in the 1920s. This initial project, which supported the action of psychoanalysis in a world marked by catastrophe, went unexamined; it is as if the study of this inaugural experiment was left to those who claimed to be Freud's direct heirs. By the time the Berlin Polyclinic opened, Freud was tendering his thoughts on the death drive. The negative therapeutic resistance he had highlighted in 1920 was at the heart of his new conceptualisation, and its unmistakeable character was not unrelated to the experience of the war and its consequences. The dualism of the drive was not only the expression of Freud's legendary pessimism. He had discovered that man does not desire his own good and that the satisfaction of the drive is what draws him to his own destruction, as the war had amply proved. There were no limits to Thanatos in the horror of the trenches, in the criminal blindness of the governments on both sides that sent men to be slaughtered. Each day that the war lasted – and it lasted 1,500 days – another 6,000 men perished. Some had hoped that, with the arrival of peace, the efforts devoted to reconstruction would prove that Freud's hypothesis of the death drive was wrong, and that it could simply be ascribed to the influence of circumstances and to his well-known pessimism or supposed depression. However, the climate of social and political insecurity in postwar Germany, along with growing demonstrations of anti-Semitism and the fact that attacks by the extreme right went unpunished, was proof of Freud's sagacity.

Psychoanalysis places itself on the side of life – it verifies empirically, in the treatment of each patient, the influence of what lies beyond the pleasure principle. From this statement, we can draw its efficacity and its value. What Freud had the courage to unveil was that the analyst reports every day the existence of the subject's strange resistance to wanting his own good and to being healed. The psychoanalyst knows that the jouissance of the subject is not an illusion. He aims at the opaque side of this enjoyment outside meaning. Ernst Simmel was not exaggerating when he confided that it was this dark force, which he encountered when he was a military doctor, that had convinced him of the need to open a psychoanalytic hospital. The aggressivity of the superego revealed itself to him as something without limits, and psychoanalysis presented itself as the only way to treat it effectively. In 1920, in the aftermath of defeat, the alternative was simple: either the psychoanalysts would manage to innovate, or they would leave the field in order to retrench in private practice, accessible only to those who had the means to pay. The general impoverishment of the population singularly restricted psychoanalysis's field of action, particularly in Germany. If psychoanalysts wanted to become more involved in society, they would have to invent a clinical instrument adapted to the postwar situation. The Berliners committed themselves resolutely to this path. They believed in the social mission of psychoanalysis. The creation of a place that offered free analysis seemed to them the best solution possible. So it is no coincidence that the first psychoanalytic institution in history established itself in the capital of a ruined country that was struggling against internal destructive forces that would eventually win the day.

In a nutshell, all the standard principles later adopted by the IPA – such as the length of the sessions, the training analysis and the practice of supervision – were devised in Berlin. In the 1930s, all analytical societies had to declare their conformity to the IPA. The IPA was based in Berlin and held supreme authority in everything concerning the teaching of psychoanalysis throughout the world. This hegemony can be dated to the IPA congress of September 1925, where it was considered necessary to create an International

Training Commission (ITC) that would be charged with '[correlating] as much as possible the methods and standards of training candidates for psychoanalysis in the various Societies, and to provide opportunities for the common discussion of the technical problems concerned'.[4] This standardisation of procedures was based on what was practised in Germany. 'Made in Berlin' became the guarantee of excellence in matters of analytical training as well as a guarantee of the immutability of psychoanalytic practice.

Berlin was truly the place where one had to go when one wanted to become a psychoanalyst. Franz Alexander was the first student of the institute. Karl Abraham, Melanie Klein and Karen Horney were part of the teaching faculty. Richard Sterba, Otto Fenichel, Siegfried Bernfeld and Wilhelm Reich left Vienna in order to go to Berlin. Alix Strachey, a student at the institute, delivered her version of the hectic life led by the analysts of this epoch. After a long day's work at the polyclinic, they sometimes went to a masked ball. The startling sight of Melanie Klein as Cleopatra and Ernst Simmel dressed as a night porter remained engraved on her memory. Her account seems compatible with that of a student who reported that, at the end of a semester dedicated to Freud's case study of President Schreber, Otto Fenichel still hadn't got beyond page two.[5] She was also greatly impressed by the courtesy of Max Eitingon, who was the supervisor of numerous analysts, including a certain Rudolph Loewenstein, the future analyst of Jacques Lacan.

Lacan, who began his training analysis in June 1932, later delivered his own testimony about the Berliners. During a 1971 intervention on the occasion of the translation of the *Écrits* into Japanese, he recalled how the American school of the 1950s had been animated by 'the compulsory methods that the German immigrants inherited through a certain German academic style'.[6] This is a valuable pointer insofar as Lacan identified the academic style that dominated the Berlin Institute. It relates to the fact that reference to the university inspired the manner in which psychoanalysis was taught at the Berlin Institute: a curriculum lasting a certain number of years, its courses, its teaching commission. In this institutional context, could one deduce that the university discourse prevailed over the analytic discourse?

Lacan's remark does not concern the existence of a privileged link between academics and psychoanalysts. It is at the level of the discourse and, more exactly, of the place occupied by knowledge in this discourse, that we must situate ourselves in order to grasp the importance of that remark. Lacan showed that the university discourse was dominated by a categorical imperative that consisted in always knowing more, never stopping, always marching further ahead on the path of the accumulation of knowledge. In this discourse, which is also the discourse of science, knowledge is in command. Lacan formulates it like this: 'It is impossible not to obey the commandment there in the place of what is the truth of science: "Continue. March on. Keep on knowing more and more."'[7] The Kantian imperative that dominates the university discourse is consonant with the imperative methods of the Berlin analysts. A strict method of organisation was taken for granted by one of the institute's founders. In 1928, Max Eitingon described the regulation of the organisation of the analytical training he had set up through the ITC as being in the 'Prussian style'.[8] Prior to the reign of Wilhelm II, the term connoted duty, altruism and incorruptibility, values with which, it seems, Eitingon identified despite his Russian origins. But with the advent of Wilhelm II, the Prussian spirit came to have a definitively pejorative connotation, referring as it did to the aggressiveness, arrogance and rigidity of the Junker military caste. Indeed, this note of self-derision evidenced a certain subtlety, since in laughing at the rigidity of his own methods, Eitingon put the bar of castration on the function of the master that he himself incarnated.

It will be a question of determining whether the emphasis on academic knowledge was an obstacle to the mission for which the Berlin Institute had been created. Was the social extension of psychoanalysis compatible with an academic course in analytic training? To try to answer these questions, we have to go back. And first of all, we have to ask: why Germany? Why Berlin?

The Weimar Republic and the psychoanalysts

In contradistinction to the clichés that have made of it a moment of pure decadence and exuberant jouissance before the arrival of the Great Depression, the Weimar Republic offered favourable conditions for the emergence of important artistic and scientific innovations. Expressionism in painting and cinematography, the architecture of the Bauhaus, the theatre of Brecht and the operas of Alban Berg constituted a major turning point in the art of the twentieth century. On the scientific level, the history of art found a new source in the publications of the Warburg Institute. We can also date from this period the step that allowed the political sciences to free themselves from the idea that they should serve to train the servants of the state through public law. If the work of Max Weber hardly benefited from a wide diffusion in Bismarck's Germany, things began to change with the creation of the Deutsche Hochschule für Politik (German Academy for Politics) in 1920. The political education of the German people was a matter of urgency in the revolutionary spirit of this school. For that reason, only a third of the students who were enrolled in 1930 had graduated from the *Gymnasium* system; the others had either not followed their cycle of studies through to the final diploma or came from the free state secondary schools, which did not usually permit them to enrol at university. Such a tendency to openness which allowed students from the lower classes to access higher education is worth emphasising. In contrast to the Deutsche Hochschule, the Frankfurt Institute, founded in 1923, anchored itself more resolutely in a Marxist orientation. Between 1931 and 1933, its *Journal for Social Research* (*Zeitschrift für Sozialforschung*) published the works of Theodor Adorno, Erich Fromm, Walter Benjamin and Herbert Marcuse.

The Frankfurt Psychoanalytic Institute, the second German institute of psychoanalysis after Berlin, was created in 1929. It was hosted by the Institute of Social Research, through which it was attached to the University of Frankfurt. Because it didn't take patients, the Frankfurt Psychoanalytic Institute did not become a training centre. Its perspective consisted of building bridges between psychoanalysis and a non-orthodox brand of Marxism. At the level of knowledge, the foundation of the Berlin Psychoanalytic Institute, at the beginning of the 1920s, was not an isolated case: the blossoming of psychoanalysis in Germany inscribed itself in a more general cultural movement. What we need to remember, nevertheless, is the fact that important research centres were created independently of the German university system, which remained under the control of the professorial old guard, which was generally anti-Semitic, revanchist and attached to the bygone values of a vanished empire. Furthermore, as Peter Gay has emphasised, the creation of institutes is neither a German speciality nor specific to the Weimar Republic:

> New disciplines, seeking to clarify their purpose, train their personnel in their own way, and propagate their findings have often created institutions separate from, or only loosely affiliated with, old centres of higher learning. What is special about the institutes of the Weimar Republic is above all the quality of the work that was done in them.[9]

Several of the most successful scientific enterprises developed outside the German university system. More generally, Weimar culture barely penetrated the academic world during this period. The professors' opposition to the republic was rooted in their attachment to patriotic values, to the fidelity that had once bound them to the Kaiser and to their belief in the power and the civilising mission of Germany. For a large majority of them, the German defeat and the revolution of 1918 had been a real disaster. Very few university teachers belonged to the centre left; most of them were reactionary, without necessarily adhering to the ideas of the extreme right. Those who did not openly attack the republic generally showed ambivalence towards it. Parliamentarianism and the unpatriotic character of the new regime were generally poorly accepted, and the annexationist tendency was predominant in academia. As Walter Laqueur has pointed out, this political orientation was accompanied by an aversion to Weimar's avant-garde culture. Thus, according to Laqueur, 'no new or revolutionary idea was born in German universities at that time'.[10] The rapprochement between psychoanalysis and the university was probably not surprising for the psychoanalysts of the 1920s. Such a relationship was in the air. Freud's article on the teaching of psychoanalysis in the university was contemporary with his discourse regarding the new ways of therapy.[11] How to make analytic therapy accessible to those who are not in a position to bear the cost? Where and how to teach psychoanalysis? The two questions appear to be linked.

For its part, the correspondence between Freud and Abraham argues that the project of creating the polyclinic was strictly contemporary with efforts to bring psychoanalysis into the university. In fact, the Freudian reference to the university corresponded to the mutation of places of transmission of knowledge, which was precisely one of the characteristics of the Weimar period. It was a question of inventing an institution with a didactic aim at the very moment when the German university system was clinging to its former autocratic functioning. A whole section of the German intelligentsia, driven by a desire for social and political renewal, was attracted by original projects. The intelligentsia longed for new democratic spaces, schools and institutes at a time when, and certainly because, the economic crisis of the postwar years was accelerating. The 1920s were particularly chaotic. On the political front, the extremists of the left and the right clashed. The political right was composed of nationalists, monarchists and elements of the army who were opposed to the young republic. The military elite had invented the *Dolchstosslegende*, a myth that held the war had been lost because civil society stabbed the military in the back by withdrawing its support. The military authorities tried to exonerate themselves by accusing the democratic leaders who were now in power. The rightwing movements were united in their opposition to the republican regime; they wanted to avenge the defeat of Germany.

On the other hand, the success of the Bolshevik revolution in Russia inspired the German Communist Party (KPD) to oppose the German Social Democratic Party (SPD), which had recoiled from the attempted German workers' revolution of 1919. In 1922, the German government declared that it was unable to pay the amount of the reparations demanded of Germany by the Treaty of Versailles. France immediately responded by occupying the Ruhr, Germany's industrial heartland. The German economy was now on its knees. To counter this, Germany printed an extraordinary quantity of money. At the end of the war, four marks bought one US dollar. In January 1923 the dollar was worth 7,000 marks. Five months later, 160,000 marks were necessary to buy a dollar. At the end of the same year, the dollar was worth 4,200 billion marks. Thousands of savers were ruined by hyperinflation and the number of unemployed continued to grow.

Five to six hundred thousand Jews were living in Germany at this time, and there had long been a rift between the Jewish refugees from Russia and Poland and the assimilated German Jews, who had been settled in Germany for many years and saw themselves as citizens of one of the most civilised countries in the Western world. 'In the socio-economic space, German Jews played an important part not so much in finance, contrary to popular beliefs, as in the press, publishing, medicine and law,' says Gustave Peiser.[12] But before Weimar, German Jews could not become senior officials or officers in the army. During his engagement in the army, someone like Walther Rathenau, the future Weimar Foreign Minister who was assassinated by rightwing extremists in 1922, could only hope to reach the rank of non-commissioned officer.[13] It was not until the establishment of the Weimar Republic that Jews could assume high office in the army and the university. Psychoanalysts of Jewish origin were obviously concerned. During the first months of the new political regime, the creation of a chair of psychoanalysis at the University of Berlin – which Karl Abraham would eventually occupy – finally seemed possible. In any case, the founders of the Berlin Institute always insisted on the courage and daring that it took to create and promote a psychoanalytic institution in the context of an almost permanent economic, political and social crisis. Could this adventure have come to pass anywhere other than 1920s Berlin?

Berlin, crossroads of expectations

There is a direct correlation between the democratic aspirations established on the ashes of the old empire and an awareness of the social mission of psychoanalysis. It was this movement that took off in Berlin. In the postwar years, the development of places dedicated to public health initiatives – offering free medical consultations to the most needy, child guidance services, the training of social workers and an interest in new teaching methods – influenced the creators of the Berlin Polyclinic. Parallel to the progressive ideals that guided the desire for social renewal, the artists of the Neue Sachlichkeit (New Objectivity) movement, who had chosen Berlin as the centre of their activities, returned to civilisation the image of a real without veil or adornment. This came at the very moment when the discourse of the time was undergoing a decisive change. The advent of the era of technology had, as its arena, the great city which had been transformed by the birth of the entertainment industry and the market for consumer goods. After the terrible financial crisis of 1923, a powerful workforce, supported by the adoption of modern organisational methods imported from North America, facilitated a spectacular recovery of the German economy in the late 1920s. The chemical, electrical and mechanical industries throughout the country were modernised. Exports went through the roof, and construction resumed on the outskirts of urban centres. This irruption of technology, which had so recently modified the relation of man to war, first manifested itself in Berlin and permeated every domain of existence. One could say that before producing the worst, the rationalisation linked to the advent of technology was incontestably one of the master signifiers of Germany in the 1920s.

Berlin's decadence, immortalised by Stefan Zweig, was especially memorable:

> Berlin was the worst sink of iniquity in the world. Bars, amusement arcades and shady dives sprang up like mushrooms. What we had seen in Austria was only a mild and gentle prelude to this witches' sabbath, for the Germans now turned their methodical methods to the cause of perversions.[14]

But Berlin, the capital of Prussia, was not only a place of debauchery; it also had a growing influence in the Germany of the 1920s. The phenomenon of centralisation made Berlin a place that brought together the governmental services and the headquarters of the political parties; many eminent personalities, often immigrants, met there. The city also became a unique laboratory of experimentation in the artistic and literary fields. 'To go to Berlin was the aspiration of the composer, the journalist, the actor; with its superb orchestras, its hundred and twenty newspapers, its forty theatres, Berlin was the place for the ambitious, the energetic, the talented.'[15]

Berlin represented the future of Germany even as the stigmata of the Great War still marked people's bodies. In Berlin, one frequently came across disfigured or limbless war veterans begging in the streets. In 1920, the fate of these war wounded was far from settled. The city was also a transit point for thousands of refugees from the Ukraine, Galicia and Hungary, who crowded into neighbourhoods in the eastern part of the capital. These refugees were hoping to make their way to the Netherlands, America or Palestine. Many of them did not succeed. Between 1890 and 1920, there were an estimated 200,000 Jewish refugees in the city. These eastern European Jews – known as *Ostjuden* – spoke Yiddish and were largely rejected by the assimilated German Jews, who feared that a new strain of anti-Semitism would be added to the secular anti-Semitism that remained a problem in Germany. Berlin thus testified to the rift between the German Jews and the eastern European Jews.

The writer and journalist Joseph Roth brilliantly described everyday life in the Scheunenviertel district. In Wiesenstrasse, the old municipal asylum had been transformed into a residential centre. The influx of refugees was such that it was not uncommon to see travellers disembarking from trains with their suitcases and going straight to the Turkish baths – which were open all night – because they had been unable to find a hotel room:

> The grotesque spectacle of a hot room at night, containing sixteen naked homeless people, trying to sweat out the soot and coal smoke of a train journey, gives rise to a positively infernal range of interpretations. A series of illustrations, say, to Dante's journeys in the underworld,[16]

wrote Roth in the *Neue Berliner Zeitung* in March 1920.

The glimpse of the future that this pathetic vision offers certainly displaces its meaning for us. In Roth's newspaper articles we also discover the troubles caused by traffic congestion linked to the modernisation of the Berlin transport system, the building of tramways and the increasing presence of cars. He also addresses the consequences of the nascent entertainment industry and the transformations brought about by the opening of large department stores. These developments heralded a lifestyle increasingly marked by the enjoyment of consumer goods. It is thus a valuable subjective testimony relating to the effects of the irruption of technology into the big city. An interesting counterpart to Roth's journalism is the work of another famous Berliner, Walter Benjamin, who was writing about art at the time of its technical reproducibility. Berlin's architecture bore witness to various influences, blends and confusions, which, he says, made the city 'an unfortunate conglomeration of squares, streets, cubical barracks, churches and palaces. A well-ordered confusion, an exactly planned arbitrariness; an absence of goals under an apparent purpose'. Berlin, then, appears as a place where the changes in a civilisation dominated by the value of images and the incessant decipherment of the tragedy of the world as headlined by the newspapers were concentrated to excess. Roth knew exactly how to capture the essence of this city, focusing not on the unity of the image, but on pieces of the real, on the infinitesimal, on the inessential: 'I no longer have the sense of the grand gesture of the hero embracing all things on the world stage. I am a wanderer.' According to the opinion of other authors, the Berlin of the 1920s presented all the aspects of a paradoxical city where the best of opera, cinema, theatre, publishing and painting rubbed shoulders with the sad world of the ghetto located near Alexanderplatz. Laqueur points out that Berlin

> was a dynamic city, populated by a neurasthenic generation (to quote Eduard Spranger), a city with a strong social conscience and exacerbated individualism, a centre that attracted the most productive and creative forces, but also, very often, the marginalised, the sick, and the failures. The Jewish community, important enough, exerted a considerable influence on cultural life; in this respect, Berlin had a certain resemblance to New York. But its position as the national capital at the head of the country was not undisputed, and some even claimed that Berlin was no longer part of true Germany.[17]

Berlin was desirable because of its very eccentricity.

The group of pioneers

'Berlin is clamouring for psychoanalysis,'[18] wrote Karl Abraham to Freud in October 1919. Freud, for his part, felt that nothing very interesting was going on in the Austrian capital. 'There is absolutely nothing to be said in favour of Vienna, no good is to be done here,'[19] he replied. At the end of the war, Freud doubted that psychoanalysis could continue to develop at the heart of the countries of the former Triple Alliance (Germany, Austria-Hungary and Italy), from which Italy had withdrawn in 1915. England, particularly, seemed to him better placed. It was simply a fact. Freud was hardly enthusiastic about the idea that German might no longer be the original language of psychoanalysis. Abraham, who was more of an optimist, was not of the same opinion. He believed that Germany still had an important role to play in the movement, to the point of proposing that the first postwar congress could be held in Berlin, where he had been an analyst since 1907. Freud considered this proposal completely unreasonable. Abraham, he felt, was totally underestimating the anti-German sentiment that would almost certainly prejudice a congress held in Berlin. They opted for Holland, much to Abraham's regret. Freud's misgivings regarding anti-German feeling proved to have been well founded. An hour before the opening of the congress, which was held in the Salon Louis XV of the Society of Artists of The Hague on 8 September 1920, the tension was palpable. In an attempt to calm things down, Freud asked Abraham, who was secretary of the IPA, to deliver his inaugural speech in Latin, which he did without the slightest difficulty.[20] This congress gave rise to Freud's communication of supplements to the theory of dreams. Abraham presented his study on the manifestations of the castration complex in women. Ferenczi explained his latest developments in the active technique.

Karl Abraham had been eager to make the Prussian capital a leading centre of psychoanalytic training since well before the war. He had studied medicine in Würzburg and Freiburg im Breisgau, and had then worked at the Dalldorf psychiatric hospital in Berlin. In 1904, he went to Switzerland, to Paul Eugen Bleuler's Burghölzli Clinic, where Jung, who was interested in Freud, was chief medical officer. In December 1907, Abraham returned to Berlin. He was thus the first psychoanalyst to settle in the city. At the beginning of his practice, Abraham was assisted by Dr. Hermann Oppenheim, who regularly referred patients to him for analysis. Oppenheim was a famous Berlin neurologist who had married Abraham's cousin. These ties of kinship facilitated a rapprochement between the two men, even though the neurologist refrained from following psychoanalytic theories. Oppenheim was a pioneer in the field of traumatic neurosis. In 1889, he published a monograph on this subject based on his observations of patients at the Charité hospital – which was attached to the University of Berlin – who had been victims of railway accidents. Despite his fame, Oppenheim, as a Jew, was only a lecturer; he was not eligible for a university chair. Undoubtedly tired of this status, Oppenheim eventually opened his own private polyclinic in the north of Berlin. He proposed that Abraham come and work there.

Freud, who paid close attention to the vicissitudes of Abraham's career in Berlin, was well acquainted with Oppenheim's work, and had not forgotten the latter's break with Jean-Martin Charcot. Oppenheim's conception from the 1880s was that post-traumatic symptoms constituted a distinct entity, a special kind of neurosis. Oppenheim did not dispute the existence of male hysteria, but he refused to equate traumatic neurosis with hysteria. Freud did not believe that it was possible to convert Oppenheim to psychoanalysis. He did not, however, object to Oppenheim's support for his cousin, who he helped to get his start in the profession. In 1909, Abraham suggested to Eitingon, his former colleague at Burghölzli, that he join him in Berlin. Oppenheim also offered a doctor's post to Eitingon in his polyclinic. So Abraham and Eitingon saw a lot of each other before the war. The two men worked in Berlin in close collaboration well before the creation of the psychoanalytic polyclinic. It may seem astonishing that, despite his public opposition to psychoanalytic ideas, Oppenheim chose to help these two pioneers of psychoanalysis in Germany. Is kinship enough to explain such support? It seems that another consideration must have come into play. This help was translated into a great deal of confidence in their value as clinicians. Might it be surmised that Oppenheim was a secret adherent to the psychoanalytic theses he openly criticised? It is not altogether absurd to think so, despite the fact that Freud thought the opposite. Indeed, a few years later, Eitingon acknowledged the contribution of psychoanalysis to psychiatry and neurology that Oppenheim had accomplished. The latter, commenting on the pathological hatred of some mothers towards their offspring, said that this disease seemed to have 'its roots in the unconscious, and it is quite possible that the impressions left in childhood, dream experiences, processes of repression, in short, Freudian mechanisms play a role in their development'.[21] Then again, does solidarity between members of the same profession who shared the same condition (being of Jewish origin in Germany) provide another explanation? There is nothing to prove this, but nothing prevents us from making the hypothesis. In any case, Oppenheim's support was tangible; it allowed Abraham and Eitingon to study cases of traumatic neurosis in peacetime.

In 1910, encouraged by signs that psychoanalysis was being accepted in Berlin, Abraham founded the Berlin Psychoanalytic Association (Berliner Psychoanalytische Vereinigung, or BPV). Four years later, when the war came and during the time of his mobilisation, he devoted himself to war neuroses as chief of a military psychiatric unit in East Prussia. As Freud later clarified, psychoanalytic research on war neuroses was decisive. The stakes were high for the analysts of the time, as traumatic neurosis was used as an essential objection to the sexual aetiology of neuroses by advocates of official psychiatry. The traumatic neuroses seemed to prove that their emergence was the result of a shock, an accident or a bodily injury, and that, consequently, they were not directly related to the sexual life of the patients who had been affected. The research conducted during World War I was used as a counter-argument. These studies focused on the nature of the conflict between the old pacifist ego and the soldier's new warrior ego. In times of war, the soldier became the seat of an authentic subjective splitting, the new warrior ego having the status of a graft. This new ego behaved like a double parasite which scorned mortal danger. It represented a danger from which the old ego was trying to save itself by a flight into illness. The originality of the psychoanalytic clinic of traumatic war neuroses corresponded to the effects of the division of the subject brought to a climax.

Abraham's prewar observations at Oppenheim's clinic emphasised the sexual signification present in traumatic neurosis, as well as in other neurotic conditions. This time, the examination of war neuroses allowed Abraham to highlight the effect of trauma on sexual life. According to him, what we see in these cases is the regressive and narcissistic modification of the libido. Abraham skilfully focused his research on the problem of individual predispositions. In his communication to the IPA's 1918 congress, he referred to the case of a soldier who had remained psychologically unscathed after four major traumas – three injuries in frontline fighting, followed by burial in rubble and a subsequent loss of consciousness for two days. Another soldier, who had stumbled into a ditch without injuring himself, later presented 'neurotic trembling of a most severe kind',[22] accompanied by an almost complete physical deterioration. This study showed that individuals suffering from war neuroses were characterised by a certain sexual instability in civilian life. They were either impotent or men who had little interest in the other sex, as Abraham pointed out. Abraham emphasised the lack of interest in sexual matters among those suffering from war neuroses. By necessity, the clinical research on war neuroses involved representatives of the male sex. In civilian life, these men were not particularly interested in women. In the army, this condition became more pronounced. This resulted in a clinical picture characterised by a huge presence of states of anxiety. For his part, Oppenheim had hypothesised that the high frequency of tremor symptoms was related to the specificity of trench warfare.

This link between impotence and anxiety echoes some of the elements mentioned by Lacan in the year following the end of World War II. In a talk on British psychiatry and the war, Lacan recalled this paradoxical but nevertheless acknowledged fact: war generally favours the dialectical evolution of human knowledge and, more particularly, that of the discipline of psychiatry. 'In this, as in other fields,' he wrote, 'war proved itself to be the midwife of progress in the essentially conflictual dialectics which, indeed, seem to be characteristic of our civilisation.'[23] Lacan explained that at the beginning of the war of 1939–1945, British specialists – there weren't very many – were confronted with the arrival in hospital of a torrent of individuals who were unfit for combat. In a well-known description, he referred to the types of individuals that military psychiatrists were confronted with:

> The subjects affected by too strong a deficit must be isolated as *dullards*, for indeed they are slowcoaches at instruction, ravaged by the feeling of their inferiority, maladjusted and prone to delinquency, not so much through lack of understanding as through impulses of a compensatory order, and consequently are the favoured terrain of depressive or anxious *raptus*, or confusional states manifesting themselves under the emotional or physical shocks incurred on the front line, natural carriers of all forms of mental contagion. Our friend Dr. Turquet … has indicated the French equivalent of the term *dullard* to be *lourdaud* rather than *arriéré* [retarded]; in other words, it refers to what our colloquial vocabulary designates with the word *débilard*, which expresses less a mental level than an evaluation of personality.[24]

In another part of his presentation, Lacan established a causal link between the decline of the virile type, at the collective level, and the social collapse of the paternal *imago*. Does not this reference point resonate with the phenomenon of sexual instability reported by Abraham among war neurotics in the aftermath of World War I? Indeed, at this time as at the other, these subjects' lack of appetite for sex was noted. From there, one may wonder whether the anxious states of war neuroses spotted by Abraham still related to castration anxiety. The sexual determinism of war neuroses was to be questioned by Freud himself.

The Budapest congress had been dedicated to the theme of psychoanalysis and war neuroses, but Freud was not entirely satisfied with the work of his colleagues. He dared to state it openly: no treatment for war neuroses had been completed, and one could not, therefore, draw a valid conclusion. It was not only a question of the impossibility – because the war had ended – of verifying whether the soldiers treated by Simmel at the military hospital had had relapses or not. Beyond the therapeutic effects, repetition of the trauma in dreams did not fit with the conception that had hitherto been taken of the function of the dream as the satisfaction of a desire. Freud could not resign himself to endorsing an objection so fundamental to his theory of the unconscious. On the other hand, he admitted that the psychoanalytic therapy of war neuroses had served to propagate psychoanalysis to the medical profession in Germany and Austria. It should be remembered that, at the beginning of the war, psychiatrists were announcing almost unbelievable rates of success (98 percent), having had recourse to authoritarian methods of therapy in order to correct behaviours deemed unpatriotic in the soldiers hospitalised in their facilities. They resorted to a whole heterogeneous arsenal, which mixed diet, hydrotherapy, faradisation, isolation, hospitalisation in special units and dosing with revolting substances, all of which were administered by force. It was to impress the soldier, to impose on him, even to terrorise him, in order to make him give up the symptom which was conceived of as a lack of willpower. Many psychiatrists took little care because they felt that the war neurotics were simply cowards and that they were malingering. If, by chance, a soldier died during electrotherapy treatment, the psychiatrists did not consider themselves responsible. In fact, since the soldiers concerned were hospitalised, the doctors sought to restore obedience by subjecting them to an iron discipline modelled on the spirit of the barracks. The practitioner based his success on the fear he inspired: the effectiveness of the treatment was founded on the authority of the master who belonged to the ruling class, in accordance with the monarchical structure of the society, which was very much reflected in the organisation of the army. It was all about suppressing the symptom by subjecting it to the will of the chief. Identification with the commander was the most powerful motor of the 'cures' obtained by these coercive means. But as the morale of the troops decreased over time, the power of this authority began to weaken as well. Worn out by the barbarity of the fighting and the manifest incompetence of their high commands, the nations of Central Europe were gradually overwhelmed by pessimism and bitterness: the disaster of a rout was looming. Quite logically, the success of treatments based on the authoritarian re-education of unpatriotic behaviour became more rare, and doctors could no longer boast about spectacular cure rates. When the war settled down for the long run, the therapeutic enthusiasm of the opening stages faded away among the military psychiatrists. The clinical material changed, the standard of the elite was lowered and the soldiers declared fit to fight were recruited from among individuals whose constitution proved to be incapable of withstanding the violence of the fighting.

During a military symposium in Munich in 1917, a psychiatrist declared himself openly hostile to the use of the coercive and degrading methods that were commonly being used:

> Then I should like to put a word in for the soldiers with nervous diseases. I simply cannot understand why we should, from the first, fling against people whose nervous system, through an unfortunate disposition, does not possess the necessary resistance against the intolerable demands of war, such accusations as took shape today, and particularly in the course of yesterday's discussion, in words like wish-fulfilment fantasies, pension addiction, defect of health conscience [*Gesundheitsgewissen*], and so on. Nor can I say I agree that if a man had done frontline duty for a long time and paid for it with his health, we should suspect him of malingering, because his symptoms happen to appear artificial, manufactured or unusual.[25]

At that time, interest shifted to new methods, including psychoanalysis. The reason why psychoanalysis aroused new hopes in 1918 relates, in one respect, to the worn-out and ineffective treatments dispensed by official psychiatry to war neurotics. While it certainly produced a rapprochement between analysts and psychiatrists during the war, this rapprochement gave rise to the hope for wider social recognition of psychoanalysis. Some key notions of psychoanalysis – the benefit of illness in resolving conflict, the flight into illness, the significance of unconscious drive forces involved in the formation of symptoms – had some resonance for the medical authorities. As Freud recognised, the war neuroses were very useful to psychoanalysis from a didactic point of view, even though the debates had mainly focused on the problem of their sexual aetiology. But the operation of disseminating this information throughout the medical corps had obscured what, for Freud, represented the essential theoretical interest of this business. The problem of the attachment of the libido to the ego itself, the narcissistic dimension identified in the war neuroses, had not been properly grasped. To put it another way, the diffusion of psychoanalytic notions to representatives of official psychiatry was based on a misunderstanding.

The end of the conflict led to the disappearance of this particular field of applied psychoanalysis. As Freud explained, it was no longer possible to carry out psychoanalytic studies because the clinical material was lacking. Secondly, it was important not to overestimate the understanding of psychiatrists. Freud soon realised this, pointing out that it was hardly necessary to place excessive importance on the rapprochement made during the war between psychiatrists and psychoanalysts. Rapprochement is not agreement. Demonstrating that the same mechanisms were in play in the neuroses of peace and war is not enough to weaken the substantial resistances of the medical profession to psychoanalysis. Freud always considered psychoanalysis indivisible. According to him, psychoanalytic practice possesses the practitioner entirely or not at all. The pragmatic use of psychoanalysis as a therapeutic method does not necessarily imply acceptance of the psychoanalytic discourse as such. But still, on the theoretical level, Freud was not totally convinced by the efforts of his pupils. On the one hand, Abraham had shown that there was some sort of predisposition to war neurosis when some men lacked the heterosexual libidinal orientation. The relation to castration and the phallus was, according to him, malfunctioning in those whose anguish reached an unbearable threshold in time of war. On the other hand, the practice developed by Ernst Simmel was based on the principle, long held in psychoanalysis, of abreaction. The liquidation of the affect turned out to be the principle of the treatments which mingled the hypnotic suggestion with the interpretation of dreams. Simmel encouraged his patient to remember his dreams in order to interpret them. Through the associative thread, he tried to provoke the abreaction of affects. Simmel considered that war neuroses were the expression of an aggressiveness that had not been able to express itself. The soldier had repressed the desire to respond to the brutality of a superior, he had suppressed the desire to defend himself from an injustice, he had repressed the desire to kill. The aggression that turned back onto the ego provoked a crushing guilt that the analyst had to strive to liberate. Simmel proposed to the patient under hypnosis to get rid of the affect by hitting dummies. Generally, one to three sessions were enough. With regard both to sexual causation, in the form of lack of libido, as Abraham had suggested, and to treating these neuroses by abreaction of affect, as Simmel did, Freud's dissatisfaction had to do with the fact that these data, arising as they did from previously acquired knowledge, left a new and inexplicable element in the shadows.

Freud believed that traumatic neurosis came close to the picture of hysteria via the presence of motor symptoms, but that it was differentiated from it by the notable presence of signs of subjective suffering that brought it closer to melancholic or hypochondriacal states. In the same way, the pronounced disorganisation of the psychic functions was not met with to the same extent as in hysteria. If war neurosis could arise in the absence of any proven mechanical shock, the traumatic neurosis of peacetime nevertheless offered some openings, particularly with regard to the fact that anxiety cannot play its role as a signal. Anxiety protects you, in effect, from fear and from the neurosis that it provokes. An attack on the body or a combat wound is not usually accompanied by a war neurosis. Prisoners of war are also protected. The element of fright is therefore an essential condition. The temporal dimension of anxiety is, in itself, a defence. Anxiety is distinguished from the fear that accompanies the sudden onset of a danger for which the individual is not prepared. Again, Freud was noticing a phenomenon that had not, until then, received sufficient attention. The dreams of those suffering from traumatic neurosis constantly bring them back to the situation of the accident. During the day, they do not think about it, but at night, the dream fixation on the traumatic event triggers fear and wakes the dreamer. On its own, this fixation is certainly not typical of traumatic neurosis; hysteria also presents the same characteristic. Simmel and Ferenczi had, moreover, endeavoured to explain the presence of motor symptoms in war neuroses by this fixation on trauma.

It is at the level of the economic function of the trauma that Freud made a distinction between traumatic neurosis and hysterical psychoneurosis. In a letter he sent to Jones in February 1919, he explained that traumatic neurosis was a narcissistic affection in the same way as dementia praecox (schizophrenia). Here, the effect of trauma on the narcissistic libido is related to the fact that the *Reizschutz* (defence against stimuli) has been submerged. This defence is not identical to the neurotic defence. The condition of the traumatic neurosis is that the psyche has not had time to resort to this protection, that it is overwhelmed, surprised without being prepared by the trauma, and 'the principal and primary function of keeping off excessive quantities of "Reiz" [is] frustrated'.[26] Anxiety is therefore a protection against shock (*Schreck*). In the case of war, a conflict arises in the ego between the habitual ego and the new warrior ideal. 'The first is subjugated but when the "shell" arrives, this old Ego understands, it may be killed by the ways of the Alter Ego.'[27] With the onset of shock, there is a reversal to the extent that the new master becomes in turn a weak and impoverished *Ich*. All this leads to the result that the whole constituted by this division between these two masters passes under the duplicity of traumatic neurosis. The difference between peacetime neurosis and war neurosis is that, in the first case, the ego is strong but surprised, whereas, in the second case, the ego is prepared but it is weak. For this reason, Freud believes, war neurosis is a case of internal narcissistic conflict similar to the mechanism found in melancholy. The conflict between two masters, between the old ego and the new warrior ego, is characteristic of war neurosis. In melancholy, the shadow of the object falls on the ego, while in war neurosis the alter ego presents itself under the aspect of an ideal with which the subject is identified. What Freud demonstrates in this way is that in times of war, the enemy is not only outside, he is also within because he is an Other that pushes the individual to sacrifice himself. At the end of this passage from the letter to Jones, Freud added that he himself had not analysed any cases of war neuroses. In *Beyond the Pleasure Principle*, Freud provided clarifications of the retrospective function of anxiety. The attachment to the trauma in the dream brings up the anxiety that had been lacking at the moment of shock. This approach to traumatic neurosis highlights the instance of repetition of displeasure. Freud came to distinguish between reproduction (*Reproduzieren*), remembering (*Erinnern*) and repetition (*Wiederholen*).

If Freud subsequently reconsidered the predominant manifestation of anxiety in war neuroses at this time, on what basis could he establish that traumatic neurosis and transference neurosis had something in common? In his 1914 article 'Erinnern, Wiederholen und Darcharbeiten',[28] Freud articulated the function of repetition in its difference with recollection. He pointed out that during the course of the treatment, repeating is a way of remembering, but in a very particular way, since it is always a repetition in action. At the beginning of analysis, the patient does not say that he remembers certain facts of his childhood; he repeats them in the act of transference. He does not remember being ashamed of certain sexual activities, but he is ashamed of the treatment, and he makes it a secret that he tries to hide from the people closest to him. Freud then emphasises that the patient repeats everything that comes from the repressed: inhibitions, inappropriate attitudes, pathological traits. This is why a worsening of the patient's condition often occurs during the course of the treatment.

In the first cathartic phase, the determination of the moment of the formation of the symptom and the sustained effort to reproduce the psychic processes of this situation should lead to the discharge by means of a conscious activity. At that time, the work of interpretation was designed to make up for what could not be remembered. The communication to the patient of his resistances should allow him to overcome them, which allows him access to forgotten situations. In the later phase, with the identification of the repetition compulsion in the transference, the analyst no longer processes a past illness. He is dealing with a current and active force, a transference neurosis. The symptom then enters the field of action of the cure as something real. Freud points out that the analytic treatment leads the patient to reconsider his own relation to his illness. The illness no longer appears to him as something despicable; on the contrary, his illness will retain his full attention. The illness becomes a part of one's being that is based on good motives, and something in which one must look for precious elements for the post-analytic existence.

The link between act and repetition was deepened by Freud in his *Beyond the Pleasure Principle.* He emphasised the function of repetition of trauma in the dreams of war neurotics insofar as it escapes the domination of the pleasure principle. Freud pursued the thread of a reflection initiated in 1916 on the economy of trauma: trauma has no other meaning than an economic meaning. Trauma is defined as a lived event which, in a short time, brings so much extra excitement that its suppression or assimilation by normal means is impossible.[29] This results in lasting troubles in the use of libidinal energy. Subsequently, Freud looked again at the problem of traumatic neurosis and, more particularly, clarified the relationship between anxiety and the formation of symptoms. In 1919, he defined fright as the sine qua non condition of traumatic neurosis. In the letter to Jones quoted above, there was talk of the function of anxiety as a signal. If anxiety has been lacking at the moment of the shock, the distancing of excessive amounts of stimuli is frustrated and the narcissistic libido subsequently receives the anxiety in the form of signs of anxiety. Which amounts to saying that after the shock, anxiety as a signal is situated at the level of the ego. It is precisely this point that will be repeated in 1926 in *Inhibition, Symptom and Anxiety.* Anxiety is defined there as the reaction to the situation of danger. Anxiety is a signal and the symptoms are formed in order to avoid the situation of danger signalled by the development of anxiety. Freud then shows that the danger concerned is always related to the danger of castration. The moment of shock confronts the subject with his own death, and that death in turn has the signification of castration. By its repetition, the dream of traumatic neurosis thus has the primary function of hooking the subject to his most intimate connection to the feeling of life.

Let us mention that Lacan commented on this crossing-over from remembrance to repetition. In his opinion, it was hardly surprising that early psychoanalysis emphasised the process of remembrance. With the hysterics, memories flooded in, and the treatment gave access to the repressed events that came to the surface. 'For the benefit of him who takes the place of the father, one remembered things right down to the dregs,'[30] he explained. However, the re-memorialisation of the biography has limits, since thought always avoids the same thing. The real is that which always returns to the same place, and it is the place where the subject, insofar as he thinks, does not encounter it. This is why Freud's discovery of repetition as a function came to indicate this relation between thought and the real. In traumatic neurosis, the real appears as the point which the subject can approach only by being divided in different instances. As Freud insists, at night, the memory of bombardment is repeated in a dream, but by day the same event usually leaves the individual completely indifferent. The division of the subject is already visible at the level of the difference between day and night, between awakening and dreaming. Freud points out that the dream fixation to trauma comes from the beyond of the pleasure principle. In the treatment, this same principle is responsible for the patient's singular resistance to getting better. The consequences of Freud's introduction of the death drive to therapeutic application in psychoanalysis turn out to be radical. It is no longer a question of what does or does not get in the way of healing and how to remedy it. Negative therapeutic resistance returns to inertia, to the patient's own resistance to interventions that aim to cure him, to normalise him.

Psychoanalysis of war neuroses had not been fully endorsed by the time the Armistice was signed in 1918 – far from it. The controversy between the partisans of psychoanalysis and its detractors also continued after the fall of the Austro-Hungarian monarchy. As soon as the war ended, the Austrian Parliament voted to create a commission to investigate military misconduct. This commission recorded the complaints of former soldiers against the psychiatrists and endeavoured to ascertain whether or not the psychiatrists had exposed the hospitalised soldiers to excessive electrical currents.

During the investigation, Freud was asked to pronounce on the case of Lieutenant Kauders, whose story was exemplary in more ways than one. This German-speaking patriot was sent to the Russian-Polish frontier as early as September 1914. All indications are that his ideal collapsed when he came face to face with the Austrian army's astonishing lack of resources. All he had in the way of equipment were a pair of antique field glasses, an old-fashioned pistol and a sabre that made marching almost impossible. He did not even have a map of the location where he had been ordered to take his men. Instead, he was given an extremely inaccurate pencil drawing of the forest and its surrounding area. To this scarcity of material was added the inconvenience that most of the men he was leading spoke only Hungarian, which was not that exceptional in the armies of the Central European powers. His regiment came under heavy Russian fire near Zamosz, and Kauders saw two of his NCOs die before his eyes. He himself was wounded. At that moment, he felt his underwear getting wet. Without realising it, he had urinated. His last impression was of a suffocating stench. He later regained consciousness at a first aid post.

Kauders was declared an invalid by an arbitration commission and sent back home to Berlin. He had the opportunity to consult the most famous German neurologist of the time, who confirmed the neurological nature of the symptoms he was suffering from. The specialist concluded that Kauders was suffering from a partial crack in the left side of the occiput, which explained his severe headache and his difficulty in walking. However, in the autumn of 1917, an Austrian doctor from a mobile military commission reversed this decision. He suspected that Kauders was malingering and sent him to Vienna. From there, the unfortunate lieutenant was taken to the garrison hospital and immediately placed in a sort of cell with a barred window. The next day he was taken by ambulance to a secure unit at Professor Julius Wagner-Jauregg's clinic, where he spent seventy-seven days in solitary confinement. He described in detail the faradisation to which he was subjected by Wagner-Jauregg's assistant:

> These unmistakable tortures were specially prepared psychologically: The patient is usually given to understand that he is about to experience a procedure which is known to be horrible. This is done once by fellow-patients briefed to do it, then by attendants and finally by the physician. Last of all, they let the candidate watch a 'brush faradisation' – as this electrical torture is called – or force him to it, even when he can no longer endure the penetrating cries of pain of those in treatment … The pains caused by brush faradisation are indescribable. It feels as though innumerable drills are being driven right into the bones at a furious speed. The most horrible thing about it is the uneven quality of the pain which consists of a huge number of heavy jabs. I concentrated all my energy on not allowing one cry of pain to be forced out of me. I was assured that this had never been seen before. These notes [which Kauders

> had been able to 'glance at by stealth' and found remarks about his having behaved 'heroically' and 'with extreme courage'] prove that the intention in giving me faradic treatment was not to improve my health but that I was quite intentionally exposed to torture. The first torture lasted over half an hour; I was taken back to my room, where I collapsed on my bed.[31]

Eissler's astute observation that, at the very moment when Kauders saw the two NCOs die, a bodily function escaped the control of the subject's ego, must be kept in mind. Eissler understood this bladder malfunction as the real trauma. The involuntary release of urine not only caused shame but was also an authentic experience of fragmentation inasmuch as, 'at that instant, his relationship to his own body had been profoundly disturbed. His body was no longer his own'. This disintegration of the unity of the body either symbolised an experience of subjective death or, via the phallic dimension that was implicated in it, constituted a body event relating to the meaning of life and thus, fundamentally, to the guilt of the survivor: why the other and not me, since one has lost his life and the other has escaped. This interpretation is made possible by all of the above – i.e. the presence in Kauders (whom Eissler met in New York later in life) of the oppressive memory of his humiliation. Eissler shows that the trauma of 1914 hid an older trauma, one dating back to the subject's childhood. It was the childhood trauma caused by the words of his authoritarian father, who had repeatedly said to him, 'You lie!' The suicide of an elder half-brother, whose existence was entirely dominated by paternal despotism, was a decisive step in the constitution of Kauders' personality. In the emotional distance in which his father's authority held him, this elder brother occupied a paternal position for Kauders. This is how this suicide confronted him with the traumatising death of a substitute for the father. One can hypothesise that the formula of his fantasy was the murder of the father by another father.[32]

Kauders had always tried to make a lie of the superegoic command, 'You lie'. He had defended himself throughout his life by obliging himself to tell the truth, the whole truth and nothing but the truth. It is therefore understandable that, during the war, the accusation of malingering formulated by the Austrian military doctor echoed the infantile trauma. This criticism probably hit Kauders with all the force of those shells that blew his NCOs apart before his eyes on the Russian-Polish border. How could one man's call for justice have mobilised so much energy and led him to appeal to an expert such as Freud, if his accusation was based only on this experience of injustice? What the lieutenant strongly defended himself against, once again, was the accusation of having lied. Freud was therefore called as an expert witness by the parliamentary commission. He wrote a report for the meeting, which convened on 14 October 1920. It argued that war neurotics were not malingerers, that medicine was in danger of losing itself by serving goals that were foreign to it. When the doctor became a functionary of war, he became the seat of a struggle between the demands of humanity and those of national conflict. Freud outlined distinct levels of responsibility:

> The physician should be the advocate of the ill first of all, not that of another. His function is impaired as soon as he starts serving someone else; at the moment when he is ordered to rehabilitate people for war duty as quickly as possible, a conflict had to emerge for which the medical profession cannot possibly be made responsible.[33]

The treatment of war neuroses was practised by doctors who were aiming not at the recovery of the sick but at the restoration of their ability to fight. But if the doctor became an official under military command like any other, he lived in fear of being accused of negligence and treason himself. Without excluding the possibility that a traumatic neurosis was formed when Kauders came under fire at the front, Freud was immediately suspicious of the neurological nature of the symptoms that he was suffering from. Freud's strategy did not, however, involve calling Wagner-Jauregg into question. He took care not to contradict the diagnosis of traumatic hysteria made by his eminent colleague. Freud declared that Wagner-Jauregg had treated Kauders according to the methods traditionally used in Viennese clinics at the time. A great specialist such as Wagner-Jauregg could not be accused of having knowingly tortured a lieutenant; it was impossible to claim that he had acted cruelly. Freud refuted the idea that Wagner-Jauregg had been able to commit any kind of crime. (We are, let us not forget, in 1920.) This episode clearly shows Freud's desire to avoid any direct confrontation with the most conservative representatives of psychiatry at the very moment when the Viennese Psychoanalytic Association (WPV) was working on opening a polyclinic on the model of the clinic that had just been created in Berlin. The Vienna polyclinic would need the approval of the medical authorities, and Freud could not afford to antagonise one of the most famous representatives of official medicine. Because of his conservatism and notoriety, Wagner-Jauregg was the adversary Freud needed, for tactical reasons, to manage.

Despite the precautions that Freud had taken when speaking of the activities of Austrian psychiatrists during the war, psychoanalysis was ferociously questioned by the opposing party during the committee's debates. First of all, Wagner-Jauregg pointed out that Freud had never been anywhere near war neurotics. Moreover, he believed that the multiplicity of languages spoken in the Austro-Hungarian Empire's army – no fewer than eleven – would have constituted a genuine obstacle to the use of psychoanalysis in wartime. To which Freud replied that psychoanalysis was usable during armed conflicts. The results obtained in Germany by doctors who had applied psychoanalytical principles in the treatment of war neurotics had proved it. Wagner-Jauregg pointed out that psychoanalysis could be used, at a pinch, to treat isolated cases, which Freud vigorously contested.

Here is the passage from the discussion that took place during Freud's appearance before the commission:

PROFESSOR WAGNER: Concerning psychoanalysis, I would like to state that this type of treatment often takes God knows how long, and that this method is not usable in war. The circumstance of foreign language has been admitted by Professor Freud.

CHAIRMAN: According to Professor Freud, treatment needs individualisation.

PROFESSOR FREUD: It has been carried out even in war.

PROFESSOR WAGNER: But only in singular cases.

PROFESSOR FREUD: In large numbers. But it was shortened by hypnosis. It took extraordinary pains, but it would have been worthwhile in especially difficult cases.[34]

Consequently, at the beginning of the 1920s, Freud reiterated what he had already stated during the war. When trauma takes on a collective dimension, psychoanalysis must make itself accessible to the masses. The Berlin Polyclinic would become the original laboratory of this experiment.

A knot between therapeutics, training and teaching

The Berlin Psychoanalytic Institute had to fulfil three essential objectives. In the first place, it had to make the therapeutic application of psychoanalysis accessible to the masses. This was the function that was devolved to the polyclinic. It was also necessary to create a place where psychoanalytic theory would be taught. The most experienced analysts would be responsible for teaching it to the students. A study programme for trainees was developed and became mandatory in the autumn of 1927. Finally, for research purposes, it was necessary to study cases that did not usually come within the field of classical indications for analysis. To satisfy this recommendation, Berlin analysts broadened the indications of analytic treatment to include so-called mild psychoses, psychopathy, criminality and abnormalities of character. To make analysis accessible to all, to create a place of teaching and to test the knowledge already acquired it was necessary to invent the knot capable of holding these three objectives together.

In order to study in detail the modalities of this knotting, we will pay attention to the main texts written by the founding members of the Berlin Institute in 1922, 1928 and 1930. Other documents – such as the later testimony of Siegfried Bernfeld, who left Vienna to train in Berlin in 1926 – will shed further light on the subject. Other information punctuates the correspondence of James and Alix Strachey and the biography of Melanie Klein. Furthermore, the leftwing Freudians found means of expression in Germany that were difficult to realise elsewhere. At that time, indeed, some analysts had tried to put psychoanalysis at the service of revolution, much to Freud's chagrin. The management of the institute agreed to hold a small seminar under the direction of Otto Fenichel. This Kinderseminar – the so-called children's seminar – was a laboratory for a new generation of students who trained in Berlin. Various leftist political opinions were freely expressed there. That the concept of character and its social implications were the subject of passionate discussions within this subgroup can be explained by the affinity of thought that existed between Fenichel and Wilhelm Reich, who was directing the seminar on psychoanalytic technique at the WPV at the time.

The most precise elements relating to the organisation of teaching, to statistical data and to the results of treatments appear in two activity reports published eight years apart. A first report was written, at Freud's request, by Max Eitingon on the occasion of the Seventh International Psychoanalytic Congress, which was held in Berlin in 1922.[35] A preface by Freud served as an introduction to this document, which first appeared in 1923 in the *Internationale Zeitschrift für Psychoanalyse* and was subsequently published in the *International Journal of Psychoanalysis.* A French translation was published by the review *Topique* in 1977, but without Freud's preface, which deserves to be studied closely.[36] The most complete amount of information can be found in the activity report written in 1930, on the occasion of the Berlin Institute's tenth anniversary. Published by the Internationaler Psychoanalytischer Verlag, this monograph was long kept under the title *Zehn Jahre Berliner Psychoanalytisches Institut* at Freud's house in Vienna, as well as at several IPA institutes.[37] The French translation of this original report was published in 1985.[38] In the translated volume, the interesting address that Max Eitingon gave at the inauguration of the polyclinic's new premises in 1928 also appears.[39] This lecture highlights Eitingon's decisive influence on the institution. From this point of view, the tribute that Freud paid him by granting him the title of founder of the Berlin Institute was entirely justified. Without Eitingon's singular desire to lead such an enterprise, which he financed until his forced departure from Germany, this institutional experiment could not have begun and developed as it did.

In the wake of the Budapest congress, Abraham and Eitingon, who had been working together for a long time, forged closer ties with the politically engaged neurologist Ernst Simmel, who was eager to insert psychoanalysis into the social field. In 1913, he cofounded a group of Social Democratic doctors with his colleague Karl Landauer, who later led the Frankfurt Psychoanalytic Institute. Through Landauer, Abraham anticipated gaining support from parliamentarians. In addition, Simmel's relations with the Ministry of Religious Affairs and Public Instruction offered the chance of access to the university faculty. The teaching of psychoanalysis in German universities no longer seemed a utopian prospect. There was no time to lose. With the advent of the Weimar Republic, a political breach opened. The time had come for the psychoanalysts to act. In the summer of 1919, Simmel and Eitingon asked the BPV to give them a mandate to establish a psychoanalytic institute.

In a letter to Freud dated 21 July 1919, Eitingon announced his decision to open a polyclinic in Berlin in these terms:

> I would like to speak to you today about a small psychoanalytic element which is perhaps not devoid of significance. Last Saturday, at my request, our Association took the decision to open, next winter, a psychoanalytic polyclinic in Berlin. We are therefore going to begin analytic 'psychotherapy for the people' without waiting for the state, which is currently undergoing reconstruction, or for the generous anthropophilic impulses of an individual in the style of Dr. von Freund to give us great resources to pursue these objectives. A polyclinic seemed to me, in its modesty and feasibility, the *ovulum* that is best suited to serve as a future research institute for psychoanalysis. We are already pretty sure we have the relatively small means for a not too small polyclinic – three doctors should be able to work together. As a first step, the quantum of daily medical treatment time will be provided by a number of experienced colleagues in our association, depending on how much time they have available. I have asked the Association, for myself and for Simmel, for the mandate to direct the polyclinic. A few meetings will still be devoted to the discussion of the details, purely practical questions, but I look forward to sending you this provisional information in order to hear your opinion, Professor – our decisions are not yet final.[40]

Freud's response to this extremely important information is not known. In September 1919, during a visit to Hamburg, he made a detour to Berlin to visit both Eitingon – who introduced Freud to his extremely wealthy parents – and Abraham. Later that same year, through Simmel, the German Parliament asked Abraham to prepare a detailed scientific paper on the BPV with a view to creating a chair of psychoanalysis in Professor Bonhoeffer's[41] department at the University of Berlin. Freud, who was very doubtful about the possibility that a chair of psychoanalysis would be entrusted to Abraham, told Eitingon of his concerns regarding the future of psychoanalysis. These misgivings dated back to the time when he had been alone in supporting the psychoanalytical enterprise. It corresponded to 'the anxiety about what the human rabble would do when I am no longer alive'.[42]

The secret committee, formed in 1912 in the aftermath of the break with Adler and Jung, had the mission of extending Freud's presence in the world. The creation of a psychoanalytic institute also inscribed itself in the temporal perspective of continuing Freud's work beyond the man himself. In addition, from the strategic point of view, the polyclinic would situate the IPA's centre of gravity in Berlin. The German language, the original language of psychoanalysis, would remain dominant. Let us not forget that Freud accorded great importance to the written vector of his thought. To publish, to disseminate, to translate, to find collaborators who would come together to take up all of these tasks – this was, for Freud, a perpetual race against the clock, a wager, a worry without respite. Finding the necessary financing for the Verlag was a constant headache; the publication of articles, the translations and the sales figures (frequently mediocre) for the journals and other works were a huge worry. But Freud was also a citizen of Central Europe and, moreover, a Jew. He had witnessed the disintegration of the civilisation that he had known, the collapse of a world where the Germanic language had become established. Perhaps we can see there the foundation of the famous bitterness that some in Freud's circle noted at the beginning of the 1920s. Wilhelm Reich, for example, believed that only a depressed Freud could have invented the death drive. The reality is that the westward orientation – towards the countries that had won the war – seemed inevitable to Freud, who nevertheless made an effort keep this evolution in check for as long as possible.

Abraham kept Freud informed of his search for a suitable place to house the polyclinic: 'You may already have heard from Eitingon that there is a possibility of premises for our polyclinic. We shall rent it if the price is within our means. Simmel will be an excellent force for the polyclinic.'[43] On 25 November the offices of the polyclinic were approved by the municipal housing commissioner. The imminence of the inauguration of the polyclinic was referenced in another letter that Abraham addressed to Freud at the end of 1919: 'Interest in academic circles is visibly increasing. The polyclinic, which will definitely be opened in January, is arousing the greatest interest on the part of the Ministry,'[44] he wrote. As we can see, the creation of a psychoanalytic polyclinic went hand in hand with the project of teaching psychoanalysis at the university. Unfortunately, the medical circles of the time, generally conservative, opposed the creation of a chair of psychoanalysis. During the Weimar period, the most educated strata of German society were largely grouped at the conservative end of the political spectrum. The Berlin establishment had little time for intellectual innovation. As the analysts could not count on financial aid for the polyclinic from a state that was practically ruined, it was necessary to find a way of compensating for this lack of assistance. Eitingon and Simmel then proposed that the polyclinic's expenses be covered by the BPV membership. In fact, Eitingon was forced to make the first downpayment. He then regularly compensated for the institution's annual losses. The analyses would mostly be free, as Freud had wished. But this principle did not exclude payment from patients who had the means. The price of sessions would not be advertised in advance. A place would be reserved for discussion between patient and analyst at the time of the initial consultation. In addition, each member of the BPV would commit to taking at least one patient from the polyclinic into analysis, either within the institution or in their own office. If they were not in a position to do so, they would pay a prearranged sum every month to support the psychoanalytic activities of the polyclinic. Once these principles had been accepted by the BPV, there would be nothing to stop the polyclinic from opening.

On 16 February 1920, the BPV inaugurated the Berlin Polyclinic for the Psychoanalytic Treatment of Nervous Illnesses. For reasons of prestige and to illustrate the close ties that existed between the BPV and the polyclinic, Abraham's name was included in the list of directors on the sign at the entrance. The programme for the inauguration placed great emphasis on the arts. After Abraham had given his welcome address, Willy Bardas played a Beethoven sonata; next, Simmel recited poems by Rainer Maria Rilke; then it was back to the music with Schubert lieder, a Chopin ballad played by Bardas and his wife, a piece by Arnold Schoenberg and another by Hugo Wolf. There followed a few of Christian Morgenstern's poems, a talk by Simmel on the writer Oskar Hermann Schmitz and, finally, a talk by Abraham concerning the link between the polyclinic and the unconscious.[45]

The new institution's premises were located in eastern Berlin, at Potsdamer Strasse 29. Freud did not attend the inauguration. Rail traffic between Austria and Germany was badly disrupted at the time, and Freud had recently lost both his good friend Anton von Freund and his second daughter, Sophie, who lived in Hamburg. 'The pressure since Sophie's death has not left us,' he wrote to Ferenczi in March 1920. In the same letter, Freud mentioned the inauguration of the polyclinic:

> The most gratifying thing at this time – apart from new editions and translations – is the opening of the Berlin polyclinic, founded by Eitingon (14 February), at which Ernst, Mathilde, and Robert happened to be present. Ernst also looked after setting up and equipping it.[46]

Most patients turned up at the clinic spontaneously, without being referred. This caused a minor sensation in Berlin's medical circles, which Eitingon mentioned to Freud. Abraham was appointed director of the polyclinic thanks to the prestige he enjoyed at the heart of the movement. Just one week after the inauguration, it was planned that his teaching activities would begin with a course on psychoanalysis for doctors and students. A delegation from the Youth Protection Service and some Berlin city councillors approached the polyclinic's management to ask about treatments for children. In March 1920, Abraham told Freud that the institution was already well attended, but he complained that his course had been poorly advertised. Only ten auditors had attended. He hoped that a regular system of teaching would be developed as soon as possible. Eitingon, who had wanted to set up a reading room, asked Freud to make copies of books on psychoanalysis available to the polyclinic's library. The project dearest to his heart was a department specialising in the treatment of neurotic children. 'I would like to specially train a woman doctor for this purpose,' he told Freud.

It is interesting to note that in 1922 (when Abraham was director of the polyclinic) Freud had asked Eitingon to write the first report on the polyclinic for that year's IPA congress, and in the short preface he wrote for that occasion Freud presented Eitingon as the true founder of the polyclinic.[47] In this preface, we can see that Freud took for granted the need to multiply therapeutic analytic institutions in order to make psychoanalytic treatments accessible to the middle classes, which had been ruined by the postwar financial crisis. A second theme referred to the fight against unscrupulous and poorly trained practitioners. Hence the urgent need to engage a policy of training analysts in an unprecedented way, through psychoanalytic institutes. Where did this last idea come from? To ask this question is not so odd because some testimonies have emphasised Freud's misgivings concerning protocols and established procedures for the training of analysts. Surprising as it may seem, in the early 1920s Freud could still advise a young colleague to embark on analytic practice without having first gone through a didactic formation at a training institute. He felt that it would always be possible to come and talk to him when there were difficulties in the treatment of a patient. Of course, Freud was also an exception. Moreover, his opinion did not prevent the younger man from going to Berlin anyway, which says a great deal about the institute's prestige. However, the need to organise training through an educational institute had yet another goal, not mentioned by Freud in the preface of 1922: to attract as many *francs-tireurs* as possible.[48] It should be remembered that the problem of wild psychoanalysis had preoccupied the analytic community well before World War I. In the year that saw the founding of the IPA, Freud wrote an article on so-called wild psychoanalysis. He took no responsibility for the practice of those who claimed to be psychoanalysts without having joined the movement he had created. Freud gave the example of a woman in her fifties who had suffered from anxiety since her divorce. She had consulted a young doctor with no analytic training who explained that her anxieties came from sexual desires and that she should satisfy them by returning to her husband or by taking a lover or by indulging in masturbation. Unable to bring herself to apply any or all of these solutions, she was speaking to Freud in utter desperation, telling him about the damage caused by the inexperience of the doctor in question. Freud explained that the clumsiness of the young colleague was due to his lack of training, since the proposed solutions left no room for psychoanalysis. Freud used the example of a physician, but the analytic community also felt threatened by the rise of 'wild' practitioners who did not belong to the medical profession.

At that time, Hans Blüher was a member of the BPV. He accurately noted that the phenomenon of the spread of psychoanalytic ideas in society was being experienced as a disturbing loss of mastery. The numerical importance of two groups – one made up of trained doctors and the other not – created a fear of being overwhelmed by practitioners who did not belong to the psychoanalytic societies of the time:

> In Berlin, Vienna and Zurich, a psychoanalytic group consisted of two circles: one restricted, medical, using a strictly medical terminology and devoted to the treatment of neurotics; the other, non-medical, much wider, seeking to interest the public in neuroses and psychoanalysis. According to Blüher, this non-medical circle was the main driving force

> of the psychoanalytic movement; its members produced an abundant pseudo-psychoanalytic literature. In their outrageous words, they proclaimed that psychoanalysis could provide a solution to all the problems of humanity, from the treatment of individual neurosis to the abolition of war. In this way, while encouraging patients to submit to psychoanalytic treatment, they discredited the movement.[49]

The members of this non-medical circle were looking for a way to engage with the general public. These practitioners were perceived as a danger to the psychoanalytic organisation. But it made no sense strategically simply to dispense with enthusiastic amateurs. Hence the question: how to attract them and persuade them to undergo analytic training? Later accounts have a similar tenor: the penetration of psychoanalytic ideas into the wider culture was often perceived as a danger. The Berlin Institute was also conceived as an essential instrument in the fight against wild psychoanalysis. The stakes were high: it was a question of capturing, attracting and training as many *francs-tireurs* as possible. It was, it was felt, necessary to approve the candidacy of individuals who had no previous medical training. This, in turn, involved supporting the principle of lay analysis. Freud was very much in favour of it in 1927: 'The important question is not whether an analyst possesses a medical diploma but whether he has had the special training necessary for the practice of analysis.'[50]

Notes

1 Hanns Sachs, 'L'analyse didactique' (1930), in Fanny Colonomos (ed.), *On forme des psychanalystes: Rapport original sur les dix ans de l'Institut psychanalytique de Berlin 1920–1930* (Paris: Denoël, 1985), p. 137.
2 Felix Boehm (1881–1958), a neuropsychiatrist, studied with Kraepelin. He was analysed by Eugenie Sokolnicka and Karl Abraham. He began teaching at the Berlin Psychoanalytic Institute in 1923 and was president of the DPG from 1933 to 1938. He was also secretary and teacher at the Göring Institute. After World War II, he participated in the refounding of the DPG.
3 Moustapha Safouan, *Jacques Lacan and the Question of Psychoanalytic Training*, trans. Jacqueline Rose (London: Palgrave Macmillan, 2000).
4 Ernest Jones, *Sigmund Freud: Life and Work, The Last Phase, 1919–1939*, vol. 3 (London: The Hogarth Press, 1957), pp. 118–119.
5 Russell Jacoby, *The Repression of Psychoanalysis: Otto Fenichel and the Political Freudians* (Chicago: University of Chicago Press, 1986), p. 35.
6 Jacques Lacan, 'The Tokyo Discourse', trans. Dany Nobus, *Journal for Lacanian Studies*, vol. 3, no. 1 (London and New York: Karnac, 2005), 130.
7 Jacques Lacan, *The Seminar of Jacques Lacan, Book XVII: The Other Side of Psychoanalysis* (1969–1970), trans. Russell Grigg (New York and London: Norton, 2007), p. 105.
8 Max Eitingon, 'Allocution prononcée le 30 septembre 1928 lors de l'inauguration des nouveaux locaux de l'Institut', in Fanny Colonomos, *On forme des psychanalystes*, p. 182.

9 Peter Gay, *Weimar Culture: The Outsider as Insider* (London: Martin Secker & Warburg, 1969), p. 30.
10 Walter Laqueur, *Weimar: A Cultural History, 1918–1933* (London: Weidenfeld and Nicolson, 1974).
11 Sigmund Freud, 'On the Teaching of Psychoanalysis in Universities' (1918), *Standard Edition*, vol. 17, pp. 171–173.
12 Gustave Peiser, 'Introduction', in *Berlin entre les deux guerres: une symbiose judéo-allemande? Actes du colloque tenu à l'université Stendhal à Grenoble* (Paris: L'Harmattan, 2000), p. 15.
13 Rathenau's assassination by rightwing militants in June 1922 marked a turning point in the history of the Weimar Republic.
14 Stefan Zweig, *The World of Yesterday: Memoirs of a European*, trans. Anthea Bell (London: Pushkin Press, 2009), p. 338.
15 Peter Gay, *Weimar Culture, op. cit.*
16 Joseph Roth, 'The Steam Baths at Night' (*Neue Berliner Zeitung*, 4 March 1920), in *What I Saw*, trans. Michael Hofmann (London: Granta, 2003), p. 70.
17 Walter Laqueur, *Weimar: A Cultural History, 1918–1933* (London: Weidenfeld and Nicolson, 1974).
18 Abraham to Freud, letter of 19 October 1919, in Ernst Falzeder (ed.), *The Complete Correspondence of Sigmund Freud and Karl Abraham, 1907–1925*, trans. Caroline Schwarzacher (London and New York: Karnac, 2002), p. 405.
19 *Ibid.*, p. 406.
20 Phyllis Grosskurth, *Melanie Klein: Her World and Her Work* (London: Hodder & Stoughton, 1986), p. 92.
21 *Zeitschrift für die gesamte Neurologie und Psychiatrie*, XLV, 18. Cited in Michael Schröter (ed.), *Sigmund Freud et Max Eitingon, Correspondance: 1906–1939* (Paris: Fayard, 2009), p. 176.
22 Karl Abraham, 'Contribution to the Symposium on Psychoanalysis and the War Neurosis Held at the Fifth International Psychoanalytical Congress in Budapest' (1918), *The International Psychoanalytical Library*, vol. 2 (1921), 23.
23 Jacques Lacan, 'British Psychiatry and the War', *Psychoanalytical Notebooks of the London Society of the New Lacanian School*, no. 33 (2019), 45.
24 *Ibid.*, 21–22.
25 Gustav Aschaffenburg, *Diskussionsbemerkung* (1917). Cited by Kurt R. Eissler in *Freud as an Expert Witness: The Discussion of War Neuroses Between Freud and Wagner-Jauregg* (Madison, CT: International Universities Press, 1986).
26 Freud to Jones, Letter 232, 18 February 1919, in R. Andrew Paskauskas (ed.), *The Complete Correspondence of Sigmund Freud and Ernest Jones, 1908–1939* (Cambridge, MA: The Belknap Press of Harvard University Press, 1993), p. 334.
27 *Ibid.*
28 Sigmund Freud, 'Remembering, Repeating, and Working-Through (Further Recommendations on the Technique of Psychoanalysis, II)' (1914), *Standard Edition*, vol. 12, p. 147.
29 Sigmund Freud, 'Fixation to Traumas – The Unconscious' (1917), *Standard Edition*, vol. 16, pp. 273–285.
30 Jacques Lacan, *The Seminar of Jacques Lacan, Book XI: The Four Fundamental Concepts of Psychoanalysis*, trans. Alan Sheridan (New York and London: Norton, 1978), p. 50.
31 Kurt R. Eissler, *Freud as an Expert Witness, op. cit.*
32 *Ibid.*, p. 222.
33 *Ibid.*, p. 58, fn. 44. Eissler points out that Freud was probably prevented from reading his expert report before the commission, as he had intended. His oral

testimony, however, provides essential data on how he handled the sensitivity of the psychiatrists; this excerpt is from page 60 of Eissler's book. For the written report, see S. Freud, 'Memorandum on the Electrical Treatment of War Neurotics' (1920), published as an appendix to 'Introduction to *Psychoanalysis and the War Neuroses*', *Standard Edition*, vol. 17, p. 211.

34 *Ibid.*, pp. 66–67.

35 Max Eitingon, 'Report on the Berlin Psychoanalytical Policlinic' (1922), *Bulletin of the International Psychoanalytic Association*, vol. 4 (1923), 254–269.

36 Sigmund Freud, 'Preface to Max Eitingon's Report on the Berlin Psychoanalytical Polyclinic (March 1920 to June 1922)' (1923), *Standard Edition*, vol. 19, p. 285.

37 Available online in German at Deutsche Psychoanalytische Gesellschaft.

38 Fanny Colonomos (ed.), *On forme des psychanalystes: Rapport original sur les dix ans de l'Institut Psychanalyticque de Berlin, 1920–1930* (Paris: Denoël, 1985).

39 Max Eitingon, 'Ansprache bei der Einweihung der neuen Institutsräume am 30 September 1928', in *Zehn Jahre Berliner Psychoanalytisches Institut* (Vienna: Internationaler Psychoanalytischer Verlag, 1930), pp. 71–74.

40 Letter from Eitingon to Freud, No. 142 E, 21 July 1919, in Michael Schröter (ed.), *Sigmund Freud et Max Eitingon, Correspondance: 1906–1939* (Paris: Fayard, 2009), pp. 182–183.

41 Karl Friedrich Bonhoeffer (1868–1948) was responsible for psychiatric services at the Charité hospital in Berlin.

42 Letter from Eitingon to Freud, No. 151 F, 23 November 1919, in Michael Schröter, *Correspondance*, p. 194.

43 Letter from Karl Abraham to Sigmund Freud, 7 December 1919, in Falzeder, *Complete Correspondence*, p. 410.

44 Letter from Karl Abraham to Sigmund Freud, 29 December 1919, in Falzeder, *Complete Correspondence*, p. 413.

45 The pianist Willy Bardas studied the psychology of pianistic technique; he published a paper on that theme in 1927. The second volume of poet Christian Morgenstern's *Galgenlieder* was published in 1905. Oskar Hermann Schmitz wrote a patriotic pamphlet on the 'True Germany'. There is no written record of the speech made by Karl Abraham during the inauguration.

46 Sigmund Freud to Sándor Ferenczi, Letter 837, 15 March 1920, in Ernst Falzeder and Eva Brabant (eds.), *The Correspondence of Sigmund Freud and Sándor Ferenczi, Volume 3, 1920–1933*, trans. Peter T. Hoffer (Cambridge, MA: Harvard University Press, 2001), p. 13. The March 1920 Kapp Putsch prevented Martha Freud from going to Hamburg. At the time of this attempted coup by the radical right, vehicles decorated with swastikas crisscrossed Berlin.

47 Sigmund Freud, 'Preface to Max Eitingon's *Report on the Berlin Psychoanalytical Polyclinic (March 1920 to June 1922)*', *Standard Edition*, vol. 19, p. 285.

48 [TN: A term that originally described people who fought skilfully and courageously for their country but were not subject to military discipline, operating as they did independently of the regular army. The term originated during the Franco-Prussian War of 1870–1871 and was still in use in the French Resistance during World War II.]

49 Hans Blüher, *Traktat über die Heilkunde* (Stuttgart: Klett, 1926). Cited in Henri-Frédéric Ellenberger, *À la découverte de l'inconscient* (Villeurbanne: Simep, 1974), p. 663.

50 Sigmund Freud, 'Postscript' (1927) to 'The Question of Lay Analysis' (1926), *Standard Edition*, vol. 20, p. 252.

Chapter 2

Asserting the authority of psychoanalysis

Enlarging the field of psychoanalytic action

The public reading of the first report on the polyclinic's activities took place in 1922, two years after the clinic opened. The document had to be concise, precise and in some ways combative at one and the same time. Eitingon introduced his remarks with an account of the sensational effect produced by Freud's declaration in Budapest:

> [Freud] recommended that we should be ready for the moment when the public conscience awakens and the state considers it an urgent duty to take measures to ensure the mental health of its citizens … Public centres and institutes would then be created to make psychoanalytic treatment affordable for a larger number of people. When Freud spoke these words – half prophecy, half challenge – we still had a man among us whose memory will always remain alive for us; he strove, by means of bold projects, to make these distant hopes begin to be realised; and it is not simply the respect due to a deceased colleague that leads me to evoke the name of Dr. Anton von Freund as I prepare to describe to you how far we have come since the founding of this polyclinic.[1]

These two terms – 'prophecy' and 'challenge' – need to be borne in mind, along with the emphasis placed on Freud's ability to anticipate which way to go. However, the statement itself emphasised the utopian aspect of the Freudian dream, and, in so doing, made it happen. We have to face the fact that the ideal would eventually be taken down a notch, that it would deflate when faced with concrete realities. We have seen that the visions of 1918 had a pragmatic origin linked to the experience of war, and it must also be remembered that the call for the creation of free clinics was in the interest of the public authorities. According to Jones, this was the only time Freud ever read from a script when speaking in public. It is known that he could talk for hours without reading from notes. In September 1918, however, this was reportedly not the case. How are we to interpret this? Had Freud read out a

DOI: 10.4324/9781003215684-4

text that was not entirely his own work? Or was a written intervention perhaps more appropriate in such exceptional circumstances? If one sticks to the hypothesis that Freud had been influenced by one or more of his colleagues and that he was expounding a programme that was not completely of his own devising, the criticisms directed at Ferenczi in the Budapest speech remain somewhat inexplicable. How might we determine which parts of the text were written by Freud and which parts were written by others? Such speculations lead nowhere. What we can see, however, is that the 1918 programme underwent a measure of revision at a later date.

In 1922, Eitingon argued that the place of psychoanalysis had been consolidated both during the war and during the troubled period that followed:

> In the early years of the war, one might have thought that psychoanalysis would be swallowed up like everything else; and yet, precisely because of the war, psychoanalysis was progressing and gaining a great deal of ground. War neuroses were the simplest demonstration of Freudian mechanisms, even for the most blind and the most sectarian; towards the end of the war, a project was born in the Austro-Hungarian army … a project to open psychoanalytic treatment centres for neurotics; our colleagues in Germany had similar intentions.
>
> The Fifth Psychoanalytic Congress seemed to confirm these hopes. When, at the end of the war, Austria and Germany were crushed, those hopes came to an end; in Germany, it was no longer possible to envisage the participation either of the state or of the governmental authorities. The old public and scientific institutions had no more money and were on the brink of extinction. The prospect of creating new institutions was completely illusory, especially in places where this system still encountered widespread and persistent opposition from the profession's scientific authorities: obviously, disaster had not brought about many changes in the administration of the old school. Freud's prediction proved to be correct. Private initiative would have to get the ball rolling. Action would have to be taken immediately if we did not want to wait too long, and things would need to be set in motion quickly so as not to miss the moment of opportunity. That such a moment of general collapse, full of so many external difficulties, was a favourable time for psychoanalysis surprised none of us. Psychoanalysis was now looking beyond the illusions that had been destroyed.[2]

Instead of asking a large number of analysts to spend a small amount of their time on the polyclinic, the project's authors were in favour of an inverse formula. Their idea was to encourage a small number of analysts to devote most of their time to the polyclinic on a regular, daily basis. This was to be done on a contractual basis, not a voluntary one. Private financing, which essentially meant the money made available by Eitingon (though Eitingon himself didn't mention it), made it possible to start up by calculating for an undertaking that would last several years.

The new institution opened with just three permanent employees: Eitingon, Simmel and Dr. Anna Smeliansky, their assistant. Each worked fourteen hours a day. They were soon joined by other members of the BPV, who offered to help by taking patients from the polyclinic for analysis. One of the special features of this arrangement was its great flexibility. The analysts would be able to see polyclinic patients either on the institution's premises or in their private offices. In addition, at the same time, didactic analyses were sometimes carried out free of charge in private offices. This was also the case at the polyclinic until Eitingon decided to put an end to free consultations at the polyclinic after a few years of operation.

At the end of 1921, the group of permanent staff members grew to seven. The first three analysts were joined by Dr. Muller, Karen Horney, Franz Alexander, Hans Lampl and, later, Melanie Klein, who arrived from Budapest. At the end of two years of operation, a few students, five doctors and a psychologist who had come to train in psychoanalysis were already conducting cures at the polyclinic.

By presenting the details of the internal organisation of the polyclinic, the report enabled Eitingon to provide some statistics. Thus, a total of 130 analyses were in progress in June 1922. Eitingon stated: 'Now, for the first time, analysis can show statistics to those who are waiting for them; they relate to a single place and a relatively short period of time.'

These statistics were indeed a turning point. Their introduction marked the beginning of the trend of wanting to quantify the results obtained by psychoanalysis, an orientation that had become particularly developed in the USA for historical and ideological reasons. The statistics compiled by the Berlin Institute in the 1930s served, for example, to measure the exaggeration of the speed of spontaneous remission in patients not treated by psychoanalysis. This use of figures seemed to prove that the validity of psychoanalysis would be acquired by accepting the methods of evaluation used in other disciplines. Subsequently, following in the footsteps of Heinz Hartmann, some authors have devoted their efforts to the obsessive distinction between data and hypotheses, to the comparison between control groups of patients treated and untreated by psychoanalysis and to the calibration of the results of cures. At the time when the first statistics were collected, however, they were only intended to serve to highlight the therapeutic effects obtained during treatments in the polyclinic. It is striking that Freud, in at least one place in his work, rejected the use of statistics in psychoanalysis. He expressed himself on this theme in 1925. In his opinion, the statistics produced at the Berlin Institute were of little use. Only a cure at the individual level could be of demonstrative value.

The Berlin Institute occupied the fourth floor of a modest building near the city centre. In this location, fitted out by Ernst Freud, five rooms were dedicated to receiving patients. The largest room served as a lecture theatre and reading room. The consulting rooms were soundproof, and their furniture was simple and functional: a rattan couch, a lamp, a table, some portraits on the walls. There were about forty chairs in the waiting room. By 1922, these premises were already insufficient, not only because of the number of patients but also because teaching activities were expanding. The budget for 1922 was quite modest. The first capital outlay, in the autumn of 1919, was 20,000 marks, corresponding to approximately $5,000 at the time. This budget included salaries, rent, maintenance costs and operating costs. Those employed by the polyclinic received a small salary. Professional recognition was presented as compensation for the low level of remuneration.

As we have seen, in the spring of 1920, about twenty analysts were receiving patients, but only three were permanent salaried employees. Despite the help provided by members of the BPV, the waiting list of patients was getting longer. Let us also remember that after only two and a half years of activity, some 600 patients had turned to the polyclinic for treatment. Some of them had seen the sign at the entrance, others came via word of mouth and more had been referred by doctors. Newspaper advertisements had also attracted many people, so much so that a decision was taken to limit the advertising campaign in order to avoid too great an influx of applications. By 1921, between fifty and sixty analyses were in progress. Eitingon's solution to the problem of handling patient numbers was to wait until demand had been regulated to the point where it became smaller but remained constant. Offering access to analysis to as many people as possible did not mean that mass therapy was necessary. This position allowed hypnotic suggestion not to be used as a therapeutic method, contrary to Freud's prediction in Budapest. Eitingon added that the polyclinic's analysts relied instead on the effects of indirect suggestion, that is, on the phenomenon of impregnating society via word of mouth. Similarly, the presence in the reception area of a multitude of patients waiting for their sessions had a special significance in that it created a situation where 'reality imposes on the neurotic the idea that he is not the only one for whom the doctor is the father'. The fact that the patient was of no material interest to the analyst could sometimes accentuate this finding. In any case, the analysts had noted that this concentration of patients alone produced beneficial effects. In such circumstances, they felt, transference was directed more to the institution than to the individual analyst. This did not, of course, preclude the possibility that the analyst himself might be perceived as a representative of the paternal function from which the patient hoped to gain favour. Not being alone in the waiting room thus took on a special significance that was very much opposed to the fantasy of being loved by the father. In 1922, most patients received by the polyclinic were neurotics, but there were still many instances of long-term organic affects as well as psychic symptoms grafted onto the remnants of organic diseases. Many patients had consulted medical specialists before coming to the polyclinic. Now they had a place where they could tell their story.

Particular attention should be paid to the social categories to which the patients belonged. The variety of patients received in the early days – 'factory workers and maidservants, the daughter of a general, the niece of a minister of state … and a very influential politician' – had evolved. Little by little, this initial diversity was replaced by an audience composed mainly of middle-class individuals and members of the intelligentsia. This might seem contradictory given the retention of the unique criterion of subjective urgency, since it was precisely and solely the level of urgency that had to be evaluated during the consultation while taking the precaution of remaining within the framework of neurosis as frequently as possible.

Moreover, in order to justify the increasing rarity of patients of slender means at the clinic, Eitingon contended that it had been a question of not 'letting ourselves get caught up in the task of improving the general condition of the country when there were so few of us'. For Eitingon, this development was ultimately explained by an arithmetical truth. Because there were so few analysts, it was impossible to deal with crowds of people. At first glance, the formula makes sense: analysts are not on a mission to change society. They simply offer treatment to those who ask for it, which, it should be noted, is not exactly in line with the project outlined in Budapest, which was intended to provide the masses with a means of accessing psychoanalytic treatment. Not getting caught up in the task of improving the country's situation effectively meant that analysts were not to get involved in politics and should confine themselves to the psychotherapeutic field. This common-sense statement refers to the enunciation of the subject who utters it. And this is where the problem lies. The fact that the working class quickly turned away from the polyclinic became a symptom.

The dilemma was a serious one. By reducing the political scope of the project, by foregrounding the ultimately therapeutic purpose of the enterprise, was Eitingon not running the risk of going down the path of the kind of therapeutics that can kill science, as Freud feared in 1926? If one sticks to purely therapeutic aims, nothing stands in the way of the mutation of psychoanalysis into a medical speciality like any other, with its diplomas, clinics and professional societies. If it becomes purely therapeutic, psychoanalysis isolates its members from the general cultural movement in order to establish itself as a profession, with its customs, codes, hierarchical structure and administrative organisation. Paradoxically, the entrenchment of psychoanalysts, their isolation from society, may very well be based on the therapeutic purpose of their discipline, that is to say its specialisation. As soon as it defines itself univocally as therapeutic, psychoanalysis can only mutate, in the long run, into a variant of the master's discourse. To remain true to itself, as Eitingon noted, it must resist the temptation to buy its respectability by branding itself as a therapeutic vocation. For this reason, the only real dispute between Freud and Eitingon concerned lay analysis.

Freud, as we know, never yielded on that principle. Right up until the end of his life, he firmly maintained his position regarding *Laienanalysis.* In 1938, in response to the rumour that he had changed his opinion concerning the practice of psychoanalysis by non-physicians, he wrote that he had never repudiated his views on the subject and that he now held them more strongly than ever before in the face of the fact that the Americans were increasingly turning psychoanalysis into a kind of maid-of-all-work psychiatry. In Berlin, another way of proceeding could have been to admit the political component of the wish to make psychoanalysis accessible to all. In return, the consequences would have to be accepted without using the fact that there were not enough analysts available to bring about any kind of change in society as an excuse. The project of inserting the discourse of psychoanalysis into civilisation is intrinsically political. It is, whether we like it or not, a calculation on a collective scale. The selection of trainees at the Berlin Institute, mainly doctors, was also part of the problem.

Preserving true psychoanalysis

Consultations were undertaken by Eitingon and Simmel for one hour a day, except on Sundays. Wednesdays were reserved for training. Soon, however, Eitingon assumed responsibility for consultations because doing so made it 'easier to get an overview of all the material'. Did his reasons for doing this relate to the other analysts' lack of diagnostic experience? This seems highly unlikely, since important figures in the analytic movement had joined the Berlin group from the very beginning of the polyclinic. The likelier case, as Eitingon in fact suggests, is that it was a purely administrative decision: a single person needed to control the whole operation. As it turned out, this trend became more pronounced over the years, which is why, at the polyclinic, the administrative organisation gradually took precedence over the 'purely democratic constitution of the medical team'.

Eitingon noted that the duration of sessions had initially been set at half an hour. He mentioned that this 'was only possible for a small class of people who could, despite their neurosis, still submit to this discipline – as is the case in Prussian Germany among civil servants and others. In general, sessions last three quarters of an hour or, classically, a full hour'. One hour was the amount of time Freud had spent daily, from the start of his practice, with each of his patients. At the polyclinic, patients came for their sessions three or four times a week, sometimes more, depending on the severity of their condition. It is obvious that a desire to take the orthodox approach prevented the analysts from limiting the duration of the cures. The Berliners tried, but without success, to change the time parameter:

> The question of speeding up or shortening analyses had been our main concern, and it is a subject to which we pay constant attention at the polyclinic – ultimately, however, without result in spite of our strong desire to make use of anything that would make things progress.

> Psychoanalysis is simply the process Freud named, the process he created. Anything else is not true analysis and cannot be counted as one of its successes.

Two tables (Table 2.1 and Table 2.2) taken from the 1922 report and relating to duration of treatment and therapeutic results are reproduced below:

Table 2.1 Duration of treatment

Time	*Number of patients*
Less than 3 months	35
3 to 6 months	49
6 to 9 months	30
9 to 12 months	13
12 to 18 months	6
More than 18 months	8

Table 2.2 Treatment outcome

(It should be noted that for many of these cases the analysis was still ongoing.)

Results	*Number*
Healing	22
Improvement	72
No progress	28
Treatment stopped	19

The first activity report of the Berlin Polyclinic contains little information relating to actual diagnoses. It simply states that the patients received were often suffering, as noted previously, from old and chronic neuroses, long-term illnesses and psychic disorders grafted onto the remains of organic diseases. Eitingon also mentions, however, that symptomatic improvement could lead to the discontinuation of the analysis, thus emphasising the therapeutic purpose of the treatment at the polyclinic. Similarly, it was not uncommon for treatment at the polyclinic to be split, with patients being re-treated in successive tranches. In addition, the end of the treatment was presented in the form of a question relating strictly to practice. At that time, it was not the subject of systematic research. It is true that this report was written just two years after the polyclinic opened, and that many analyses were still in progress. It is therefore likely that there was a lack of hindsight and, more importantly, a lack of accurate data relating to the termination of treatments. Did the therapeutic effects last? Were there times when patients treated in this way wanted to go further? This was not specified. Treatment results were recorded on a graduated scale from 'stable state' to 'recovery'.

The most astonishing part of this presentation, which must surely hold our attention, is the remark that the pure gold of analysis was not mixed with the copper of suggestion for the simple reason that one can hardly 'find a metal capable of such an alloy'.[3] Was it the effect of a certain desire for conformity, for adjustment to established technical rules – or does it represent a desire to harmonise and standardise practice within the IPA? The Berlin Institute was at the centre of this issue in the 1920s. If there was a desire for standards, what was its origin? Did the visionary project that Freud had proposed in Budapest already seem out of reach? Was it felt that the Budapest programme related to conditions that were now out of date? That it was possible to dissociate the project of free treatment centres from the new paths of analytic technique? The claim that it was hardly possible to change the traditional analytic technique probably reflected the influence of the medical model. Ideally, the quality of care provided in the public sector would not be inferior to that offered in private establishments. It was less internal necessities, linked to the evolution of psychoanalysis as such, than the respect for an implicit deontology that could explain this attachment to 'true psychoanalysis' as opposed to the mass therapy contemplated only four years earlier by Freud. In a surprising way, the polyclinic wanted to be more Freudian than Freud himself. For the sage of Vienna, it was a matter of treating a crowd of people, implementing popular psychotherapy and massively applying analytic therapy – which would mean adapting the initial technique to this expansion. As far as the Berlin Institute's founders were concerned, however, the offer of free treatment was not to be allowed to degrade the method developed by the creator of psychoanalysis. The principles of the standard cure were to remain unchanged. For this reason, Eitingon defended the orientation according to which the principle of free association should be the only one applied in Berlin and therefore insisted that suggestion not be used.

Consequently, the immutability of the analytic technique could be summarised as follows: to remain true to itself, to be 'true', psychoanalytic practice had to remain unchanged. It is impossible to deviate from this rule without being viewed as guilty of heresy, falsification, error and treason. In other words, it is not because an institution wants to make analytic treatment accessible to the masses that its exercise should differ from what is practiced in the analyst's private office. There should be no difference – no method other than free association – as long as there is no discrimination against the indigent patient. The right of all to receive psychoanalytic treatment presupposed respect for this implicit deontology. The problem was, however, that the inventor of psychoanalysis had seen things differently. Freud's interest in active technique had shown that the invention of new ways of therapy was not only inevitable but desirable. Ferenczi had explained that it was a question of breaking down resistance, of making the patient who was stagnating in his treatment move forward by provoking an overflow of symptoms, with the occurrence of anxiety serving to bring new repressed material to the surface.[4]

The last part of the 1922 report concerned the training policy for the Berlin Institute's students. This policy was the institute's second goal. In Eitingon's words, the establishment's most urgent concern was 'the propagation of the psychoanalytic species'.[5] A teaching system had been created and directed by Karl Abraham, who was still the director of the institute at that time. He had been giving introductory courses in psychoanalysis since 1920. Later, he was in charge of classes for advanced students, with an average of twenty to thirty students per course. Hanns Sachs, who was not a medical doctor and who had been brought in from Switzerland, was the first person to be appointed as a tutor. Sachs' course dealt with questions relating to the application of psychoanalysis to the human sciences and the interpretation of dreams. Karen Horney and Ernst Simmel lectured on the psychoanalytic attitude of the medical practitioner. Simmel also lectured on psychoanalytic technique. Students were required to have completed a personal analysis if they wished to become analysts. Thus, the Berlin Institute used the weight of its influence at the heart of the IPA to impose this requirement on the rest of the analytic community. In the same way, it succeeded in imposing the idea that didactics should be considered 'an independent branch of psychoanalysis'.[6]

From the beginning, most of the students in training were doctors. Many came from Austria, Hungary, the Netherlands, the USA and England. Once they had completed their personal analysis, they could become members of the analytic society and start receiving patients from the polyclinic. The transition to practice was duly controlled, and only cases suitable for beginners were referred to them. They were required to write detailed notes. Care had to be taken, and risks and errors had to be limited. The practice of these beginners had to be controlled. Eitingon provided little detail as to how the errors made by trainee analysts were corrected, except to emphasise the dimension of control over the treatments conducted by these students, who were sometimes removed from working with a patient so that Eitingon could take over the treatment himself. Eitingon freely admitted that the Prussian spirit, the spirit of discipline and organisation based on respect for hierarchy, had prevailed. 'The growth of the Institute brought about a change: while maintaining the purely democratic constitution of the medical team, the organisation became much stricter. I am now in control,' he said bluntly.[7] The results showed, a posteriori, the validity of the teaching system, whose rigour could be measured in terms of the satisfaction of each individual. The note that concluded this first report was almost tautological: 'For two years, our students have studied hard and well, which proves that our method is the right one.'

The use of free treatment

As Ferenczi pointed out in 1928, the question of money in the context of psychoanalysis deserved to be taken seriously. Following Freud's recommendations fifteen years earlier, Ferenczi wished to address the discipline's financial aspect openly:

> Psychoanalysis is often reproached for attaching too much value to financial matters. I don't think we're concerned enough yet. Even the wealthiest man is reluctant to give his money to the doctor; there is something in us that seems to take medical assistance – first given in childhood, in fact, by those responsible for care of a child – for granted; at the end of each month, when patients receive their fee statements, the patient's resistance only fades when everything hidden, all hatred unconsciously aroused, all mistrust or suspicion has been brought to the surface again. The most characteristic example of the distance between concealed displeasure and conscious consent to sacrifice was given by a patient who, at the beginning of his interview with the doctor, declared: 'Doctor, if you help me, I will give you my entire fortune.' The doctor replied: 'I will be content with thirty crowns per session.' The unexpected answer to that statement was as follows: 'Isn't that a bit too much?'[8]

The 1922 report addressed the matter of payment with some caution. Its aim was to echo the formula employed by Freud in Budapest, according to which treatment in future psychoanalytic centres would be free of charge. Free treatment was linked to the catastrophic economic situation in the postwar period and to the ruin of the middle class, many of whom turned to the polyclinic. It should be noted, however, that this economic argument repressed another posture relating to the revolutionary position. Won over by the ideology of class struggle, the young generation of analysts who clustered around Eitingon in Berlin had developed another conception of the link between economics and psychoanalysis. For them, social conditions were at the origin of neuroses. Free psychoanalytic treatment had political significance. Eitingon, reasoning like a clinician, said nothing about this. According to him, free psychoanalytic treatment was problematic in relation to the question of anal erotism. From a theoretical point of view, could one ignore the equivalence between money and the drive object, to which Freud and Abraham had devoted extensive research? This explained why the principle of completely free treatment could not be applied to the polyclinic, for both economic and theoretical reasons.

The Berliners chose an alternative solution, proposing that patients should pay in accordance with their means. Those who were not in a position to pay anything would be treated free of charge. However, other patients who felt they could afford it would have to pay a lot for their analysis. In 1922, payments for sessions represented about 10 percent of the polyclinic's budget. In order to justify his refusal to apply the principle of completely free treatment, Eitingon relied on a remark he had previously made to Freud concerning the disadvantages of free treatment. He gave no further details, however. These arguments were most likely similar to those developed by Freud in his 1913 study on the beginning of the treatment, in which the question of payment or nonpayment of fees was discussed. In that study, Freud noted that patients tended to treat money and sexual matters in the same way. The advice he gave to practitioners was to approach both of these issues quite openly and with as much candour as was necessary. The patient should be told that the payment made to the analyst would directly reflect the difficulty of the work; this was a way of saying that analytic work was at least as indispensable and worthwhile as that of a surgeon. Consequently, the emphasis was placed on the value that the analyst himself placed on his work.

For this reason, Freud calculated that if the analyst undertook two free treatments a week for a month, his loss of income could correspond to the effects of a serious traumatic accident. This, he said, was precisely why it was possible to refuse to treat a patient for nothing – the benefit to the patient would not compensate for the sacrifice made by the analyst. Freud explained it precisely in the following terms:

> I may venture to form a judgement about this, since for ten years or so I set aside one hour a day, and sometimes two, for gratuitous treatments, because I wanted, in order to find my way about in the neuroses, to work in the face of as little resistance as possible. The advantages I sought by this means were not forthcoming.[9]

According to Freud, free treatment favoured the patient's resistance. Women interpreted it as a sign of love; men were mired in the debt they owed to the father figure. He presented payment for the session as something that was likely to correct certain transferential effects. According to this reasoning, free treatment would prove detrimental to the conclusion of the analysis in that it would increase the de-realisation of the analytic situation. In contradiction to this, we do know that Freud took patients into analysis free of charge. We can also see that if he decided to proceed in this way, it didn't necessarily have anything to do with a patient's financial means. He treated Marianne Kris on a nonpaying basis between 1931 and 1938.[10] However, Kris had no pecuniary difficulties and later confided that Freud would not let her pay for her treatment because her own father, Dr Oscar Rie, had not been paid for his services to the Freud family. She made a direct connection between her father and her analyst, but she immediately defended herself by denying it. She considered the situation of the doctor who does not get paid for his visits not to be comparable to that of the analyst.

Freud's 1913 reference to trauma indexes the fact that a certain real is at stake. When the cure does not give rise to remuneration for the analyst, the lack changes its meaning. The analyst is the seat of a subtraction; he takes something at his charge. Freud suggests that it is up to the analyst to pay a certain subjective price for the analytic operation to take place. Under what conditions can the analyst agree to bear such a burden? Does it depend only on the context? How are we to understand this? Is this subtraction the equivalent of castration? We find in Lacan a development that is likely to shed light on the notion of the analyst's assumption of responsibility. There is a point in his teaching where he stresses that fantasy is not articulated in the same way in neurosis, psychosis and perversion. The place of the drive object (object *a*) that is at stake in fantasy differs in each of these structures. Insofar as the position of the subject with respect to the object (which causes the inherent lack of desire) is not the same in these three structures, Lacan states that this involves an appropriate handling of the transference. With regard to psychosis, in order

> to handle the transferential relation, we do indeed have to take within us the *a* at issue, like a foreign body, like an incorporation of which we are the patient, because the object in so far as it is the cause of his lack is utterly foreign to the subject who is speaking to us.[11]

In this passage, Lacan stresses that in order to separate the subject, the analyst must take within himself the object *a* of the analysand. This object is totally foreign to the analysand; the subject is unable to have the idea that it can come from him, that it is in him. This object does not have the status of the lost object; it only appears on the side of the Other.

The position of the analyst in the transference with a neurotic subject is not equivalent. In the construction of the fantasy that takes place during the treatment of a neurotic patient, the image of the object will appear on the side of the subject. That is to say, the patient will be able to recognise that this image of the object is his, that it comes from him, that it is situated in him. For all that, however, this object is not real; it is a semblant of real because, by definition, the drive object does not have a specular image. The paradoxical expression that Lacan uses here corresponds to the fact that the psychoanalytic cure is a device that allows something of the real to appear at the level of the imaginary. This is obtained by recourse to speech, to the symbolic, as Freud reminds us:

> Nothing takes place between them except that they talk to each other … The analyst agrees upon a fixed regular hour with the patient, gets him to talk, listens to him, talks to him in his turn and gets him to listen.[12]

Can a loss of jouissance, a symbolic castration, occur in free treatment? Would the relationship to desire, which is supported by the dimension of lack, be articulated to castration in a logically different way? When Freud compared the cost (to the analyst) of free treatment to the effect of an accident, that is to say, to the trauma from which the analyst would suffer, he indicated that the subject who suffered was, in fact, the analyst. Moreover, if the analyst bears the cost of the treatment, he must take it into account in the transference. Free treatment can threaten the cure insofar as the analyst does not appear de-completed. If he does not seek payment, it means that he is without desire. His satisfaction becomes enigmatic. This enigmatic meaning can encourage the erotomaniacal postulate: if he listens to me for pleasure, it is because he loves me. When Ruth Mack Brunswick analysed the Wolf-Man in 1926, she was grappling with a patient whose erotomania had been fostered by the gift of money from Freud's own hands. In this case, the actual gift expected from the father coincided with the allowance that Freud was willing to give to the Wolf-Man to save him from destitution. The gift of money reinforced the Wolf-Man's certainty that he was Freud's favourite patient. Brunswick uncovered the persecution that had been redirected from the analyst to the doctors that the Wolf-Man had consulted when suffering from extraordinary hypochondria. Although she agreed to treat the Wolf-Man without charge, Brunswick managed to help him by convincing him that Freud did not love him, that Freud had not chosen him as an object of love and that he was just one patient among many others. To achieve this result, she took the position of an authoritarian counsellor rather than that of the subject supposed to know. So when the analyst does not get paid, does he not risk appearing like an other who lacks nothing? What happens when money does not intervene as an object of separation between the analyst and the patient? In psychosis, the meaning of getting something at no cost can be interpreted in terms of the will to enjoy. The patient finds himself in the place of the object of the Other; he is confronted, without any possible third party, by the jouissance of an Other who does his utmost to make him speak. When the analyst himself assumes the cost of the cure, he must know in advance the traps and errors to be avoided. He has to present himself as a place cleansed of jouissance, cleansed of any desire for the good of his patient. The institution where the cure takes place, the limited time and the teamwork involved contribute to the establishment of a third object: the analyst simply does his work and gets paid by the institution where he works voluntarily for a cause that is beyond him. The transference this brings about is therefore caught up in a network of normalised and ordinary significations.

With regard to the modulation of the free treatment provided by the Berlin Polyclinic, the principle that the patient should pay for his analysis according to his means – or, rather, to what he thought he could pay – was therefore fixed from the outset. The analyst approached the question of payment or nonpayment from the beginning in all simplicity, quite openly, as Freud had recommended. This meant that prior discussion of payment between the analyst and the patient was an integral part of the consultation. It involved a subjective assessment by the patient of what he or she could afford and, more importantly, whether he or she was actually able to do so. If only the economic criterion had been taken into consideration, a different procedure would have been applied, with, for example, a fee scale based on income. This implies that both free and paid analyses were carried out simultaneously at the polyclinic. According to Eitingon, a comparison of the results showed that there was no essential difference between the two procedures. He also made the surprising assertion – on which he did not elaborate – that payment or nonpayment for an analytic treatment had no influence on the course of the treatment. This would tend to prove that, at the beginning of a treatment, the question of payment or nonpayment was a valuable diagnostic indicator for the polyclinic's analysts. Variability in payments for treatment would also have had another advantage. Eitingon associated it with the importance that analysts placed on the active technique at that time. This reference to the active technique suggests that it was seen as a means for analysis to reach an increasingly wide audience. However, Eitingon did not go into details on this point either.

We do, however, need to pause on the fact that Eitingon did not consider Ferenczi's bid to overcome resistance and thus shorten the duration of the cures to be 'real psychoanalysis'. The assertion that no means could be found in Berlin to shorten the duration of treatment contradicts this reference to the active technique. In fact, it is quite probable that Eitingon's allusion to Ferenczi's invention was used here to show the points of agreement between the vision developed by Freud in 1918 and the programme set up by the polyclinic. It was still a question of making it understood that the utopia envisioned in Budapest had become reality. Eitingon then made another important point: the patients treated free of charge at the polyclinic were not seen solely by students in training. No distinction was made between paid and unpaid treatments. The presence in the same place, at the same time, of nonpaying patients, patients who paid a little and patients who paid a lot was desirable. And because the analysts also saw polyclinic patients in their private offices, the mix was truly complete.

The desire to be an authority

After a few years of operation and in response to growing demand for treatment, Max Eitingon bought new, larger premises at Wichmann Strasse 10, and once again Ernst Freud was invited to fit out the premises. On the occasion of the inauguration, which took place on 30 September 1928, Eitingon addressed his colleagues. Eitingon had officially become director of the Berlin Institute following Abraham's death on Christmas Day in 1925. His comments began with a heartfelt tribute to his colleague Ernst Simmel. At the time when Eitingon had had to take over the IPA's delegated presidency from Karl Abraham, Simmel had assumed the presidency of the DPG. He was not only an important collaborator; he also had a vision of the social responsibility of psychoanalysis and of ways of spreading it through the founding of a psychoanalytic hospital service.

In paying tribute to Simmel's creative optimism, Eitingon praised the spirit of sacrifice and selflessness of all the teachers at the polyclinic. He summed up the first eight years of the institution's existence by recalling that it had been necessary to start modestly, never yielding to discouragement in the face of the immense task of making psychoanalytic treatment accessible to as broad a section of the population as possible. Eitingon insisted that the needs of the populace had been at the origin of the of the polyclinic's creation. After the war, people had been clamouring for psychoanalysis. It had been necessary to respond to the demands of citizens dealing with abandonment, trauma and ruin. Psychoanalysts had been unable to back down in the face so much psychological distress and misery. It was their sense of responsibility that had forced them to respond to the collective demand emanating from this social other, which Freud referred to as the mass. It must also be noted that this was the essential argument of the founders of the Berlin Institute: the social extension of psychoanalysis was a matter of duty, and analysts were under an obligation not to avoid it.

In spite of this, there were, entirely due to force of circumstance, limits to the extension of treatment to all classes of society. According to Eitingon, the numerical factor could not be ignored. How many analysts would be needed to make analysis accessible to all? Analysts would have to be trained on a scale never seen before. At that time, it was not known whether the extension of the field of analytic therapeutics could lead to new possibilities. Nevertheless, more clearly than he had done in 1922, Eitingon felt that it was hardly possible to modify the technical rules of classical analysis:

> We could not hope to make any changes to the method, even though we were anxious to tackle the problem of reducing the time it took. The larger numbers of people coming to the clinic and waiting to use it put us under much greater pressure than had been known by the individual analyst.[13]

Freud had conjectured that a modification of the technique would be inevitable when it came to applying psychoanalysis to the masses. Nevertheless, the management of the polyclinic felt that it was unrealistic to treat a large number of patients while simultaneously modifying the technique traditionally used. How was the problem of reducing treatment time to be tackled in order to treat a crowd of people? That went right back to the problem of the influx of patients. It was actually an institutional problem, a headache that had no solution. As Otto Fenichel was to point out in a report drawn up in the early 1930s, the only option was to select patients carefully at the time of initial consultation. Eitingon made no mention of this. If the social extension of psychoanalysis forced the analysts of the polyclinic to think seriously about the question of treatment duration, the practice developed by Freud in his private practice was set up as an absolute model in Berlin. This apparent paradox needs to be examined. The management of the Berlin Institute focused on the modalities of classical treatment not only out of pure orthodoxy and for reasons of principle but, more fundamentally, because the technique developed by Freud was perceived as solid and assured. The major point, on which Eitingon had no intention of giving way, was respect for the rule of free association. His reasoning was that when one goes into something experimental, one can't be sure of anything. One needs visible markers, solid reference points, predetermined routes, tools that one is used to. It was a matter of prudence. It was necessary to strive to preserve the rule of free association at all costs, and it was also necessary to banish and challenge the use of hypnotic suggestion, which was something that Freud had not totally rejected in 1918 except in the treatment of traumatic neuroses.

It is true that, on this subject, one could throw Freud's own words back at him, since in 1912, in an address to doctors, he had written as follows:

> In practice, it is true, there is nothing to be said against a psychotherapist combining a certain amount of analysis with some suggestive influence in order to achieve a perceptible result in a shorter time – as is necessary, for instance, in institutions. But one has a right to insist that he himself should be in no doubt about what he is doing and should know that his method is not that of true psychoanalysis.[14]

Eitingon firmly believed that anything deviating from the technique invented by Freud could not be called psychoanalysis. To remain in the dimension of true psychoanalysis necessarily disallowed any recourse to suggestion. The transformation of psychoanalysis into an adapted and devalued practice for the purpose of tailoring it to institutional treatment was a pitfall to be avoided. The creators of the Berlin Institute assumed that strict adherence to certain technical principles would enable them to advance towards the uncertain horizon of psychoanalytic practice applied to the masses. It was not only the Prussian spirit, on which Eitingon prided himself, that was at issue. His attachment to the rule of free association was linked to his anxiety about the enthusiasts. As paradoxical as it may seem, the rule of free association had a landmark function that the Berliners clung to in order to move forward in the dark. Of course, there were also other rules applying to analysis that had to be respected, such as abstinence, the prohibition on making essential decisions during the course of the cure and regularity of sessions. There was also the rule of having the patient lie on a couch. But none of them carried as much weight as the rule of free association, which was rightly considered to be the fundamental principle of the analytic technique. In order to argue that psychoanalysis could be applied on a wide scale at the polyclinic, one had to be able to argue that the proposed treatments were firmly within the framework of true psychoanalysis, that what was being offered was not a diminished, overused or degraded form of psychoanalysis aimed at crowds. In a way, this position is the opposite of the option proposed by Ferenczi, who wanted the technique to evolve.

Should psychoanalysis be defined by the application of – and respect for – technical rules? This question was constantly raised by certain innovations introduced in the decades that followed. The most famous example of this tendency to denounce a lack of respect for standards in psychoanalysis relates to the IPA's rejection of the variable-duration session originated by Lacan. As is well known, Lacan's innovation caused a scandal; he was ordered to stop training analysts and ejected from the French branch of the IPA. But can we ignore the fact that Freud himself advocated allowing the analytic technique to evolve? It had to be adapted to the traumas of war, to the real of its time. Or should we distinguish institutional analysis for large numbers of people from a private psychoanalysis, which would be the real, authentic one? Freud had asserted that psychoanalysis is one and does not permit itself to be decomposed. But were there not already two possible applications of psychoanalysis: one with a therapeutic aim, the other with an emphasis on the training of analysts? Lacan showed that even if the analyst assumes some detachment vis-à-vis therapeutic effects and the desire to cure, there remains the question of whether introducing technical modifications goes beyond the limits of psychoanalysis. Freud's flexibility where standards were concerned was also questioned by his contemporaries.

Freud could recommend going about analysis in such and such a way without being constrained by his own indications. On another level, concerning the initiatives introduced in order to shorten the duration of the cure, Freud was content to state that the best way to shorten the cure was to carry it out correctly from beginning to end. He did not a priori situate these experiments outside the limits of psychoanalysis, contenting himself with indicating that efforts to accelerate the progress of the analytic cure had been failures. The unity of psychoanalysis is not established by rules; it is based on psychoanalytic concepts.

Yet another problem remains: did Eitingon always speak in the first person? This is a less obvious question than his position as director of the Berlin Institute would lead one to believe. One could easily deduce a certain immodesty from a sentence like, 'The real risk was that we had the courage to want to be an authority.'[15] Yet it is possible to demonstrate that these two notions of risk and authority relate to two different subjects of enunciation. It is quite certain that Eitingon took considerable risks on a financial level. As Ernst Simmel pointed out, the establishment of a psychoanalytic institute in times of economic misery was an extremely treacherous undertaking. In addition to having the financial wherewithal necessary to ensure the institution's survival, it was necessary to demonstrate the tenacity, the will to endure and the extraordinary capacity for resistance that Freud and his colleagues recognised in Eitingon. The notion of risk thus refers to the daring and courage displayed by the founder of the Berlin Institute. The term 'authority' (*Autorität*), on the other hand, is, in Freud's language, a signifier that always relates to the place that psychoanalysis should, he felt, occupy in culture. For Freud, the term referred to an ideal beyond himself, an authority beyond his own person. It concerns the authority of psychoanalysis as such, its mission in civilisation. The term also connotes Freud's concern about what would happen to psychoanalysis after his death. The authority of psychoanalysis thus designates the origin and the temporal projection involving the time of its foundation and what it becomes. Establishing the authority of psychoanalysis in society was one of the three objectives of the psychoanalytic enterprise that Freud set out at the Nuremberg congress of 1910, at the time of the creation of the IPA. He stated that the improvements to be expected from psychoanalysis had to move along three different paths. These were the acquisition of internal progress in knowledge and technique; the increase in the authority of psychoanalysis within civilisation; and the general effect to be expected from the disclosure of the secret of neurosis. 'Society will not be in a hurry to grant us authority. It is bound to offer us resistance, for we adopt a critical attitude towards it,'[16] he wrote. What Freud actually foresaw was a clash between psychoanalysis and civilisation. Psychoanalysis denounced the intense effort of repression that civilisation imposed on the individual. In return, civilisation took its revenge by characterising psychoanalysis as mere charlatanism. Time would, however, favour psychoanalysis insofar as the truth of the discoveries made by psychoanalysis would, despite its unpleasant character, eventually prevail. The authority of psychoanalysis corresponded to this truth, which would end by imposing itself on civilisation and being accepted by it.

A strong proponent of analysis

Was Max Eitingon guided by ideals of social justice? Was he seduced by the revolutionary theses of class struggle? Nothing could be less certain. His aversion and indifference to the workers' uprisings and popular demonstrations that took place in Germany immediately after the war suggest otherwise. Did he want to regulate the training of analysts according to his 'Prussian' formula, by imposing – by force or by trickery – the principal standards first developed in Berlin and then extended throughout the IPA? In short, was Eitingon a visionary, a tyrant, an upstart, a man of ambition? Those who knew him praised the sharpness of his organisational skills rather than any kind of penchant for domination. He does seem to have been a very caring person. His helpfulness, his appreciation of beautiful things and his wisdom and cultivation left pleasant memories in people's minds. Was he, rather, a builder, an inventor, a man of desire misjudged by history, a herald unjustly disparaged?[17] This is the opinion of those who recognise him above all as a pioneer of the implantation of psychoanalysis in the land of Israel. Was Eitingon, as Jones claimed, an impressionable man of unfailing faithfulness who was despised by Jung from the outset, someone Freud no longer esteemed particularly highly and, to put it bluntly, someone who was simply Freud's factotum?

It goes without saying that the nature of the bond that bound Eitingon to Freud has to be grasped at the level of transference. In a certificate written at

Eitingon's request in 1933, Freud outlined the work of his colleague, who was then setting up a medical practice in Palestine, as follows:

> Dr. Max Eitingon, until recently resident in Berlin-Dahlem and president of the German Psychoanalytic Society, is one of the best known, most influential and most meritorious persons in the psychoanalytic movement of his time. I made his acquaintance in 1907. He came from Zurich, where he had trained as a psychiatrist under Professor Bleuler. After moving to Berlin in 1919–20, he founded, using his own resources, the Berlin Institute of Education, which remained under his direction until his emigration. This institute became a model for all other institutions of its kind and did much for the establishment and propagation of psychoanalytic theories. Within its framework, it has also been possible to make analytic therapy accessible to large sections of the population without means. Dr. Eitingon became the central secretary of the International Association in 1922 and its president in 1925; confirmed by several congresses, he remained in that position until September 1932. During these years, he had ample opportunity to prove himself as an organiser, to mediate in difficult situations, to defend … the interests of psychoanalysis as a science and as a practical activity. I am convinced that his remoteness from the scene of his current business represents only an episode, and not the end, of his invaluable work in the service of our cause.[18]

Despite the conventional character of the style of this certificate – 'a rather ridiculous assignment'[19] – which Freud was forced to concoct in order to help Eitingon flee Nazi Germany, these lines do emphasise Eitingon's personal involvement in the creation of the Berlin Institute. According to Freud, the creation of this first psychoanalytic institution was Eitingon's life's work. Not surprisingly, we learn that Eitingon's unfailing devotion to Freud's person resulted in his being portrayed rather unkindly by Ernest Jones. In his biography of Freud, Jones commented that Eitingon's main distinguishing feature was his possession of a personal fortune. This was unique in the world of psychoanalysis. Entirely devoted to Freud, Eitingon carried out the master's every desire and considered even the slightest of his opinions eminently worthy. Despite these qualities, Jones considered him quite impressionable. Eitingon made no attempt to hide his Jewish origins and reacted very strongly to anti-Semitic prejudice. According to Jones, Eitingon's first trip to Palestine, in 1910, was already an indication of his future choice to move there. Eitingon, he says, had three specific qualifications that Freud never forgot:

> Firstly, he was the first foreigner who, attracted by psychoanalysis, came to see him. Then he brought invaluable material help to the master's enterprises, especially, for example, in the creation of the Verlag. Finally, his devotion to Freud was such that the latter could count on his

> friendship in all circumstances. Nevertheless, it was impossible to believe that Freud had a particularly favourable opinion of his intellectual abilities.[20]

This remark suggests that Freud's unwavering confidence in Eitingon offended Jones.

According to Michael Schröter, editor of the correspondence between Freud and Eitingon, Eitingon was essentially an auxiliary as well as a supporter. He was, according to Schröter, 'an operative in direct contact with Freud who cautiously but surely built up his position within the psychoanalytic movement and was especially called upon in situations where Freud's work appeared to be under threat'.[21] Schröter also sees a recurring pattern in Eitingon's existence. In most of his functions at the highest level, Eitingon did not play the role of instigator. He was not a leader, a first choice. He was a follower, a substitute, a reliable source of assistance in times of distress. As we have seen, Eitingon first of all replaced Anton von Freund on the secret committee. He then implemented von Freund's plan to found a psychoanalytic polyclinic. He also took over from von Freund in the matter of raising funds for the Verlag. In 1922, he replaced Hans Liebermann as secretary of the BPV, but he was not entirely satisfied. Similarly, in 1924, at the time of the disagreement with Rank, Eitingon took over from Rank as secretary of the IPA and director of the Verlag and its journals. When Abraham died in 1925, Eitingon took over both the presidency of the IPA and the leadership of the BPV. As Schröter points out, it is not exactly easy to distinguish between selflessness and the quest for power in this progression.

Finally, according to Olivier Mannoni, the translator of the voluminous Eitingon-Freud correspondence into French, a striking asymmetry, making itself apparent at the level of style, characterised the relationship between Freud and Eitingon.[22] The deference Eitingon showed when addressing his elder and master was so marked that it made the task of translation particularly difficult. The asymmetry did not only manifest itself at the level of written expression – Freud had an exceptional mastery of the German language, which was not the case with Eitingon, whose first language was Russian. The difference was expressed in the latter's phraseology, which multiplied polite formulas whose length and rate of repetition were very unusual compared to the far less elaborate German and Austrian conventions of the time:

> The sentences at the end of his letters are in themselves a veritable anthology of epistolary reverence as Eitingon progressively augments the instances of verbal admiration: from the simple 'Your devoted one' in the first letter to the 'Warm greetings from your cordially devoted one' of the last few years – and let us not forget 'She thanks you cordially for your question and joins me in sending you a very warm greeting,' which

> appears in a letter he wrote with Lou Andreas-Salomé in February 1925. They strike the reader all the more because Freud generally contented himself with dry, concise formulas like 'I greet you cordially.' Neither are these cascades of veneration confined to the endings of his letters. Everywhere – and this was one of the main difficulties encountered in translating these texts – Eitingon multiplies carefully phrased remarks and qualifying clauses. It's particularly flagrant when he talks about psychoanalysis.[23]

What we know for certain is that the relationship between the two men was protracted and continuous. Eitingon's first letter to Freud dates from 1906, when he was working as an assistant psychiatrist in Bleuler's department at the Burghölzli Clinic. The young practitioner was seeking Freud's advice about a hysterical patient of Russian origin whom he wanted to bring to Vienna for analytic treatment. His last letter to Freud was written in Jerusalem on 20 June 1939, three months before Freud's death. Curiously enough, Eitingon is also the least known of Freud's immediate pupils in that, unlike Ferenczi and Abraham, he was not a theorist. Eitingon often complained about his inhibitions where writing was concerned, and Freud regretted that the younger man failed to make more frequent use of his pen as a tool and a weapon. Freud certainly appreciated the effectiveness of his writing, however. Eitingon devoted himself to administrative problems, not to scientific matters. He was a man of action rather than a researcher. Despite his relatively unassuming character, though, he was by no means a man of the second rank in the history of the psychoanalytic movement.

The eldest of four children from an Orthodox Jewish family, Eitingon was born in Mogilev, Russia, in 1881. When he was twelve years old, his parents moved to Leipzig. His father, Chaim Eitingon, had made a fortune in the fur trade; he was so rich, in fact, that he was nicknamed the Rothschild of Leipzig. A leading patron of the community in which he lived, Chaim financed the construction of a synagogue in 1922 and, later, a Jewish hospital, which opened in 1928.[24] The Eitingon-Schild Company was run by Max Eitingon's brother-in-law, Motty, from offices in New York. There were branches of the company in Leipzig, Paris, London, Moscow and Stockholm. This international company was, for a time, the official supplier of Alaskan furs to the American government. Until the Wall Street Crash of 1929, which precipitated the Great Depression, its annual turnover reached colossal sums of up to 15 million dollars a year. Members of the Eitingon family had shares in the company that provided them with a very comfortable living. None of them had to work. Until the late 1920s, therefore, Max Eitingon was largely sheltered from want; since he was receiving dollar dividends at the time of the German financial crisis, his income became even greater. Up until the time when the American crisis directly affected the family business, Eitingon had no need to rely on his medical activities to make a living. Consequently, nothing except his identification with his father's philanthropic activities had prepared this heir of a wealthy merchant family to take an interest in the social mission of psychoanalysis. And yet the Jews found themselves in all the vanguard positions in the most innovative of the movements that flourished under Weimar. Among them were Expressionist poets and writers, theatre producers and filmmakers:

> They owned the great liberal newspapers such as the *Berliner Tageblatt*, the *Vossische Zeitung* and the *Frankfurter Zeitung*, whose directors and editors were frequently Jewish. They owned many of the major liberal and avant-garde publishing houses (S. Fischer, Kurt Wolff, Cassirer, Georg Bondi, Erich Reiss, Malik). Many of the great theatre critics were also Jewish and they dominated the entertainment world.[25]

Eitingon, who financed and directed the two principal instruments of the analytic movement during the 1920s, was part of the Jewish-German cultural symbiosis which was foundational to cultural activity in Weimar.

His years of apprenticeship were rather difficult, hampered in his studies as he was by a stutter that forced his parents to enrol him in a private school that specialised in languages. There, he learned about ten languages, which enabled him to write his medical observations in many languages and dialects. He terminated his secondary school studies before he obtained his baccalaureate but still managed to achieve an equivalence that allowed him to start a university course. During those years, whose details are a little hazy, he hesitated, in all probability, between medicine and philosophy. His first studies took him to Leipzig and Halle, following which he succeeded in enrolling in medicine in Heidelberg and then went on to Marburg, where he attended the lectures of the neo-Kantian philosopher Hermann Cohen, who lectured on the subject of the possible assimilation of Judaism and German culture. In the winter of 1904–1905, Eitingon finally enrolled at medical school in Zurich. He then worked as an assistant at the University Psychiatric Clinic at Burghölzli. There he met Jung, who was the senior doctor, and Karl Abraham, a Berliner who, like him, was working as an assistant. It was Bleuler himself who sent Eitingon to Freud to find out everything a young psychiatrist should know about psychoanalysis.

Let us look at the details of Eitingon's first visit to Freud, in January 1907, when he accompanied the Russian woman whose case he had previously submitted to Freud by mail. As a young psychiatrist, he felt an irrepressible need to meet the inventor of psychoanalysis:

> I came one Monday, if I'm not mistaken. I visited him at his office between three and four o'clock. I was too bewildered and overwhelmed by my first impression to get a clear idea of the man. I only remember that he was wearing a black frock coat, a dark waistcoat with a flower

> pattern, buttoned up to the top, and I remember that face that everyone who saw Freud then or later knows, a face that hasn't changed since, even though that grey head has now become silver. He invited me to come back that evening and the following evening, and he spoke of the difficult situation of analysis in the world. He was confident as to the value of what he had created, but not without bitterness about the strong positions that the scientific world had begun to take at the time.[26]

Eitingon then referred to the scandal caused by the publication of the Dora case. On the evening of the third day, Eitingon was invited to attend the Wednesday meeting of the select group of psychoanalysts who surrounded Freud. His memory of the occasion proved imperishable. The various members of the audience were asked to answer questions about the specific mechanisms of the neuroses, about the aims of analytic therapy and the manner in which it proceeds, and about what a patient looks like after a completed and successful analysis. Once everybody had given their answers, Freud took the floor. He explained that the criteria of illness were defined by the characteristics of the symptoms, not by their intensity and quantitative increase. Freud also stated that analytic therapy does not pretend to eliminate the symptom because that is, in itself, an impossible task. The cure, he said, must lead to the elimination of resistance and repression, to the abolition of the repressed, to free passage between the unconscious and the conscious. He also alluded to the fact that obsessive neurosis was more common among Jews, that the Jewish religion was an obsessive neurosis that had been in the making down through the centuries. The energy capable of overcoming resistance was called transference. Similarly, the secret of the psychoanalyst's action is that healing is healing through love. At that time, Freud believed that no relapse could occur after the cure because it was the unconscious that created the symptoms. If the repressed (that is to say, the infantile) is what attracts and has been expelled, repression can no longer occur.

On the other hand, Freud said, therapy had its limits. Eitingon was greatly impressed by the formula Freud employed on this occasion, and also later on, regarding therapeutic success. With his inimitable style, Freud argued that 'with great personal effort one could perhaps overcome these limits, but one would leave one's skin behind'. Later, Freud said: 'You can get more during the treatment, but then you'll have to cut some strips in your own skin.'[27] In Eitingon's opinion, these were phrases to be carved into the marble of the secret tablets of analysis. But how can situating the end point of a successful analysis in the motifs of the illness be kept secret? Freud's enigmatic comments about gashes in the skin could be understood in two different ways. First, to go beyond the limits of the current indications of analysis (meaning the neuroses to which he had just alluded) in order to extend the field of application of analysis, it would be necessary to sweat blood and water in the near future. Analysts will have to work tirelessly. Their technique will have to evolve, and innovative theoretical and clinical research will be required. All this work will have to be undertaken in order to push back the current limits of therapeutics.

But these things can also be understood in a different way, inasmuch as Freud emphasised the new limits of a successful therapy, meaning those of a particular analysis. One can, of course, object that this comes to the same thing, since these limits also apply to the motifs of the disease. Nevertheless, this emphasis on the particularity of a cure draws attention to a crucial point. From the point of view of therapeutics, when an analysis does not lead to the expected results, when the denouement and the expulsion of the repressed have not occurred, Freud would contend that it is not possible to make the symptom disappear because it simply can't be done. But when the analyst wishes to obtain more in terms of therapeutic success, when he wishes to push the analysis to the point of healing, then, says Freud, he must pay the price with his own flesh. This was the secret lesson: in relation to the therapeutic dimension, the desire to heal at any cost induces a masochistic position in the analyst. It is a question here of a threshold, of a beyond, of a crossing. It's a warning. In order to say that, Freud had to have known something about it, to have experienced what it cost to push back the limits of a cure in order to obtain therapeutic effects at all costs. If Eitingon concluded his evocation of Freud with this admonition, it is probably also because he himself never shrank from making any kind of sacrifice in order to help his fellow man. This first lesson in psychoanalysis was decisive for Eitingon's involvement with the discipline. It was unforgettable for him, as were each of his subsequent encounters with Freud. Emotion, amazement – these were the terms he used.

Eitingon's doctoral thesis, which he completed in 1909, was titled 'Effect of an Epileptic Attack on Mental Association'. Its objective was very much in line with the style of the research projects that were being carried out at that time by the Zurich group. Eitingon then decided to return to Abraham in Berlin to complete his specialisation in neurology. Through Abraham, Eitingon worked at Hermann Oppenheim's clinic. We have already mentioned the time when, from 1910 onwards, Abraham and Eitingon were involved in the refounding of the BPV.[28] In the end, after their meeting at Burghölzli, Abraham and Eitingon continued to work together. From that time on, this collaboration placed Eitingon in the position of a follower of Abraham, the leader of psychoanalysis in Germany.

By the beginning of the 1909 academic year, Eitingon had had an opportunity to visit Vienna again. He was invited to participate in the Wednesday meetings of the Vienna Psychoanalytic Association (Wiener Psychoanalytische Vereinigung, or WPV), and became one of the first people to learn about Freud's study of one of Leonardo da Vinci's childhood memories. Between October and November of the same year, Freud offered to accompany him for a walk twice a week after dinner, which gave Eitingon the opportunity to be analysed. There were about ten sessions, twelve at the most. Part of the content of this ambulatory analysis, as Freud called it, is known. Eitingon talked about the difficulties he was having both with his family and with his love life. Ernest Jones raised this analysis to the level of myth by defining it as the first didactic analysis in history. When Abraham brought him to Berlin, Eitingon did not throw himself wholeheartedly into the task of developing the BPV. The reason for this was his relationship with Mirra Jacovleina Raigorodsky, a Russian actress from the Moscow Art Theatre to whom Eitingon became engaged in 1912 and married the following year. Freud believed that Eitingon's choice of spouse was dictated by his neurosis. Mirra was, in his opinion, too troublesome a symptom. In truth, Freud detested Mirra, blaming her for never leaving her husband in peace. According to him, this spendthrift woman couldn't bear anything that might separate her from her husband. She selfishly wanted to keep him close to her.

Arnold Zweig referred to Mirra's imaginary torments. Freud confided to him late in life what he really thought of his colleague's wife:

> I don't like her. She has the nature of a cat, and I don't like them either. She has much of the charm and grace of a cat, but she's no longer an adorable young kitten; she's older than him and insipid in the way she uses what's left of his life. What was authentically human in her has remained stuck in her previous existence, or has been consumed there. She was a popular actress, it seems; she had a husband and two sons, one of whom is dead – the other is, I believe, in Siberia, and pretty much lost to her. Our friend has certainly conquered her under neurotic conditions of love. She shows not the slightest sympathy for his interests, his friends or his ideals, and what she displays in my company is pure pretence. She is very jealous of everything Max gets up to because it disturbs her exclusive possession of her husband. I don't know if Max amounts to anything more in her eyes than the doorman who opens the door to every useless luxury and the satisfaction of her singular moods and distractions. Is it absolutely necessary for an old woman like her to have at hand a crate containing exactly a hundred pairs of low-heeled shoes, as she once showed me?[29]

Freud was obviously upset by the fact that he had failed to relieve Eitingon of this hysterical and amorous tyranny. Eitingon's attachment to his wife at times raised doubts about his ability to fulfil his obligations to the analytic movement. For example, in order to reassure his colleagues and obtain the IPA's delegate chairmanship, which he demanded after Abraham's death, Eitingon had to promise that his wife would give him some respite. For his part, Freud identified the symptomatic character of Eitingon's willingness to satisfy the insatiable needs of this feminine other to the detriment of his own. Eitingon first visited Palestine in 1910. During the war, he opted for Austrian nationality. Later, he took Polish nationality, as did his father. This resulted in his working as an assistant in various military hospitals, where his wife assisted him as a volunteer nurse. Eitingon was appointed chief doctor of the observation section at Kassa (in Slovakia), and then became chief doctor in charge of the psychiatric department of the reserve hospital at Miskolc, in Hungary. This earned him the highest military decorations.[30] When he was stationed in Hungary, he proposed Ferenczi as an expert in a military trial. The two men then met at meetings of the Budapest Psychoanalytic Association. In 1918 they began to think about opening a psychoanalytic polyclinic in Budapest. From 1919 onwards and following his acceptance into the secret committee, Eitingon's ties with Freud and members of his family, especially Anna Freud, grew closer. While working hard to establish the polyclinic, Eitingon rendered many services to Freud's sons. He helped Ernst to set up as an architect in Berlin at the time of his marriage, and he also had many conversations with Oliver, whose depression and instability were giving Freud cause for concern in 1920. In 1921, Eitingon moved into a beautifully decorated multi-storey residence where he established an important philosophical library. The Freud family usually stayed at what they called Hotel Eitingon whenever they travelled to Berlin. Alix Strachey fell under the spell of the house at the end of 1924:

> I had the impression of being in a *real* house for the first time in Berlin. It was almost Mid-Victorian, so solid & un'Wohnung'like. Of course the Grunewald houses are specially gim-crack & villa-like; but I suspect the man of having taste … It was heavenly to lean back & look at … thick carpets & 2 or 3 almost passable pictures. I daresay all this is comparative.[31]

Max Eitingon spent a great deal and travelled a lot. He often took his wife, who was frequently unwell, to rest in the grand hotels of the Riviera. His lifestyle was that of a *grand bourgeois* who appreciated beautiful things and did not deprive himself of them. His salon was open to renowned artists and writers. Rilke and Pirandello were frequent visitors. More than 55,000 Russians were living in Berlin in the wake of the Bolshevik Revolution, and Max and Mirra had many contacts in the city's Russian circles. Despite his devotion to the analytic cause, Eitingon was, in fact, living between two worlds that did not communicate with each other: psychoanalysis and the Russian émigré community of artists and intellectuals. Freud disapproved of Eitingon's opulent and fashionable way of life, which, he felt, did not fit in with the way a psychoanalyst should conduct himself in civilisation.

During the war and thanks to his means, Eitingon became accustomed to supplying Freud with cigars and food. Whenever he went on his travels, he regularly sent parcels to Vienna. Freud sometimes had to put the brakes on him: the customs duties for Austria were extremely high, and the tangerines

Eitingon sent from Italy were often spoiled by the time they arrived. Freud did, however, call on him in a wide variety of situations. In 1922, Eitingon sent Freud, at Freud's request, some money to keep the Wolf-Man alive after he had lost everything in the Russian Revolution. At that time, Sergei Pankejeff was surviving as best he could in Vienna by selling the few precious items he had managed to retrieve from his homeland. But because he was a Russian – 'that is to say, basically a savage',[32] Freud wrote – Freud feared that he would end up sinking into alcohol, gambling and misery. Hence the idea of finding employment for him with the Eitingon concerns in Leipzig or Russia. We know, however, that that solution came to nothing. One might wonder if Freud quite had the measure of Eitingon's constant efforts to please him. What did he think of Eitingon's total dedication to him? How did Freud interpret the place he held in his colleague's life? It should not be forgotten that, above all else, Freud was Eitingon's analyst. There is at least one letter in which Freud openly refers to the contents of Eitingon's ambulatory analysis in the autumn of 1909. It was written in January 1922:

> You know what a role you have won for yourself both in my life and in the lives of my family. I know that I was in no hurry to tell you this. For many years I noted your efforts to get closer to me, and I have kept you at a distance. It was only when you found those particularly warm words, when you told me that you wanted to be part of my family – in the strict sense – that I let myself go with all the free and easy confidence of my youth, that I adopted you, and accepted your giving me all kinds of help and performing all kinds of services for me.[33]
>
> I confess, today, that at the beginning I did not value your sacrifices as much as I did later, when I came to understand that you were taking care of a loving and much cherished woman who was not willing to give up a part of you and that you were connected to a family that, deep down, had little sympathy with what you were accomplishing or with the fact that you actually overburden yourself with every offer you make. Do not, however, draw from this remark the conclusion that I am ready to set you free. The sacrifices you have made are precious to me, and it is up to you to tell me if they have become too burdensome for you.
>
> I therefore propose that you maintain this relationship, which has progressed from friendship to a father-son relationship, throughout the time that may yet separate me from the end of my life. Since you were the first person to come to me in my isolation, you can bear to stay with me until the end.
>
> Things will no doubt always have to remain thus: that I, for my part, need something and that you, for your part, strive to find it. That is the fate you yourself have chosen, the one that I so deplored in Berlin. But I know, from our ambulatory analysis, that you are in a state of love from which you have not yet freed yourself.

> In the last fifteen years, my situation has changed radically. I find myself freed from material worries, hemmed in by a popularity that repels me, engaged in undertakings that deprive me of the time and leisure to carry out quiet scientific work. What I need now is support to keep the psychoanalytic movement alive, particularly with regard to the Verlag. The next thing you could do for me to this end is to write an eloquent and detailed report on the activities of the polyclinic – the polyclinic that you brought into the world – so that I can, on the strength of that text, go elsewhere to ask for support for the [Berlin] Institute and encourage the foundation of similar institutions. The prospects in this field seem favourable in America.[34]

Eitingon's reply to this letter was written the following month. It states that all the money made available to the analytic movement by Eitingon came from the family business. Taking up Freud's assertion that his family had never understood the value of his efforts, Eitingon explained that his parents themselves had never considered it necessary to calculate the soundness of their charitable donations. Right from the outset, this extremely wealthy family had agreed to provide the financing necessary for the Freudian enterprises without asking too many questions. At some point, however, it had to be shown that the eldest son was reaping some benefits in terms of social status. The people who were financing the project had to be reassured in some way. There is nothing ambiguous about the following extract from one of Eitingon's letters to Freud:

> Please be assured that I would not be denied any specific request to support our cause if I put my personal stamp on it. I have, of course, had neither the opportunity nor the right to do so, and it seems to me to be less and less necessary now. That is why it was also very opportune that I did something myself; it brought them closer to your cause and ours, even if it was only, at first, through my person.[35]

The Berlin Polyclinic project was a response to Max Eitingon's need to attach himself to a personal undertaking. His family would thus be reassured that the funds donated to the psychoanalytic movement would also be used to settle the position of a family member. While there is nothing shocking in this reasoning, it is nonetheless a pointed reminder. In times of crisis, the creation and durability of the Berlin Institute would hardly have been possible without a substantial and constant flow of funds. Unlike his compatriot Sergei Pankejeff, Eitingon wanted to prove that he was the kind of son who could assume a symbolic place in society, that he had a destiny.[36] In embracing a medical career, he had distanced himself from the world of business. He was, however, always at ease with numbers and the most modern means of communication. Moreover, tragedy had struck when his parents lost one of their sons in April 1919. In a letter written in June 1919, Eitingon mentioned the heavy shadow cast by his brother Waldemar's death from septicaemia. Waldemar had managed the New York branch of Eitingon-Schild until his death. Later, Motty Eitingon took over the management of the company in the United States. When Max spoke of his desire to undertake something on his own and when Freud pointed out that his parents did not recognise the endeavours of their eldest son, it must be understood that the plan to create an institution in Berlin was intended to reassure highly placed people and potential donors at a particular time. Freud could not ignore this conjuncture of the familial and the subjective: by agreeing to the realisation of the polyclinic project and, at the same time, keeping himself to some extent in the background, he allowed Eitingon to occupy the symbolic position of director of the enterprise. Freud supported Eitingon's desire in action. In contrast, the Eitingon family agreed to finance the psychoanalytic undertaking not so much to ensure the development of a field that didn't much matter to them as to further the personal interests of one of the Eitingon tribe. Now that Waldemar was dead and Motty was running the New York branch of the business, it was time for the eldest son, whose studies had been both protracted and a source of anxiety, to finally achieve something.

Friend Eitingon

When the relationship with the father figure unravelled – or threatened to unravel – Eitingon's reaction was at the level of the body. In the spring of 1923, following confirmation of the cancerous origin of the tumour on the soft palate for which Freud had just undergone surgery, Eitingon remained silent for two months. Anna Freud reproached him severely for this. Eitingon, however, could probably have done little else, given the fact that Freud was being kept in the dark as to the true nature of his condition by those around him. Eitingon was in no position to pen anodyne letters when he himself was in shock. Soon after hearing the terrible news, he fell ill. First, he suffered from heart problems, and then, in December 1923, he was stricken with facial paralysis. At the same time, Freud was struggling with intolerable pain in his palate. Early in 1924, Eitingon reported that hemiplegia was hampering his speech. (A colleague who was aware of Freud's health problems actually laughed at Eitingon's identification with Freud.) Both men were experiencing discomfort in the same area of the body.

Eitingon was looking for a father in Freud, and he made no secret of it. He referred to the 'great paternal kindness' that Freud showed him. As a responsible son, he was not just the director of Freud's 'subsidiary' in Berlin – he was also responsible for settling any problems that might hinder the development of Freud's global enterprise. Freud made great use of Eitingon's talents as a skilled mediator. He appreciated the younger man's strengths as a conciliator in times of heightened tension between the various psychoanalytic societies. When the Swiss analysts wanted to create a psychoanalytic association that would be purely medical, Eitingon handled the situation with great dexterity. He also worked tirelessly to avoid a split with the Americans during the stormy debates about lay analysis that preceded the IPA's 1927 congress. He served as Freud's personal secretary, writing the somewhat unpleasant letters required to call people to order. In this way Freud and Eitingon were able to complement each other. When Freud went on the offensive, Eitingon confined himself to the register of conciliation. At the time of Jones's hostility to Anna Freud and the threat of a split in the New York group, Freud spelled out the strategy that had to be adopted:

> I've always been the tolerant one, the one who wants to calm things down. It didn't do me much good; it was others who felt the need to attribute to me a dose of intolerance and aggression that was never mine. I now wish to give them this pleasure: from now on, I intend to be the demanding one, the severe one, the one who is never satisfied … We will then correspond to the typical father figure that we wish for.[37]

As the Freudian enterprise took on an international scope, Eitingon became Freud's adviser on all economic matters. He also assumed the task of raising funds to save the international psychoanalytic publications from bankruptcy. Numerous letters exchanged between the two men concerned finance and the problems that needed to be solved regarding the management of the Verlag. For Freud, these publications represented the most important organ of the psychoanalytic movement – he considered them 'even more vital than the polyclinics'.[38] In 1924, Otto Rank, the Verlag's director at the time, published his book *The Trauma of Birth*. This aroused deep emotion in the analytic community, especially among Eitingon, Abraham and Sachs.[39] Freud immediately came to Rank's defence and let it be known that he still trusted him. He firmly opposed the idea that texts that diverged from his own ideas should necessarily be submitted to the institute's committee to be read in advance, as Eitingon had requested. Rank, however, persisted in his wish for emancipation and asserted that he still wanted to settle in America. Freud eventually realised that Rank's strange behaviour was linked to the effects of the previous year's cancer diagnosis, which Rank himself later admitted. Freud and Eitingon agreed that these intrigues probably pertained to a manic episode on Rank's part. Despite his repentance, Rank was considered lost to the cause, and Freud was forced to let him go. Josef Storfer was chosen to replace him at the helm of the Verlag under Eitingon's supervision. Since the Verlag was an SARL (a limited company), Eitingon simultaneously acquired a stake in its capital and became co-responsible for the publishing house's scientific direction.

The only real disagreement between Freud and Eitingon during this period concerned the training of analysts. The IPA's International Training

Commission (ITC), which Eitingon had masterminded and whose principles he had outlined at the IPA's Bad Homburg congress in 1925, was intended to promote the extension of the standard training established in Berlin to all the other IPA member societies. There were, however, obstacles to this attempt at homogenisation. For example, the French group felt that the development of psychoanalysis required the collaboration of non-physicians and that they should be given the opportunity to have a therapeutic practice. They found the training of American and Dutch lay analysts in foreign institutes problematic because it seemed to them contrary to the statutes of the IPA. On the American side, the possibility that they would not be allowed to select their own candidates at the national level was definitely not an option. The Americans remained inflexible and refused to admit candidates who were not already psychiatrists. They flatly rejected the kind of analysis practiced by laymen.[40]

In a circular letter to the members of the secret committee, Freud expressed his disapproval of the restrictions that were to be introduced at the Vienna Institute of Education. Freud wanted to make analytic education accessible to all those who wanted it, even in cases where candidates could not meet the requirements of the full curriculum.[41] Many people in Vienna did not want to become therapists but still wanted to be trained in psychoanalysis. Eitingon, on the other hand, demanded that students in training should commit themselves to a so-called in-depth training, corresponding to the triptych of didactic analysis, theoretical courses and practical training. In the end, Eitingon decided to ask Freud what should be done with students who could only attend the Institute of Education for a short period of time. He reminded Freud of the need for greater supervision of students who were completing their training in an institute of psychoanalysis:

> We must ask of them a little more than their simply wanting to learn something – all our severity is ultimately aimed at demanding that our great association, by creating teaching opportunities in as many places as possible, should help these people to learn little by little, in temporal and geographical succession, the whole, or at least more than a small fragment. Whether a fragment is more than several fragments does not always depend solely on the quality of the teacher. Shouldn't we also rely on the material brought in by the pupils?[42]

To defend his point of view, Eitingon, who was vacationing in Italy when he wrote this letter, used a metaphor. He compared the training regulations to the Renaissance wrought-iron grills, doors and windows he had in front of him. These creations in metal, he said, defied time. Their secret was that they were not too high to cross with one good stride. Eitingon believed that 'nothing is forbidden to exceptions of greater value. There is no need to raise higher barriers to transmission by making it difficult to define exceptional character'. The training he envisaged had to have the same function as good, solid barriers. It should not be insuperable for a determined and consistent candidate. According to this conception, sustained effort over the long term is what counts. An exceptional candidate's character is not predicated on a few specific individual abilities such as intelligence, logic, tact, a high level of cultivation and, above all, a relationship with the unconscious. Eitingon favoured what withstands the test of time, meaning endurance. In other words, he emphasises willingness to complete the entire course. Furthermore, he believed that the regulation of training would make it possible to curb the rivalry between the Europeans and the Americans. Indeed, each of the groups was accusing the other of being less capable of analysis. Using the same training standards on both sides of the Atlantic would have the advantage of putting an end to competition between the old and the new. Such was his conviction. Freedom of movement, the ability to learn wherever one wanted, would be guaranteed by the standardisation of analytic training procedures throughout the world: 'Without overoptimistically underestimating the weight of jealousy and material considerations, we can and must, in the present circumstances, constantly defuse the ever-increasing subterranean conflicts in our great association while demanding something essentially objective.'

In short, Eitingon genuinely believed in the virtues of a centralised system of regulation capable of managing the conflicts and jealousies that characterised relations between the different branches of the IPA. He relied on the objectivity of the universal standard in dealing with imaginary rivalries. He called for impersonal regulation, a regime that would be identical for all. His attachment to standards and his desire for norms were linked to a belief in the virtues of universal regulation that would be applicable to everyone. He felt that definitive training regulations would limit personal ambitions. They would make it possible to support and consolidate the international character of the movement and also make it unassailable. Relying on the universal of the law, the regulation of training was an attempt to apply a regime of 'all being equal and alike' to analysts throughout the world. Unfortunately for Eitingon, the governing body of the ITC wasn't written in the sky of ideas. He failed to perceive that the ITC's presidency was installing a European in the position of chief legislator, which was something the Americans would not forget. Despite his undoubted negotiating skills, Eitingon did not understand that the international character of the movement required a kind of training that would be neither uniform nor standardised. He did not understand that there were certain American and European specificities. Using puzzles as a metaphor would probably have been more judicious than referring to Quattrocento architectural details. The scattered pieces are all the better fitted and held together when their sizes, colours and contours are irregular and differentiated and cannot be compared to one another.

Eitingon's idea of making an exception for bringing in some unusually persevering recruits testified to his sincere belief in the virtues of hard work and endurance. But he did this without taking into account the fact that his chairmanship of the ITC and the multiplicity of management functions he had assumed were propelling him into the position of leader. This 'exception', which he defined precisely by hard work and endurance, is not unrelated to certain obsessive characteristics of seriousness, stubbornness and willingness to work hard. If we really want to define Eitingon's wish-to-be, we could say that it was about embodiment of a superior entity from a lower order, about becoming the representative of the 'at least one', who would stick to marching upward from below and who would become the only one capable of occupying that place. So it is not the place of the master – it is, rather, that of the foreman or the chief petty officer, that is to say, that of the performer who has technical know-how and who leads the teams. What happens when the chief petty officer thinks he is authorised to speak in the place of the master even when the master is still speaking? Eitingon's plan to establish a centralised body under his personal control was not unrelated to his position as Freud's heir and follower. His lack of foresight concerning the powers of the ITC was almost predictable. Neutralising imaginary rivalries by imposing rules that were intended to be valid for all was not going to work. Instead of building solid barriers over time by means of rules, the ITC, which was supposed to take on the task of standardising the training of analysts around the world, turned instead to pretence, to semblant. It had no real power and gradually became simply a place of interaction for people of differing opinions who occasionally met up at major congresses. In any case, who, in Freud's lifetime, could have ventured an opinion on psychoanalytic training without the full endorsement of Freud himself?

In the eyes of Freud and the analysts of the period, the Berlin Institute was Eitingon's greatest creation. But his ambition to create centralised conditions for the training of analysts ended in failure. This grandiose dream could not win the support of those who challenged the Europeans' right to interfere in their affairs. First of all, Eitingon did not dare to thwart Freud concerning the possibility of accepting students who had no prior medical training. He adopted an intermediate position, according to which the rule could permit certain exceptions. Laymen could, under certain conditions, be admitted by the ITC to undertake their training in an institute. Eitingon drafted a resolution to this effect in June 1927. Ferenczi, who steadfastly defended Freud's position on lay analysis, felt that Eitingon was essentially a supporter of the Anglo-Saxons. 'Friend Eitingon is an absolute friend of physicians, with a decided guild mentality. As a favour to you, he decided in the end to demand the recognition, in principle, of lay analysis (by the Americans).'[43] The Americans rejected Eitingon's resolution at the IPA's Innsbruck congress in 1927.

In this difficult struggle on behalf of lay analysis, Freud considered that he had already given his opinion in writing – in his 1926 defence of lay analysis – and that there was no need to return to the subject. He felt that his position as an outsider did not allow him to do more, and he threatened that he would be the first person to resign from the IPA if any concessions were made to the Americans. In fact, though, he did not take a completely negative view of the threat of a schism. Group autonomy seemed inevitable to him. In the spring of 1927, he wrote:

> There is no doubt that my text on lay analysis was a sword stroke in the water. I tried to arouse a common analytic feeling that medical corporatism had to be opposed, but I failed. There will be consequences, and they will not be favourable.[44]

Eitingon, strenuously rejecting the idea of splitting the IPA, continued his efforts at conciliation. A precarious compromise was finally reached at the dreaded Oxford congress, which was held in July 1929. The Americans duly accepted the principle of lay analysis, and the Europeans, in exchange, undertook not to train foreign candidates in the absence of a favourable decision from the national training commission of their country of origin. Eitingon was convinced that the issue of lay analysis would not be a problem in the future and that the unity of the IPA was no longer threatened. His hard-won reconciliation with the Americans was short-lived, however. Above all, it had the effect of gradually emptying the Berlin Institute of its substance, given that it led to the logical need to open training institutes in the United States. Leading personalities in Berlin began to leave. Franz Alexander accepted an invitation to take up the first chair of psychoanalysis at the University of Chicago. Sándor Radó, who had been Eitingon's right-hand man for years, moved to New York. These and other defections took place, it should be noted, before the Nazi Party came to power in Germany. The heyday of the first psychoanalytic institution came to an end before 1933.

Eitingon's mother died on 30 November 1929. He noted both the continuation and the end of a mental process that had already been going on for a long time and during which his relationship with his mother had gradually changed. From then on, he was willing to countenance the finite nature of existence without asking himself too many questions. With his mother's demise, his obsessive fantasy of working to the point of exhaustion altered, giving him a glimpse of the prospect of his own departure from the world.[45] Freud's response was to say that one should always pay and atone for all the love that one has received, and especially for the love that one's mother gave. (Freud lost his own mother the following year.) Eitingon's prestige within the IPA declined precipitously in the late 1920s. He was accused of having mishandled disputes between members of the Berlin Institute. Three years later, the international psychoanalytic publications of the Verlag were on the brink of bankruptcy. Eitingon was held responsible for mismanagement. It has to be recognised that Eitingon's economic difficulties were not unrelated to the disgrace into which he had fallen. It was well known that his wealth had enabled him to gain access to a high position and to undertake projects no one else could have carried out. Within the IPA, this was sometimes laughed at. His counterpart at the Vienna Psychoanalytic Institute, Eduard Hitschmann, made a play on words about the origin of his fortune: 'The best *Fälle* [cases] of psychoanalysis were the *Felle* [furs or skins] of old Eitingon.'[46]

When Eitingon was no longer in a position to make good the losses generated by the Berlin Institute and the Verlag, his position in the IPA changed. Should we be surprised by this? Or should we condemn the attitude of the analysts who were gradually turning away from him because he had lost all his money? After all, Eitingon had built his position on his personal fortune, his prodigality matched only by his desire to help his fellow man. He was not a theorist, he had published little and he did not teach. For his part, Freud had something to say to his colleague about the problem of giving. For Freud's seventy-fifth birthday, Eitingon wanted to organise a fund-raising campaign among the members of the IPA in order to bail out the Verlag. Freud, however, refused to take part personally in the remittance of the funds concerned because he was opposed to the use of a sum of money that confused him with the publishing company. Thanks, however, to Eitingon's great efficiency in this instance, the damage had already been done; the money had been collected. Freud asked Eitingon to make the money available for the day when he would come to collect it himself, and he commented on this episode as follows:

> The aggression bound up with the tenderness of the giver requires satisfaction; the one to whom the gift has been made must allow himself to be bothered, annoyed, and plunged into confusion. The elderly and the weak who, on such occasions, learn to their surprise how much their younger brothers and sisters value them, pretend to be overwhelmed by the plethora of feelings and to succumb soon afterwards to the side effects. Nothing is free, as we all know, and you have to pay high taxes for a life that lasts too long.[47]

Freud reminded Eitingon that the aggressive impulse always went hand in hand with the gift. By this time, after undergoing another operation in April 1931, the inventor of psychoanalysis had lost all hope, nurtured for eight years, of a cure for his cancer. He complained that he was only an unhappy remnant of reality and that he had taken a step outside the circle of life.[48]

Two months after the Nazi Party's seizure of power and the advent of the first legislative measures aimed at removing Jews from leadership positions in medical associations, Eitingon considered closing the Berlin Institute:

> Since I cannot see who, in such altered circumstances, could keep it going in the spirit that ought to characterise it, I would prefer not to leave it to anyone – if this aberrant situation should arise – to ensure that the

> institute would continue to exist while I, being both a foreigner and a foreign doctor, could no longer work ... I may well have the right to identify myself with the Institute or, conversely, to identify the Institute with myself.[49]

It should be recalled that after World War I, Eitingon had taken Polish nationality. Moreover, it is likely that he did not possess a German medical licence. In relation to the censorship that had just been introduced in Germany, his reference to his status as a foreigner was actually an allusion to his Jewish origins.

Freud considered three possibilities regarding the fate of the Berlin Psychoanalytic Institute in Hitler's Germany. In the first case, psychoanalysis would be banned in Germany and the institute would be closed by order of the administration. Eitingon would have to hold out until the last moment before the ship sank. This possibility, the simplest case, did not lend itself to any comment. In the second case, Eitingon, as a foreigner, would not be able to continue as director but could remain in Berlin to run the institute unofficially and it would therefore not have to be closed down. Since the institute, which had been established by Eitingon, belonged to the DPG, it would be necessary to fight for its preservation. A non-Jewish analyst could formally assume the leadership of the institute. In that case, the institute would simply have to tick over, and Eitingon would stay in Berlin. The third possibility was that Eitingon would be forced to leave Berlin. This would entail a greater danger of dubious types taking over the institute, in which case the DPG would have to abandon it. It would have to part with it by disavowing it, Freud wrote, 'excluding it until it could be cleansed of its faults'.[50]

Eitingon disagreed with Freud's view of the institute's legal status. He had not offered the Berlin Institute to the DPG, as Freud claimed: he had merely taken it under his wing. Eitingon considered the institute to be his personal property and wanted to stay in place until he was absolutely forced to give it up. In the spring of 1933, his attitude was guided by a concern not to act hastily. He tried to moderate the fervour of those who wanted to reorganise the German psychoanalytic movement without delay. Eitingon defied many passages to the act by his colleagues. He wanted to prevent the analysts from throwing themselves into the wolf's maw, as Boehm had done when he had approached the authorities to find out whether the institute would be affected by the measure forbidding Jews from serving on the boards of medical associations. He felt above all that it was unnecessary to respond in advance to the new government's demands that Jewish staff members be barred from the institute. When Eitingon took this position, it was already well known that Boehm had ambitions to replace him. After consulting with the authorities, Boehm immediately went to Vienna to seek Freud's support and Eitingon's resignation. He eventually decided, however, to follow the formalities and simply comply with the decisions of the general meeting of the DPG, which was scheduled to be held in May. Aware of the dangers now threatening the institute and its staff and patients, Eitingon began to sort through the files of all the institute's patients, removing any documents that could have seemed compromising. Driven by the unshakeable conviction that 'haste and subjective indignity must be avoided',[51] Eitingon emphasised that what he owed to the analytic cause could not come into conflict with his Judaism.

While doubting the reliability of Boehm and Müller-Braunschweig, Freud obtained from the former a promise that Schultz-Hencke, whom he greatly disliked, would be kept out of the new organisation. He also demanded that Wilhelm Reich be expelled from the DPG. Eitingon then reassured Freud on one point. Schultz-Hencke, he said, would only become dangerous if he held an important position in the German General Medical Society for Psychotherapy (Deutsche Allgemeine Ärztliche Gesellschaft für Psychotherapie, or DAÄGP). Founded in September 1933, the DAÄGP was entrusted not to Schultz-Hencke but to Matthias Heinrich Göring, a psychiatrist who was a cousin of the powerful Nazi leader (and future Reichsmarschall) Hermann Göring. Matthias Göring then became the mastermind of the outlandish enterprise of cleansing psychoanalysis of Freud's work. With the help of an adviser from the Ministry of the Interior, Göring and his fellow psychotherapists finally got their hands on the Berlin Institute in 1936.

On the second point, Eitingon was not in favour of expelling Wilhelm Reich from the DPG. In his view, it would be better simply to disown him. Boehm, however, obeyed Freud's express request and demanded that Reich's name be removed from the list of members of the DPG in July 1933. Reich was formally expelled from the organisation at the IPA's Lucerne congress in 1934.

In conjunction with the terms of the Reichstag Fire Decree of 28 February 1933, the 'Law to Remedy the Distress of the People and the Reich' (also known as the Enabling Act) passed in the Reichstag on 23 March 1933 and turned Hitler's government into a legal dictatorship. As Eitingon wrote, it was Germany that was now sick. Shortly after delivering the eulogy for Sándor Ferenczi, who died on 22 May 1933, Eitingon prepared to leave Germany. His choosing to live in Palestine came as no surprise to his colleagues, who were aware of his extreme sensitivity to the anti-Semitism prevailing in Germany. His unshakeable decision to leave was met with little sympathy. At the end of November, Eitingon went to Vienna. Anna Freud reported to Lou Andreas-Salomé that Eitingon was far from happy about leaving but felt that moving to Palestine was the only solution for him. She wrote 'that this amounts to the departure of one of those people who had been counted on to support the work here – that side of things escapes him'.[52]

Freud himself said that from now on one should no longer count on the help of others but should rely on oneself exclusively. According to Lou Andreas-Salomé, Eitingon's departure was a cruel disappointment to Freud, whose entourage suspected that Mirra Eitingon's baleful influence had much to do with the situation. Mirra had always dreamed of seeing her husband freed from all professional commitments. In Vienna, Eitingon's departure was experienced as an abandonment for which his wife was responsible: it was Mirra's choice, they felt. Max Eitingon was seen as the author of his own misfortune.

Over the next four years, despite Eitingon's regular visits to Europe in connection with his settlement in Palestine, Ernest Jones quickly took his place at the central management level of the IPA.

Notes

1 Max Eitingon, 'Report on the Berlin Psychoanalytic Polyclinic', *Bulletin of the International Psychoanalytical Association*, no. 4 (1923), 265.
2 *Ibid.*
3 In the original German text of the Budapest conference, Freud spoke of copper (*Kupfer*) and not of lead. In Europe, copper was used up until the second half of the nineteenth century as an alloy that could be mixed with gold to mint coins. Freud's metaphor was monetary, not alchemical.
4 See Sigmund Freud, 'Lines of Advance in Psychoanalytic Therapy' (1918), *Standard Edition*, vol. 17, pp. 162–168; Sándor Ferenczi, 'Technical Difficulties in an Analysis of Hysteria' (1919), in *Further Contributions to the Theory and Technique of Psychanalysis*, trans. Jane Isabel Suttie (London: Karnac, 1980).
5 Max Eitingon, 'Report', *op. cit.*, p. 266.
6 Hanns Sachs, 'L'analyse didactique' (1930), in Colonomos, *On forme des psychanalystes, op. cit.*, p. 136.
7 Max Eitingon, 'Report', *op. cit.*, p. 265.
8 Sándor Ferenczi, 'Élasticité de la technique psychanalytique' (1928), in *Psychanalyse 4, Oeuvres complètes, 1927–1933* (Paris: Payot, 1982), p. 58.
9 Sigmund Freud, 'On Beginning the Treatment', *Standard Edition*, vol. 12, p. 132.
10 In his second instalment of analysis, the Wolf-Man stated that Freud also treated Eva Rosenfeld, Bruno Goetz and Sergei Pankejeff free of charge.
11 Jacques Lacan, *Seminar X, op. cit.*, p. 139.
12 Sigmund Freud, 'The Question of Lay Analysis: Conversations with an Impartial Person', *Standard Edition*, vol. 20, p. 187.
13 Eitingon, 'Allocution', in Colonomos, *On forme des psychanalystes, op. cit.*, pp. 179, 182.
14 Sigmund Freud, 'Recommendations to Physicians Practising Psychoanalysis' (1912), *Standard Edition*, vol. 12, p. 118.
15 Max Eitingon, 'Allocution', in Colonomos, *On forme des psychanalystes, op. cit.*, p. 182.
16 Sigmund Freud, 'Future Prospects', *Standard Edition*, vol. 11, p. 147.
17 Maurice-Moshe Krajzman, 'Max Eitingon, 1881–1943, Construire l'entreprise psychanalytique', *Ornicar?*, no. 48 (1989), 103.
18 Freud to Eitingon, Letter 772 F, 5 October 1933, in Michael Schröter, *Correspondance, op. cit.*, p. 802.
19 Freud to Eitingon, Letter 770 F, 5 September 1933, *ibid.*, p. 801.
20 Ernest Jones, *Sigmund Freud: Life and Work, Years of Maturity, 1901–1919*, vol. 2 (London: The Hogarth Press, 1955), p. 182.
21 Michael Schröter, 'Le Timonier: Max Eitingon et son role dans l'histoire de la psychanalyse', in Michael Schröter, *Correspondance, op. cit.*, p. 13.
22 Olivier Mannoni, 'Freud et Eitingon, les rouages de la machinerie psychanalytique', in Stéphane Michaud (ed.), *Correspondances de Freud* (Paris: Presse de la Sorbonne Nouvelle, 2007), p. 49.

23 Stéphane Michaud, *Correspondances de Freud, op. cit.*, pp. 50–51.
24 The synagogue was destroyed by civilian and Brownshirt mobs in November 1938.
25 Walter Laqueur, *Weimar, op. cit.*
26 Max Eitingon, 'Max Eitingon: des premiers temps de la psychanalyse (Document I)', in Michael Schröter, *Correspondance, op. cit.*, p. 874. This report was presented at a meeting of the Palestine Psychoanalytical Association on 6 May 1937.
27 *Ibid.*, p. 877.
28 The Berlin Psychoanalytic Association (Berliner Psychoanalytische Vereinigung, or BPV) was the first local psychoanalytic group, founded in 1910. The BPV changed its name to the German Psychoanalytic Society (Deutsche Psychoanalytische Gesellschaft, or DPG) in April 1926. This change of name was due to the creation of new psychoanalytic groups throughout Germany.
29 Sigmund Freud, 'Freud à propos de Max et Mirra Eitingon (1937), avec commentaires (Document XIII)', in Michael Schröter, *Correspondance, op. cit.*, p. 909. This relates to an extract from a letter from Freud to Arnold Zweig, dated 10 February 1937.
30 Karen Brecht, Volker Friedrich, Ludger Hermanns, Isidor J. Kaminer, and Dierk H. Juelich (eds.), *Ici, la vie continue d'une manière fort surprenante…, Contribution à l'Histoire de la Psychanalyse en Allemagne*, text established by Alain de Mijolla and Vera Renz (Paris: International Psychoanalytic Association, 1987), p. 26. Originally published as *Hier geht das Leben auf eine sehr merkwürdige Weise weiter…, Zur Geschichte der Psychoanalyse in Deutschland* (Hamburg: IPAC, 1985).
31 Perry Meisel and Walter Kendrick (eds.), *Bloomsbury/Freud: The Letters of James and Alix Strachey, 1924–1925* (London: Chatto & Windus, 1986), p. 144. ('Wohnung' means 'apartment'.)
32 Freud to Eitingon, Letter 206 F, 10 April 1921, in Michael Schröter, *Correspondance, op. cit.*, p. 261. Pankejeff eventually found employment in the insurance business.
33 Freud alludes here to Eitingon's amorous feelings towards his daughter which subsequently became close bonds of friendship. Jones entertained similar hopes, and Freud interpreted this thwarted ambition as the reason for his aggressiveness towards Anna.
34 Freud to Eitingon, Letter 229 F, 24 January 1922, in Michael Schröter, *Correspondance, op. cit.*, pp. 285–286.
35 Eitingon to Freud, Letter 230 F, 16 February 1922, in Michael Schröter, *Correspondance, op. cit.*, p. 287.
36 Laura Sokolowsky, 'La désinsertion de l'Homme aux loups', *La Cause freudienne*, no. 71 (June 2009).
37 Freud to Eitingon, Letter 467 F, 23 September 1923, in Michael Schröter, *Correspondance, op. cit.*, p. 529.
38 Freud to Eitingon, Letter 264 F, December 1922, *op. cit.*, p. 316.
39 Eitingon to Freud, Letter 323 E, 26 December 1924, *op. cit.*, p. 380. The three Berliners were Abraham, Eitingon and Sachs.
40 Freud to Eitingon, Letter 548 F, 3 July 1929, *op. cit.*, p. 608.
41 Freud, circular letter of 20 October 1925, *op. cit.*, p. 411, fn. 6.
42 Eitingon to Freud, Letter 352 E, 29 October 1925, *op. cit.*, p. 410.
43 Ferenczi to Freud, Letter 1100, 13 July 1927, in Falzeder and Brabant, *The Correspondence of Sigmund Freud and Sándor Ferenczi, Volume 3, op. cit.*, p. 317.
44 Freud to Eitingon, Letter 499 F, 3 April 1928, in Michael Schröter, *Correspondance, op. cit.*, p. 566.
45 In a letter to Anna Freud written in November 1920, Eitingon declared: 'I am hoping, one day, to die on the job.'

46 Richard Sterba, *Réminiscences d'un psychanalyste viennois* (Toulouse: Privat, 1986), p. 115.
47 Freud to Eitingon, Letter 633 F, 8 February 1931, in Michael Schröter, *Correspondance, op. cit.*, p. 671.
48 Max Schur, *Freud: Living and Dying* (New York: International Universities Press, 1972).
49 Eitingon to Freud, Letter 754 E, 19 March 1933, *op. cit.*, p. 784.
50 Freud to Eitingon, Letter 755 F, 21 March 1933, in Michael Schröter, *Correspondance, op. cit.*, p. 785.
51 Eitingon to Freud, Letter 760 E, 21 March 1933, in Michael Schröter, *Correspondance, op. cit.*, p. 791.
52 Anna Freud to Lou Andreas-Salomé, Letter 383 A, 26 November 1933, in Lou Andreas-Salomé and Anna Freud, *À l'ombre du père: Correspondance, 1919–1937* (Paris: Fayard, 2006), p. 546.

Chapter 3

The original 1930 report

Handling public opinion

Two years after the Berlin Polyclinic's move to its new premises, a monograph, with a new preface by Freud, was published to mark the institute's tenth anniversary. He wrote:

> The following pages describe the founding and achievements of the Berlin Psychoanalytic Institute, to which are allotted three important functions within the psychoanalytic movement. First, it endeavours to make our therapy accessible to the great multitude who suffer under their neuroses no less than the wealthy, but who are not in a position to meet the cost of their treatment. Secondly, it seeks to provide a centre at which analysis can be taught theoretically and at which the experience of older analysts can be handed on to pupils who are anxious to learn. And lastly, it aims at perfecting our knowledge of neurotic illnesses and our therapeutic technique by applying them and testing them under fresh conditions.
>
> An Institute of this kind was indispensable; but we should have waited in vain for assistance from the State or interest from the University in its foundation. Here the energy and self-sacrifice of an individual analyst took the initiative. Ten years ago, Dr. Max Eitingon, now President of the International Psychoanalytical Association, created an institute such as this from his own resources, and has since then maintained and directed it by his own efforts. This Report on the first decade of the Berlin Institute is a tribute to its creator and director – an attempt to render him public thanks. Anyone who, in whatever sense, has a share in psychoanalysis will unite in thus thanking him.[1]

With striking economy, Freud here summed up the institute's three objectives: therapy for the masses; analytic research; and the teaching and transmission of analytic theory and experience. It should be noted that a previous reference to the protection of citizens from unscrupulous practitioners has disappeared. This reference, which appeared in the preface published in 1923, pointed out

DOI: 10.4324/9781003215684-5

that psychoanalytic practice considered itself threatened by the spread of wild psychoanalysis. Was the threat that analytic practice might be appropriated by new generations of social workers and psychologists now less pressing? One of the aims for which the institute was created was precisely to encourage as many of them as possible to train in accordance with a procedure gradually developed in the course of a decade. The deviationist currents, which took their inspiration from psychoanalysis by borrowing some of its elements while disregarding its indivisible unity, were as much a cause for concern as ever. We will have an opportunity later to demonstrate this with regard to a specific situation. An instrument for combating these deviations would be in place from now on.

The original 'Report on *Ten Years of the Berlin Psychoanalytic Institute*', written to mark Eitingon's fiftieth birthday, included the following articles:

- an unpublished preface by Freud;
- an article by Ernst Simmel: 'On the History and Social Significance of the Berlin Psychoanalytic Institute';
- a 'Statistical Report on Therapeutic Activity between 1920 and 1930' by Otto Fenichel;
- a 'Historical Account of Teaching and its Organisation and Management' by Carl Müller-Braunschweig;
- an article on 'Consultation at the Polyclinic' by Hans Lampl.

A series of articles on teaching arrangements followed, including one by Karen Horney on organisation and one by Hanns Sachs on didactic analysis. There was also an article by Franz Alexander on the theoretical curriculum and one by Sándor Radó on the practical curriculum. Siegfried Bernfeld dealt with practical teaching for pedagogues. Felix Boehm addressed the issue of scholarships. An article by Jenö Hárnik dealt with the institute's means of dissemination. There were also testimonies relating to the interest that the institute had aroused overseas – one by Gregory Zilboorg on the response in America, another by Ola Raknes on the response in Norway. The appendix contained the address that Eitingon had given at the inauguration of the institute's new premises in 1928.

Of all these contributions, only the articles by Simmel, Fenichel and Lampl – dealing, respectively, with the institute's integration into the social fabric, statistics relating to outcomes, and protocols for patient selection – provide clinical data. These three documents are of particular interest.

Simmel's article stood out from the others by virtue of its polemical tone. It was essentially an appeal to the public authorities. Simmel defended the idea that inscribing psychoanalysis at the heart of public health policy was a necessity. He emphasised the notion of social hygiene by raising questions about the country's health insurance funds. Simmel explained that the medical consultants at these organisations were unaware of the results obtained by psychoanalysis in caring for people from the disadvantaged social strata. The Berlin Polyclinic had been established in a time of economic crisis. It had committed itself to making 'psychoanalytical treatment accessible to those who saw their neurosis reinforced by economic misery or who were even more exposed to material impoverishment because of their neurotic inhibitions'.[2] Through psychoanalytic treatment, the individual could be freed from an irrational attitude towards reality and thus provided with the resources to integrate himself into society. However, the wider social benefit of psychoanalytic treatment also had to be considered, since, through this integration, the patient's family and friends would also, in their turn, profit from the beneficial effects of the analytic treatment. For this reason, he said, the analyses undertaken at the Berlin Polyclinic were at the centre of a continuous psychoanalytic penetration of society. The process began with treating the individual and then moved outwards into the social sphere. According to Simmel, the private financing of the clinic by the DPG would, because of its public utility, be neither fair nor tenable in the long term. From an economic point of view, public funding of the polyclinic was justified. Indeed, he said, it was decidedly abnormal to have psychoanalysts themselves bearing the cost of an enterprise capable of providing such a service to citizens. Simmel's argument was essentially based on the notion of the need for psychological healthcare: 'The need for this treatment has become so obvious that in the near future the insured, whose representatives sit on the health insurance committees, will themselves demand psychoanalysis.'

Eventually, the insured themselves, Simmel believed, would claim reimbursement for psychoanalytical treatment. The resulting savings for the health insurance system would be significant, since substantial sums of money were being spent unnecessarily on the treatment of misdiagnosed neurotic conditions. Occupational medicine was a particular concern. Enormous costs were being incurred in the treatment of retirement-related neuroses, psychological trauma resulting from accidents and relapses suffered by people who had been sent back into the world of work too hastily. Simmel's entirely pragmatic argument was that psychoanalysis would therefore be highly advantageous from the point of view of healthcare expenditure. Indeed, the ignorance of the medical consultants – who were reimbursing patients with neurotic symptoms for ineffective hydrotherapy, electrotherapy, and radiotherapy treatments, as well as providing them with unnecessary medication – was costing society a great deal of money. Which was why, he said, government funding of the psychoanalytic polyclinic would result in substantial savings for the public authorities. A certain amount of dramatisation was evident in his arguments:

> The indignation of the insured, who, for the time being, are obliged to beg for psychoanalysis as a charitable act of the Berlin Polyclinic – and especially the indignation of those who are on our waiting lists and who often miss out, due to the lack of timely psychoanalytical help, on the

> most important decisions of their lives – will, in a short period of time, lead those concerned to accept as consulting physicians only those doctors who are capable of adequately treating both their physical and their psychological illnesses.

Max Eitingon was presented by Simmel as the model of the enlightened doctor, as someone who had held his own in the context of economic stagnation and near-continuous political crises. The great social merit of the creator of the polyclinic was, he said, to have financed it in such difficult times. In addition, the polyclinic had a decisive function where knowledge was concerned. It had the merit of being capable of making the poverty-stricken patient more knowledgeable concerning the origin of his illness. Before the existence of this institution, the poor person – or, as we would say today, the precarious individual – was at the mercy of all sorts of ineptitude where care was concerned.

It wasn't only the ordinary citizens of Berlin who were crying out for psychoanalysis. The doctors themselves wanted access to the training provided by the institute; they needed to be offered the possibility of undertaking internships at the polyclinic. The training of analysts was also an urgent requirement. In this particular regard, Simmel introduced an ethical differentiation between medical training and analytic training. He argued that, in medicine, patients were generally used merely as a kind of equipment in hospital wards. Wealthy patients could afford to be seen by doctors in private practice, whereas proletarians on public wards were used as 'training aids'. The nobility of psychoanalysis obliged it, he said, to prevent this type of discriminatory treatment, insofar as 'a psychoanalytical treatment is no different from the treatment of a wealthy private patient'. The risk of entrusting analytical treatment to a novice analyst was presented as almost nonexistent insofar as the practitioner would himself have been analysed. As previously mentioned, the motion obliging psychoanalysts to have undergone analysis themselves had been put forward five years earlier at the IPA's Hamburg congress at Eitingon's instigation.

Simmel was proud to be able to announce that this little university had its own library, lectures and seminars. Its courses had attracted so many people (both students and the public) that its premises had become too small, necessitating the move in 1928. The Berlin Psychoanalytic Institute was now at the centre of the psychoanalytic movement in Germany and its example had permitted its diffusion throughout the world – in Vienna, London, Budapest, and The Hague. A new institute was soon to open in New York, and another, which did not yet offer therapy, had been created in Frankfurt.[3] If all these institutions were privately funded, there would, Simmel concluded with considerable fervour, come a time when the state would sense the urgency of its obligations to the poor in the field of psychoanalytic treatment. It was, he said, a question of obtaining 'a partial liberation in relation to the disastrous mechanisms necessarily existing between culture and the creatures who are themselves its creators'.[4]

Ernst Simmel and the psychoanalytic hospital

Three years earlier, Simmel had opened a psychoanalytic clinic at Schloss Tegel, in western Berlin. The emphasis he placed on financing the Berlin Polyclinic in 1930 echoed the considerable problems that he had encountered in running the Tegel sanatorium. In appealing to the people who were in a position to finance the Berlin Polyclinic while, at the same time, admonishing the doctors who worked in the health insurance system, he was also defending his own ailing business. On the strength of his experience with the military authorities during the war, Simmel had initially hoped to obtain public subsidies for the establishment of a psychoanalytic hospital. But that was not to be. He had found it necessary to set up a company with three other administrators: an insurance company director, a Viennese doctor who had been analysed by Freud, and a minister of state.

A psychiatrist and neurologist by training, Simmel was born in 1882 in Breslau, a German city in present-day Poland. He was the youngest child of a Jewish family. His father was a banker and his mother ran an agency for domestics. He studied psychiatry in Berlin and Rostock and wrote his thesis on the aetiology of dementia praecox. He was already politically active before the war. He began his analysis with Karl Abraham in 1919 and was chairman of the Society of Socialist Physicians (SVÄ) between 1924 and 1933. During the war, he was chief doctor of the hospital in Posen. His application of psychoanalysis to the treatment of war neuroses brought him sudden fame. As we have seen, his book on war neuroses, published in 1918, attracted the attention of the military authorities and earned him an invitation to discuss the topic at the IPA's Budapest congress alongside Abraham and Ferenczi. Subsequently, Abraham, Eitingon and Simmel were joint directors of the Berlin Polyclinic from 1920 onward. In spite of its success, the creation of this first institution, where the patient-selection process gave precedence to the psychoanalytic treatment of neuroses, did not seem to be enough for Simmel.

As early as 1924, Simmel confided to his Berlin colleagues that he was considering the possibility of curing psychotics.[5] The Tegel sanatorium, which opened on 10 April 1927, was the first institution in the world to offer psychoanalytic treatment to hospitalised patients. Fitted out by Ernst Freud, it was located half an hour's drive from the city centre in a park near Lake Tegel. It had seventy-four inpatient beds and was open to patients suffering from severe neurosis, drug addiction and mental or organic diseases that were difficult to treat conventionally. Simmel would have liked to treat other types of mental ailment, but he met with opposition from State Councillor Reinhold von Heinz, the owner of the premises, who refused to create a closed unit for patients suffering from serious mental illnesses. At Tegel, each patient was followed by an assistant psychoanalyst. Psychoanalytic principles were applied to diagnosis as well as to treatment. Psychotherapy was offered to all patients with organic diseases. All staff members had received analytic training and their support had to be linked to the ongoing analytical work.

In an article published in 1937, Simmel, who left Germany in 1934 and moved to Los Angeles, reviewed the few years of Tegel's existence:

> The German Psychoanalytic Hospital existed for only four and a half years. Its functioning was greatly hampered throughout that period by the gradual political destruction of Germany. The financial needs and the difficulties concerning the adjustment of the hospital to external economic reality often made it difficult for us to take care of the inner psychic economy of our patients. At the end of 1931, it became a painful necessity for me to close this institution which had been operating under the aegis of Professor Freud. From the very beginning, Freud had agreed to the project of founding such a psychoanalytic hospital. He was very interested in its development and he had helped us very generously with his own funds.[6]

Simmel added that the need for such a place had occurred to him in the early 1920s, in the immediate aftermath of his practice with people traumatised by war. What had guided him had been the discovery of the destructive force that inhabited human beings. As a military psychiatrist, Simmel directly witnessed the psychological degradation that war had brought about in his fellow citizens. Neurosis appeared to him to be the ultimate bulwark against moral and physical disorder. In other words, according to him, neurosis was a defence against madness. He had used cathartic hypnosis in order to offer a possibility of diverting inhibited aggressive tendencies. The neurotic patients concerned had to be allowed to kill, in fantasy, the people whose existence they found intolerable. 'I gained the impression that the quantity of aggressive destruction is decisive in determining the threshold beyond which an individual can remain healthy.'[7]

At that time, Freud had not yet worked out his theory of the death drive. The experience of war had a truth-value that anticipated and confirmed the soundness of this Freudian discovery. The tragedy of World War I led Simmel to believe that there was a terrifying internal force exerting unceasing pressure on individuals. This certainty that the individual is inhabited by a drive towards destruction and self-destruction was the primary reason compelling him to set up a psychoanalytic hospital.

The principles that had guided Simmel at Tegel were made explicit in the 1937 article. First of all, he wrote, it was advisable to give priority to the possibility of establishing transference between the hospitalised patient and the analyst. However, this process was complicated by the proliferation of caregivers as the patient tended to diffract love and hate onto the caregivers around him. It was therefore necessary to operate in such a way that the transference, in its ambivalence, could be addressed to a single person. Sometimes, the presence of a superegoic transference to the head of department was noticed at the outset, before a transference to the psychoanalyst had been established. This first type of transference to the head of department could be used to set up certain initial measures of a therapeutic order. On the other hand, it was more complicated to reduce the influence that patients had on each other, and this could disrupt the smooth running of the analytic treatment undertaken. Occupational therapy workshops were developed to address this difficulty.

In any case, Simmel's practice was guided by the question of the superego and feelings of guilt, including in the analytic treatment of psychoses. The emphasis he placed on the transgression of a limit shows that he was apprehensive about this clinic with respect to the effects of disturbances in moral conduct, i.e. he situated its origin at the ethical level. The overcoming of a barrier created by the unconscious aggressivity that the subject turns against himself relates to the core of the superego. Once this process began, there was no longer any limit. As Lacan put it later, such a phenomenon engenders ever-heavier aggressivity on the part of the ego. Simmel had the idea that this auto-aggression could engender madness; beyond a certain amount of aggression turned against himself, the subject could become insane. In other words, Simmel's conception of psychosis took its inspiration from the model of melancholia. He gave the example of a young psychotic patient who had retreated into a catatonic stupor. He hypothesised that this stupor was consistent with the patient's unconscious fear of killing his mother. The patient's wish to be punished for such a misdeed was no less important. Simmel then informed him that the court would not fail to punish him severely for this. The effect of this intervention was immediate, and the patient exited his stupor. The analytic treatment could then begin. He gave a second example of the treatment of the self-destructive tendency in one of his female patients. Her need for punishment had been satisfied by placing her in a room that resembled a solitary-confinement cell. In this room, the patient had a dream that allowed her to access a tragic incident from her childhood. At the age of three, she had killed her newborn brother. Simmel explained that she was no longer afraid of remembering her act because her superego had been soothed by her incarceration. This memory was corroborated by her family, who were later questioned. The neutralisation of a pathological superego was the orientation that guided Simmel's psychoanalytic work with the patients at Tegel. In addition, his assessments of perverts and of addicted neurotics had led him to believe that such patients had to sacrifice satisfaction – a gain in pleasure – in order for the treatment to have any chance of succeeding. For change to occur in an addicted person, it was necessary to bring about a change in character at the narcissistic level. Simmel had found that this objective could only be achieved by compensation through transference. The aim was to draw the attention of his fellow psychoanalysts who were training at Tegel to the link between addiction and introjection: 'It is only through the introjection of drink that the alcoholic becomes the person he wants to love. It is, in the final analysis, his mother.' One of Simmel's alcoholic patients had taken up caring for a small cat in his hospital room, giving it milk several times a day. Simmel felt that the figure of a seductive and easily seduced mother, with which the patient was identified, was frequently at the root of the addict's superego.

Freud stayed several times at Tegel when he went to Berlin for his cancer treatment. This peaceful place offered him a pleasant refuge. He wasn't remotely bothered by the patients in the hospital, who were greatly intimidated by the presence of the famous professor among them. Freud considered Tegel an important research centre. He also felt that analytic training should include an internship as an assistant in a psychoanalytic hospital. In 1929 he launched an appeal for the creation of private funding for the hospital, and Marie Bonaparte, Raymond de Saussure, Dorothy Burlingham, René Spitz, Franz Alexander and Max Eitingon responded. However, the funds raised were insufficient. The financial crisis was so bad that patients could no longer afford to pay hospital fees. In spite of all the efforts made to preserve it, the sanatorium was forced to close in August 1931. After the Nazis came to power, the Brownshirts took over the premises at Tegel. Simmel, who was Jewish and a member of the SPD, barely managed to escape from Germany, via Belgium and England, to exile in the United States. Simmel's experience both at the military hospital in Posen during the war and at Tegel convinced him that the treatment of the death drive was a public health problem. He argued that access to psychoanalysis was the most suitable means of remedying it.

The Fenichel report

The principal clinical information in the 1930 monograph accompanied Otto Fenichel's comments relating to statistical data.[8] This first attempt at clinical classification heralded the typological rigour that Fenichel would later bring to his famous book on the theory of neuroses, which was published in the USA in 1945.[9]

Fenichel was a man of lists. In fact, it seems that he spent his entire life making lists, each of which had several entries. The lists themselves were compared with each other, set out in alphabetical order and numbered. Fenichel estimated the number of shows he had seen in a year and (by country) where he had seen them. The films listed were tagged with the name of the person who had accompanied him. There was also a list of trips made by car as well as by train. Russell Jacoby calculates that there were 'scores of other lists, catalogs, and enumerations, often completely private and opaque, including – possibly – a list of the women he slept with'.[10]

Meticulousness and a taste for classification were thus two highly developed components of Fenichel's personality. The statistical report he drew up in 1930 for the Berlin Institute is a model of its kind, pleasant to read and clearly presented. His presentation of the figures is accompanied by clinical comments on the symptoms encountered. The report began with an introduction stating that the influx of patients with modest incomes very quickly exceeded the polyclinic's reception and treatment capacities. In 1930, 117 analyses were in progress, which seemed to be a not insignificant number. Nevertheless, it also appears that, at the time, this figure was not considered to be particularly important. In fact, in the first instance, the consultations made it possible to select the patients most likely to benefit from an analysis. Fenichel described this selection process as an 'unpleasant triage' necessitated by the indications for analysis, which took precedence over all other considerations.

Above all, he outlined the crux of the problem facing the institute's members. How could analytic training and therapeutic applications be made to coexist without harming each other? Furthermore, if the two options of teaching and research were decisive in a patient's admission or non-admission to treatment following his or her initial consultation, what might the contra-indications be? It will be remembered that the question of indications dated back to 1922, when Eitingon, without providing any further details, insisted that the only criterion for admitting a patient to treatment was urgency. In 1930, the notion of selection was defined in a positive way. Fenichel did not draw up a list of symptoms that would have prevented the commencement of a treatment. He specified that it would be possible to propose a trial analysis when a regular analytical treatment was not immediately available. At the end of the trial analysis, the analyst would be permitted to make a negative decision. This, of course, explained the relatively high number of analyses interrupted by the analyst. Thus, as of 1 January 1930, 241 analyses had been interrupted out of a total of 721 analyses started since the beginning of the polyclinic's activities a decade earlier.

As the respective interests of the training and teaching options were frequently at variance, the task of patient selection became considerably more difficult. The scientific vocation of the institute encouraged risk-taking with cases that could not be helped in any other way and that did not fall within the domain of the classical indications for analysis: mild psychoses, psychopathologies, criminality or character anomalies. The interests of teaching required the most classical forms of neurosis possible in order to entrust treatment to the students in training. Fenichel noted, however, that classical forms of neurosis were becoming increasingly rare. In his view, this scarcity was consistent with what could be seen in the private practices of contemporary analysts. However, it was sufficient that an adequate number of so-called classical neuroses be present in the polyclinic's consulting rooms for the training activity to continue satisfactorily.

The number of cases considered 'not cured' had to do with complex situations. It had been noted that improvement could occur after a long period of time, i.e. more than a year. In other words, the severity of the cases meant that either thc trial analyses would be interrupted or the long-term analytical treatments continued if it was judged that, following the trial analysis period, there was no contra-indication to continuing the cure. In addition to this clinical classification for statistical purposes, the duration of treatment was also recorded. Very often, the cures were split up or interrupted several times. This factor, in turn, caused problems in calculating treatment duration, as the number of months a patient spent on the polyclinic's books did not necessarily correspond to the actual time spent in treatment. This number would only represent a maximum. The solution then settled on was to calculate the duration of the treatments in months and years. By January 1930, 363 analyses had been completed, 241 had been abandoned and 117 were still in progress. Of the 363 completed analyses, 70 had lasted six months, 108 had lasted a year, and 74 had lasted a year and a half. Only sixteen analyses had lasted more than three years.

A whole series of neuroses was characterised by the prevalence of a bodily localisation that was distinct from the conversion mechanism traditionally associated with hysteria. Conversion neurosis was defined as a condition where the symptoms corresponded to fixations or regressions in the pre-genital stages. Thus, bronchial asthma, stammering and convulsive tics were separated from hysteria itself. Fenichel classified these symptoms as pre-genital conversion neuroses. In this regard, we should mention the dominant influence of Karl Abraham's teaching on a whole generation of Berlin analysts. For example, when Melanie Klein arrived in Berlin to undertake her analysis with him in 1922, she was authorised to undertake analyses of children at the institute. Klein's proximity to Abraham was immediately reflected in a clear emphasis in Klein's work on the notion of the pre-genital stages of the libido. Fenichel's pre-genital conversion neuroses would therefore seem to have come from the same source.

Similarly, Fenichel distinguished between organ neuroses and so-called classical hysterical neuroses. The former corresponded to neuroses in which psychogenic anomalies of bodily functions that did not respond exactly to the hysterical conversion mechanism were dominant. Instead of the expression of a conflict, a substitution mechanism in a narcissistic mode was detected. In other words, the bodily localisation did not correspond to the converted expression of displaced object relationships, as in hysteria. These organ neuroses did not involve a single organ, or even a system of organs, leaving open the question, which was not raised at the time, of whether some of these symptoms were not also phenomena of bodily fragmentation of a psychotic nature.

A third form of so-called neurotic inhibitions was defined as the non-functioning or restriction of certain functions, particularly sexual functions. Frigidity, vaginismus and impotence were classified in this category. In this case, the disorder of sexual function had to be the only symptom identified. It must also be noted that enuresis, hypochondria without associated psychotic phenomena and neurosis of traumatic origin were classified under the heading of neurotic forms. In order to be able to list all cases, Fenichel specified that he had given priority to the most serious condition. Thus, in cases of phobic symptoms associated with obsessive neurosis, only the diagnosis of obsessive neurosis was retained.

Perversions were divided between three subheadings. The category of homosexuality was isolated as such, but only from the moment that this sexual orientation had become the subject of the patient's complaint. Infantilism was conceived as a perversion in which no well-defined partial drive dominated. The perversions without any other details included all the other perversions. Cases of neurosis with features of perversion were classified under the heading of neuroses. Thus, if a homosexual patient did not complain of his homosexuality and did not make it a symptom, the diagnosis of simple perversion was assigned to him. For a patient to be classified as homosexual, a question about his or her sexual position had to be present in the patient's discourse from the outset.

The majority of the psychosis cases at the Berlin Polyclinic were schizophrenic and manic-depressive. While Fenichel noted that 'asylum-ripe' psychoses were rare, it was common to find schizophrenic symptoms in many patients. Besides genuine schizophrenic cases, there were many patients suffering from psychotic symptoms, depersonalisation, paranoid reactions, delusional productions, bizarre ideas and derealisation. Also separated from the category of character disorders were people with childish behaviour, those who were not coping with life because of too much fixation on their family. However, infantilism was also associated with the perversions, which seems to confuse things a little. In fact, Fenichel made a distinction between patients whose sexual choice was left to chance encounters and fluctuations and whose libido was not guided by a well-defined fantasy and those who were unable to form a social bond or who could not manage to live outside the family cocoon. It is clear that the term 'infantilism' actually referred to two distinct situations that were not part of the same phenomenon. Next came the category of kleptomaniacs, which included the unstable, the bizarre and the impulsive. The psychopathic group included the antisocial, the abandoned, the runaways and the mythomaniacs. And then there were the so-called unclassifiable cases, which fell into the category of character disorder. This undefined group included, without further definition, cases dominated by moral masochism or cases that, faced with life, presented neurotic difficulties. Fenichel was not completely satisfied with the latter category. The presence of the category of character disorders can be explained by his marked interest in contemporary work on this theme. Indeed, this was an extremely important area of investigation within the IPA thanks to the research of Abraham, Ferenczi and Reich. The concept of character was articulated to the analysis of resistance. It was a key notion in the great debate on technique that occupied the analytical movement from the early 1920s onwards.

Fenichel's interest in historical materialism led him to openly defend the soundness of a political, cultural and social orientation of psychoanalysis in the early 1930s. This orientation made him all the more sensitive to the importance of social determinants. The relative disappearance of classical neurotic forms and their replacement by character disorders and psychopathologies was in the air at the time. Fenichel shared this observation with other leftwing Freudians for whom the social and cultural dimension of psychoanalysis had to carry over into its therapeutic application. Fenichel believed that character structures should be studied according to historical conditions.

Fenichel's system of classification already included the category of organic diseases. This was a grouping of cases of disorders of nervous origin, endocrine disorders or other organic illnesses that had turned up at the polyclinic in error. When a psychological aetiology was evoked in these cases of organic illness, with the patient seeking to be healed by means of psychoanalytic treatment, the diagnosis was nevertheless based on the neurotic mechanism initially detected. Fenichel made reference to the misdirection that had led patients to turn to the polyclinic by mistake.

It will be remembered that in addition to this clinical classification carried out for statistical purposes, the duration of treatment had been recorded. Very often, cures were split or interrupted several times. In fact, the duration of analyses underwent a rapid evolution during the 1920s. In 1919, a six-month analysis was common. Around 1920, Freud sent a patient to a colleague with the following note: 'For psychoanalysis, impotence, three months.'[11] In 1923, one year was a minimum; two or three years was preferable. We previously referred to Freud's 'History of an Infantile Neurosis', written on the basis of a case he had analysed for five years. Karl Abraham, for his part, believed that it took years to grasp the reasons for a melancholic depression. In Vienna, the extension of the duration of the cures became the object of jokes. When the patient failed to make associations, Freud had to frantically inhale his own cigar smoke in order not to fall asleep. Or, when the patient was silent for months, the analyst had to stoically remain equally silent. It was said that one analyst, waking up suddenly, found himself confronting an empty couch. As a result, while the assessment of the short or long duration of analyses varied greatly over time, a one-year course of treatment was below average in 1930.

As Fenichel relates, out of 721 analyses begun, 241 had been stopped prematurely. Of the 363 completed analyses, 47 cases had not been cured, 116 cases had been improved, 89 cases had been significantly improved and 111 cases had been cured. The change had to be sustainable over time and, most importantly, the change had to be analytically explicable. Therefore, cases that showed improvement but which lacked a theoretically satisfactory explanation for their having done so could not be considered cured. This is an important point: a very clear improvement that lacked a valid explanation was considered an analytically imperfect result. Thus, the knowledge obtained from the psychological aetiology of the symptoms and the change in character was an integral part of the therapeutic result. Such a result required the analyst to structure the knowledge derived from it.

Gender distribution was balanced, with 969 consultations for men and 986 consultations for women. The age distribution indicated that the vast majority of patients were between sixteen and forty years of age. There was a peak in the twenty-one to twenty-five group, which alone accounted for 184 of the 721 treatments. While the influence of Melanie Klein could lead one to believe that the development of analytic practice with children was very important at the Berlin Polyclinic, the statistics for child analyses enumerate just seventeen cures in the space of ten years. The number of cures effected with adolescents between eleven and twenty years of age was considerably higher, with a total of 116 treatments. The number of treatments for patients over forty-five was decreasing rapidly. Senior citizens over sixty years of age were represented by a single treatment case.

Based on the information contained in the 1930 report, we can draw up a profile of the patients received at Eitingon's polyclinic. They were generally neurotic young adults, male or female, and were mostly from the middle class. Their analyses were generally interrupted or split over the course of a year. These patients often obtained significant therapeutic benefits from their treatment. Their morbid state was significantly improved by the analytic work. There is little clarity, though, as to how these treatments were carried out and what the criteria were for judging that a treatment had led to a cure or improvement. Of course, it was only a statistical report. And, as Lacan pointed out, analysts tend to exhibit a certain carelessness concerning even the most elementary rules of statistics. In those rare surveys where results are presented, he noted in 1955, the analyst is satisfied with relatively summary assessments such as 'improved', 'very improved' or 'cured'. Lacan saw this as an indication of the psychoanalyst's detachment from therapeutic urgency.[12] As might be expected, however, Fenichel's statistical report nevertheless provides a certain number of indications concerning the theory of the technique then in use.

The old dragon and the criminal

It should first be noted that there are few clues as to how psychoanalysis was actually practiced in the period covered by the original 1930 report. There is, for example, no reference to the technique used in treating children. In fact, the great innovation was Fenichel's discreet but insistent introduction of the notion of character. The category of character disorders, which appeared alongside other more classical categories, was, he said, difficult to establish. Is it not astonishing that he should have reserved a consistent place for a notion whose use seemed to him so inconvenient from the point of view of diagnostic classification? Moreover, the equivalence between symptom and character may also seem surprising. As mentioned previously, Fenichel used the notion of character in two different places in his report: as a diagnostic category and as something that was to be permanently modified by the cure. At the time when he was writing his statistical report, the institute was taking part in the great debate on psychoanalytic technique that was going on within the IPA. Given his prodigious knowledge of the analytical literature of his time, Fenichel was obviously aware of the heated discussions that had been taking place within the Vienna group since the end of the war. There were, inside the WPV, some who wanted to perfect the basic doctrine of psychoanalysis, based on the Oedipus complex and the theory of libido, and others who considered it vital to transform psychoanalytic practice on the basis of a revision of its initial postulates. This crisis concerning technique led to a turning point that was considered decisive in the history of the analytic movement. This moment constituted, in fact, a 'before' and an 'after'. Before this turning point, material was being deciphered. Afterwards, attention was concentrated on the analysis of the ego and the analysis of resistance. The character research carried out in Berlin, as well as in Vienna and Budapest, by Abraham, Ferenczi, Reich and Fenichel played a decisive role in this major transformation of psychoanalytic practice.

The use of the concept of character was not specific to psychoanalysis. For example, as a young doctor writing his thesis in the early 1930s, Lacan highlighted the extremely problematic worth of the systems of characterological classifications used at that time in the field of psychiatry. He felt that the attempt to relate psychosis to a defined personality type, such as the cases of paranoia he was studying, had proved futile, involving as it did the establishment of a hierarchy between dominant character traits and the more variable elements of personality. Lacan pointed out that these characterological criteria could very well belong to quite different psychological registers – the resemblance could be formal, not structural. He resorted to metaphor in order to make the problem easier to grasp: 'Such, in botany, are the rays of composite flowers that may represent, depending on the case, the petals of the single flower or the leaves of the envelope.'[13] In order to obtain a valid classification of individual differences, was it necessary to resort to the use of the doctrine of constitutions? Could taking innate differences into account overcome this difficulty? The question inevitably comes up against the ancient problem of innate and acquired knowledge, of psychological heredity and the influence of the environment. Notwithstanding the theoretical impasses that one never fails to reach by dint of such reasoning, Lacan maintained that one could not deny the recurrence of certain 'clinical complexes in the field of psychoses'. Despite their contemporaneity, psychiatric and psychoanalytical works on character took divergent paths because they had different ends. The search for the influence of psychiatric science on psychoanalytic elaboration – the kind of influence one always ends up finding, if one takes the trouble – seems superfluous, to say the least. And for good reason: the psychoanalytic theory of character was linked to the discovery of partial drives, and research on character formation was to be used to prove their existence. This is why Freud and his students devoted so much attention to it. Beginning in 1926, Wilhelm Reich developed his theory of character in order to transfer his ideas about the function of the orgasm into practice with his colleagues at the Vienna Institute. From this perspective, he argued that characterological armour caused an emotional blockage (*Affektsperre*) that hindered the release of sexual energy.

In psychoanalysis, the notion of character was first associated with the field of neurosis. Freud was interested in the origin of character in its link to the life of the drives. In the summary at the end of *Three Essays on Sexuality* (1905), in the paragraph on sublimation, Freud argued that character was the result of infantile drives derived and transformed in order to make them socially acceptable. He referred, in particular, to the field of artistic creation, where the mechanism at play is that of repression through reaction formation. Such repression was defined as a kind of sublimation, he added. Then, in 1908, he published a short article titled 'Character and Anal Erotism', which he introduced by mentioning a recurring clinical fact. In some patients, there regularly appeared a correlation between their character traits and an erogenous zone that had been particularly invested during childhood. These people were distinguished by their concern for order, their thrifty attitude and their stubbornness. During their early childhood, there was a trace of the pleasure they had taken in playing with or holding their faeces: 'From these indications, we infer that such people are born with a sexual constitution in which the erotogenicity of the anal zone is exceptionally strong.'[14] Freud concluded that these traits were the result of a sublimation of the drive that occurred during the latency period, between the age of five and the first manifestations of puberty. These traits were, therefore, a direct result of early anal erotism.

In a 1913 article on the disposition to obsessional neurosis, Freud drew a parallel between character development and the formation of neurosis. Identical drive forces were at work in both cases, he said. However, character formation lacked the decisive action of repression that was characteristic of neuroses. What is specific to the mechanism of repression is that 'the failure of repression and the return of the repressed are absent in the formation of character',[15] Freud noted. The process of character formation was less accessible to analysis than that of neurosis because of this absence of repression. Conversely, character was also less accessible to analysis by virtue of the paradoxical fact that repression could occur smoothly, without obstacles. In this case, the replacement of the repressed by the reaction formations and sublimation took place without leaving any trace. Character formation thus appeared as a confirmation of the existence of sadistic-anal pre-genital organisation. Freud mentioned the quarrelsome and petty character of women who had renounced genital sexuality. Characteristic features of sadistic-anal organisation resurfaced as a result of this regression of their drive life: 'Writers of comedy and satirists have in all ages directed their invectives against the "old dragon" into which the charming girl, the loving wife and the tender mother have been transformed.'

With regard to such an alteration of character in women, Freud thought that it was not impossible that this regression to the sadistic-anal stage could be systematic once the function of the genitals had been fulfilled. It was as if the faded roses only showed their thorns, to use Lacan's botanical metaphor relating to this character trait.

In 'Some Character-Types Met with in Psychoanalytic Work', a study published in *Imago* in 1916, Freud argued that psychoanalytic investigation met with resistance that had its origin in the character of the patient. This point, which was taken up and developed by Reich ten years later, shifted the emphasis from character formation to the ability of character to counteract the course of treatment. 'What opposes the doctor's efforts is not always those traits of character which the patient recognises in himself and which are attributed to him by people around him',[16] Freud wrote. The rest of the article distinguished three situations where character traits took centre stage. The first of these categories related to the exceptions. Sometimes those who had suffered physical disgrace or real deprivation in early childhood felt the demand for future compensation. The immorality of the wronged person who felt that he was a victim of injustice was illustrated by William Shakespeare's Richard III. Similarly, the fact of having been born a girl, a reproach regularly attributed to the mother, could give rise to the female claim of being a privileged person. The daughter might believe that she was exempt from the obligations of life:

> As we learn from psychoanalytic work, women regard themselves as having been damaged in infancy, as having been undeservedly cut short of something and unfairly treated; and the embitterment of so many daughters against their mother derives, ultimately, from the reproach against her of having brought them into the world as women instead of as men.

Next came the category of those who fail in the face of success. Freud used Lady Macbeth to explain the origin of the change of character marked by the irruption of an impregnable sense of guilt in this character endowed with the extraordinary will to achieve her ends: 'And now we ask ourselves what it was that broke this character which had seemed forged from the toughest metal', Freud wrote. Macbeth himself underwent a character transformation during the play by becoming a bloodthirsty character. Freud preferred the idea that the playwright often shared a single character between two different characters. Lady Macbeth and her husband embodied two positions of the individual after the crime: remorse and defiance. Rebecca West, a character in Ibsen's *Rosmersholm*, allowed Freud to illustrate another character shift. Rebecca had planned to get rid of her rival – the wife of John Rosmer, who was Rebecca's adoptive father – by forcing her to commit suicide so that she could live with John. Her sense of guilt arose just as the realisation of her happiness finally became possible. This reversal sent her back to her Oedipal history. Rebecca had been her adoptive father's mistress in the past. When she learned from the brother of the woman she had driven to suicide that her adoptive father was probably her biological father as well, she collapsed, plagued by a sense of guilt over having committed incest, and forbade herself to enjoy the actual results of her wrongdoing.

The emphasis on the action of moral conscience established a link to the third category, that of criminals from a sense of guilt. These unfortunate people, who had done something wrong, found themselves relieved of an oppressive and earlier sense of guilt that assailed them and whose cause they did not know. The origin of this feeling of guilt came from the Oedipus complex, the generator of the two great criminal intentions: parricide and incest. The unconscious feeling of guilt appears to be the driving force of the passage to the act among criminals in search of punishment. The 'wickedness' of some children is said to have the same origin because 'after the punishment, they are calm and satisfied'.

Freud's students made use of the data he had compiled on character development. In 1913, Rank and Sachs argued that character formation depended less on intellectual factors than on a particular psychological economy, made up of affects, satisfaction, repression and sublimation. Reaction formations were capable of transforming the wicked child who martyred animals into a brilliant surgeon or, conversely, by a reversal that denoted the action of repression, into a protector of animals. In the simplest cases, one was able to isolate an unambiguous drive satisfaction. Both Rank and Sachs mentioned the existence of more complicated cases where the combination of several partial drives was attested. It therefore had to do not with a well-defined character resulting from the transformation of a single drive but with the combination of several drives that gave rise to various character traits.

Karl Abraham in turn devoted himself to the study of character formation. Three of his character studies were published in the *Zeitschrift* in 1925. Abraham extended the study of Freud's earlier obsessional character, typified by the transformation from anal erotism to the oral character and to the character form corresponding to the genital stage. The oral character is characterised by the libidinal investment of the mouth. The origin of this drive excitation explains why it is not repressed and sublimated as intensely as that emanating from anal erotism. Character formation in a child who is too spoiled or, conversely, too disappointed during the sucking period seems to be marked by a clear ambivalence. Envy and jealousy are frequently found in such children. Abraham also mentions that, when breastfeeding has been carried out satisfactorily, it can leave one with a deep conviction that life will go on in a happy way. Conversely, some subjects who have been fulfilled in this way cannot detach themselves from the expectation of a protective and caring maternal substitute: 'Their whole conduct in life shows that they expect the mother's breast to flow for them eternally, so to speak.'[17] Abraham adds that the attitude of the subject in society depends on the stage of development of the libido from which their character originates. Thus, those who were satisfied in the oral period are kind and social, whereas those who are fixed in the sadistic-oral stage are hostile and cutting; sullenness, inaccessibility and reticence remain associated with the anal character. This depreciation of anal character did not meet with unanimous agreement, and some psychoanalysts were offended by the intrusion of the moral order into the study of character. Abraham maintained that genital character depended on the fate of the Oedipus complex. In the Oedipal moment, the interests of the subject became compatible with those of others. Emphasis was placed on the existence of feelings of sympathy and tolerance deriving from the tenderness and feelings of love arising from the ambivalence characteristic of the earlier stages. When emotional deficiencies had occurred in childhood, the individual's ability to fit into the social bond and to support community life could be compromised. There was frequently a risk of the development of antisocial behaviour. 'We see the same thing happen with the neurotic patient who, though born and educated in the usual circumstances, feels that he is not loved, that he is the "Cinderella" of the family,'[18] he added.

This brings us progressively closer to the field in which we are interested – that of the technical use of the notion of character in the cure. Abraham gave the example of a young man whose character traits had evolved in the course of analysis. The patient was initially endowed with character traits that were not particularly attractive. He was presumptuous, miserly, defiant and unkind. The gradual disappearance of these traits during the course of the treatment greatly facilitated his integration into society. From time to time, however, when resistance to the treatment arose, the patient would relapse into the earlier, abandoned stage of the evolution of his character: 'On those occasions he would become disagreeable and hostile in his behaviour, and overbearing and contemptuous in his speech. From having conducted himself in a friendly and polite manner he became suspicious and irritable.' During the entire phase when resistances to analytical work arose, his previous characteristics of hate and refusal regained the upper hand. In such circumstances, the patient began to covet inanimate objects that he absolutely wanted to acquire by buying them. He was assailed by the idea of owning and stealing. When resistance receded, these two traits, oral and anal, of greed and determination to keep the object disappeared. The theme of gain and loss then receded, and the patient again became capable of socialising. We note that in this clinical vignette, published shortly before his death, Karl Abraham established a direct link between the treatment of antisocial character and the analysis of resistances. The episodic reappearance of the symptom of lust during the treatment was understood as a character trait. Abraham emphasised the patient's ability to insert himself into the social bond, which, in turn, depended on a particular type of object relation.

Make the patient understand that he is defending himself

For his part, Reich criticised this tendency to dissociate character and sexuality. He was struck by the fact that characterology and morality were often mixed in the WPV. Character often seemed to be an undesirable factor; no distinction was made between the moral evaluation of character and its scientific investigation. Among other examples, Reich mentioned that psychoanalysts considered anal character to be a defect. Oral character was regarded as more lovable – but that, he felt, would make one a big child. These considerations were extra-scientific, he declared. The study of character had to be cleansed of all moral judgements because they had turned into genuine counter-indications for the psychoanalytic cure. Reich discussed this tendency as follows:

> The view was held that there were certain 'bad characters' who were unsuitable for psychoanalytic treatment. It was said that psychoanalytic treatment required a certain level of psychic organisation in the patient, and that many were not worth the effort. Besides, many patients were so 'narcissistic' that the treatment was not capable of breaking through the barrier. Even a low IQ was considered an obstruction to psychoanalytic treatment. Hence, psychoanalytic work was limited to circumscribed neurotic symptoms in intelligent persons capable of free association and having 'correctly developed' characters. This feudalistic conception of psychotherapy, which, by its very nature, is extremely individualistic, naturally came into immediate conflict with requirements of medical work when the Vienna Psychoanalytic Clinic for destitute persons was opened.[19]

It is obvious that Reich's research on character was linked to the need to adapt the accessibility of analysis to the patients he received at the Vienna Psychoanalytic Institute. This institute, modelled on the one in Berlin, had opened its doors on 22 May 1922. Reich worked there for eight years as first assistant and then as head physician. His practice with the patients of the psychoanalytic community clinic reoriented his practice. He published a study of the impulsive character in 1925. During the previous year he had obtained the approval of the WPV to found the Vienna Seminar for Psychoanalytic Therapy, and this project served as his laboratory for the next six years. The method he advocated was systematic case study, with a particular view to compensating for the lack of elaboration of diagnostic criteria and to developing a true *theory of therapy*, which was also lacking. He asked, '*Why was a cure obtained in one case and not in another? The solution would give an indication for a better selection of patients. At that time, no theory of therapeutics had been formulated*',[20] he noted. Reich then suggested creating another seminar for young analysts. These trainee analysts would be able to express their questions, opinions, or doubts by learning to converse freely. This idea of a seminar for younger people was, of course, echoing the similar project that Fenichel had set up in Berlin in November 1924. Thus the two capitals of psychoanalysis each had their own Kinderseminar. Bearing the same name, the two programmes were similar. The debates on character analysis found a privileged place of expression there. The notion of antisocial character was combined with Abraham's analysis of resistances, but Reich wanted to take things even further by demonstrating that the form of the social bond was involved in the formation of character. He was inspired by the prewar Freudian thesis concerning civilised sexual morality. For Reich, capitalist sexual morality was at the origin of neuroses. Mental health depended, he said, on orgasmic power, which was hindered by authoritarian and anti-sexual education. It was the Oedipus, in its version of patriarchal authoritarianism, that had to be suppressed. It is known that Reich was fascinated by certain educational experiments that were being carried out in Russia, where children were raised communally, far away from their parents. Without a family, these children would not develop an Oedipus complex. In the absence of the nuclear complex responsible for the prohibition that generates guilt and symptoms, their sexuality would be unfettered. There would be no need for repression: neurosis would be overcome. Communism, Reich said, would put orgasm within everyone's reach. He did not, however, heed Freud's warning that certain drives cannot be fully discharged. He did, though, have the idea of a remnant whose existence hindered proper psychological functioning, but he conceived of it as a libidinal stasis that occurs in the absence of direct genital satisfaction and produces destructive effects. According to Reich, antisocial behaviour was caused by secondary drives resulting from the repression of this genital sexuality. Above all, the resistances that arose in the treatment were related to the patient's refusal to change anything in his or her unhappy life. The masses, he held, basically resisted modifying the capitalist order that enslaved them and deprived them of the sexual happiness to which they were entitled. Unbeknownst to them, the neurotics were propping up the authoritarian and patriarchal order that exercised its implacable domination over them. The characterological anchoring of the social order was, Reich contended, the basis for fascism and dictatorship. In 1934, following his expulsion from the KPD and the IPA, Reich was able to verify the validity of the persecution he felt he was being subjected to. He then embarked on a series of experiments whose unbalanced nature became increasingly pronounced. In Norway, he tried to capture the Freudian libido using a chain of electron tubes. During the time he subsequently spent in America, he worked on cancer and the formation of atmospheric orgone before ending his singular trajectory in prison.

Before that, among those who attended the technical seminar in Vienna in the 1920s, the testimony of Richard Sterba deserves to be remembered. Sterba reports that Reich's intelligence and clinical knowledge greatly impressed his younger colleagues. For that generation, he truly embodied a form of authority and prestige. His character research prompted enthusiastic discussions in the two German-speaking cities of the psychoanalytic movement. There was much interest in their political significance. Without sharing Reich's certainty, which they considered excessive, as to the human capacity for jouissance, the most politicised analysts followed his character elaborations closely because they reinforced their own vision of the social and revolutionary mission of psychoanalysis. Although it had been recognised that Reich was suffering from mental disorders, the attraction that his strong personality radiated had long exerted a profound influence on some analysts. In 1930, Reich left Vienna in the hope of finding a new audience in the German capital. In Berlin, he took part in private meetings of a group of analysts who met on the fringes of the institute. This group embodied a second level of dissidence, coming as it did from Fenichel's Kinderseminar, and brought together the most politically committed leftwing Freudians. It included Edith Jacobson, Eric Fromm, Wilhelm and Annie Reich and Otto Fenichel. They talked about character analysis and psychosociology.

In fact, studies of character were linked to the difficulties that had arisen within the psychoanalytic movement after World War I. At that time, analysts realised the limitations of trying to heal the symptom by means of speech and interpretation. Jacques-Alain Miller has indicated that the analysts were disappointed by the fact that they had not been able to realise all the wonders that Freud had described.[21] At a meeting of the WPV circa 1920, Freud himself introduced a decisive correction by pointing out that the symptom *could* disappear, but that it did not *necessarily* disappear when its unconscious meaning was revealed. In Berlin, where their geographical distance from Freud seemed to permit a step to the side, the analysts gradually detached themselves from their attachment to what the patient had to say. Increasing emphasis was placed on the analysis of resistance and behaviour at the expense of the elements of speech. As Jacques-Alain Miller has noted, the focus was now on what 'surrounded' speech rather than dwelling on the field of language itself. This analysis of character led to an attempt to divine, from attitudes and behaviours, the resistances that the patient was trying to conceal. Cunning, subterfuge, artifice, fakery: the patient was now viewed as a deceptive subject. It was the analyst's job to detect any signs of silent disobedience on the part of the patient concerning the fundamental rule. Reich stated that 'the patient must first find out that he defends himself, then by what means, and, finally, against what'.[22]

Some authors trace the origin of the paradigm shift that was to lead the IPA to focus on the analysis of the ego and resistance to the publication of two prewar studies by Freud. In his 1913 article on beginning the treatment, Freud had shown that transference could suppress symptoms, but only temporarily. In other words, healing lasted as long as the transference itself was prolonged. Freud explained: 'In this case the treatment is a treatment by suggestion, and not a psychoanalysis at all. It only deserves the latter name if the intensity of the transference has been utilised for the overcoming of resistances.'[23] The members of the Berlin Institute must have had this passage in mind when they claimed that a momentary and provisional resolution of symptoms could occur during treatment at the polyclinic. It should not be forgotten that Fenichel defined this improvement as successful therapeutic transference. To speak of healing proper, it was necessary to go beyond this suggestive effect of transference; it was necessary to act on another level. But which one? In that same 1913 article, Freud gave an element of an answer that was not exploited to its full potential. The nature of healing depended, he said, on its link to knowledge. Freud had realised that the conscious communication of the conditions of the trauma affecting the patient brought about no change at all. The fact of making something conscious was entirely compatible with the refusal to know. Contrary to what he himself had previously argued, knowledge did not remove the effects of repression. Knowledge, in the sense of what becomes conscious, does not produce the expected effect of eliminating the symptom. Freud pointed out that what such a revelation did induce was an increase in the patient's resistances. This was an essential shift; the interpretation that was made of this change had decisive consequences for the future. It called into question the very beginnings of psychoanalysis, where it was believed that healing could be obtained through the revelation of what had been repressed and forgotten. The original cathartic definition of psychoanalysis was now replaced by the dynamic conception of psychological processes. It no longer sufficed to make the unconscious conscious. The traumatic event could be known or recalled, but it was not symbolised for the simple reason that the refusal to know had not been removed. As a result, making conscious what had been repressed was insufficient. Resistance to healing via defence mechanisms was held responsible for the negative affects that arose in the transference despite the suffering that the symptoms caused and the demand for healing that the suffering itself entailed. A year before this article appeared, Freud explained that transference could itself become a resistance in the course of an analysis. In a study on the dynamics of transference, published in 1912, he described the phenomenon where whenever

> the investigations of analysis come upon the libido withdrawn into its hiding-place, a struggle is bound to break out; all the forces which have caused the libido to regress will rise up as 'resistances' against the work of analysis, in order to conserve the new state of things.[24]

From 1926 onwards, the meetings of the WPV's technical seminar focused on the study of resistances. Reich, who was interested in the early stages of treatment, concentrated on the effects of negative transference, to which he felt insufficient attention had been paid until then. Transferential resistance was considered to be the first phenomenon, latent or manifest, to show itself during the cure. This resistance usually found expression in the patient's assertion that he did not know what to talk about. The initial attitude of mistrust arising from the idea that it is never easy to confide in a stranger could turn into resistance. Negative transference was conceived as the expression of a conflict that had its origin in a fact of structure. The patient could do nothing but loathe the analyst, who was always an enemy, no matter what. At a meeting of the Vienna technical seminar, Reich said:

> As the disturber of the neurotic equilibrium, the analyst automatically becomes the enemy, no matter whether the projected impulses are impulses of love or of hatred; for in either case there is, at the same time, defence against these impulses.[25]

The patient was seen as a fugitive who had to be tirelessly led back to the starting point of the first transferential resistance.

In his presentation, Reich distinguished two principal phases of analytical treatment, namely the healing of the patient and his immunisation. The first healing phase was divided in turn into two others: the preparatory phase and the treatment phase. The preparatory phase was intended to discover the energy sources of the symptoms and of the neurotic character in order to begin the healing process. Since the resistances resulting from the transference struggle could hinder the progress of the cure, it was necessary to make the patient aware of them so that he or she could interpret them and eliminate them. Otherwise, the patient could put the analysis at the service of the resistances. Early interpretation of the meaning of the symptoms without taking into account the structure of the neurosis was doomed to failure. Indeed, the negative transference was not always expressed; it could be latent. It could be expressed either by an excessive tendency to satisfy the analyst and to cooperate with him, which would be characteristic of the hysterical character, or by a courteous and respectful attitude, which was typical of the obsessional character. Thus, the notion of character was linked to the apprehension of the different latent manifestations of the negative transference. As Lacan pointed out, this led to paying attention to the patient's behaviour, the way he spoke, his tone, his interruptions, his presentation, his approach, his thought processes, the affectedness of his manners, and the way he says goodbye. This meant that an attitude could count for more than a syntactical error.[26]

Freud had shown that symptoms impeded free association. Reich noted that character resistance also generally manifested itself in a failure to observe this basic rule: the difference between the trait and the symptom was no longer so perceptible. Such an orientation had a direct impact on the technique of interpretation. Character analysis and the systematisation of the interpretation of resistances pointed to the need for a true analytic strategy capable of responding to the defensive strategy developed by the patient's ego. This led to the establishment of strict rules for interpretation. Reich recommended that resistances should be carefully analysed one after the other, without skipping steps, so as not to reinforce transferential resistance. It was necessary first to start from the psychic surface, from the transferential resistance, and, if necessary, to push back the materials that were too close to the repressed arising from dreams. The interpretation of resistance should, he said, always precede the interpretation of content, and the interpretative work should be methodical, systematic and consistent. Reich put it this way:

> Our principle is: *No interpretation of meaning when a resistance interpretation is needed.* The reason for this is simple enough. If one interprets the meaning *before* eliminating the corresponding resistance, the patient either accepts the interpretation for reasons of the transference, or he completely depreciates it at the first appearance of a negative attitude, or the resistance comes afterwards.[27]

The technical problem of latent negative transference gave rise to the establishment of a typology based on four main types of characterological resistances. This typology was the outline of a psychoanalytic characterology that distinguished the following categories:

- The *good patients*, whose positive transference is characterised by submission and unlimited trust in the analyst. They are generally passive-feminine characters and hysterical women with nymphomaniac tendencies.
- The *courteous patients* with an impulsive character who have transformed their hatred into exaggerated politeness by means of reactive formation.
- Patients with *weak affectivity* whose aggressiveness is blocked and whose character is equally impulsive. It is common for hysterical women to exhibit this attitude.
- Patients suffering from *depersonalisation*, who complain about a lack of genuineness in their feelings or who have the impression that they are 'play-acting'. One finds in this group the narcissistic neuroses of the hypochondriac type. The ironic attitude that characterises them finds expression in an *inward smile*. These are very difficult cases to analyse.

Reich also used the metaphor of the strongpoint under siege from all sides to describe resistance analysis:

> It is important to undermine the neurosis from the cardinal resistance, from a definite strongpoint, as it were, instead of focusing one's attention on detail resistances, that is, attacking the neurosis at many different points which have no immediate connection. If one deploys the resistances and the analytic material consistently from the strongpoint of the first transference resistance, one never loses sight of the total situation, past and present.[28]

This image of the strongpoint was consistent with the idea that character traits were armour worn by the ego to protect itself.

The great turning point in analytic technique in the 1920s led to the confusion of the two notions of resistance and defence that Freud had distinguished. For Freud, defence was linked to the constitution of the ego, whereas resistance was defined as a phenomenon that arose during the cure and signalled the emergence of the repressed in the patient's speech. By conceiving the cure as an attack to which the ego responded with a succession of defences that had to be fought one by one, the post-Freudians came to centre the analysis on the ego and aggressiveness. Lacan denounced this deviation from practice in which the subject's defences were conceived as a real strongpoint. This led, he said, to making the ego something that existed outside all reference to speech:

> By reversing the correct choice that determines which subject is welcomed in speech, the symptom's constituting subject is treated as if he were constituted – like material, as they say – while the ego, as constituted as it may be in resistance, becomes the subject upon whom the analyst henceforth calls as the constituting agency.[29]

If Lacan criticised the attack on a strongpoint of the subject's defences recommended by Fenichel, it is important to remember that Fenichel had originally borrowed the metaphor from Reich. Referring to the artifices elaborated by the ego in order to protect what would be the nucleus of the drive, the mental projection of the ego's defences transformed the analytic dialectic into a veritable palace of mirages.

Reich's first paper on the technique of the interpretation and analysis of resistance was published in the *Zeitschrift* in 1927. It was later included in his book on character analysis, which appeared in 1933. In December 1926, Reich had had the opportunity to give a talk to Freud's inner circle on the theme of the analysis of resistance. It was a question of reflecting on the following problem: in the presence of a latent negative attitude, should the patient's incestuous desires be interpreted or should one wait until the patient's mistrust has been eliminated? Freud then interrupted Reich:

> Why don't you want to interpret the material in the sequence in which it appears? *Of course*, it is necessary to analyse and interpret the incest dreams as soon as they appear.[30]

Reich was extremely surprised by this statement. He realised that the idea of following the line of resistances instead of that of the material was completely foreign to Freud. The atmosphere of the meeting was unpleasant, and Freud's criticism of him allowed Reich's opponents to preen themselves a little. Nevertheless, Reich managed not to lose his temper.

The technical seminar that Reich conducted in Vienna focused on analytic therapeutics. In addition to the analysis of resistances, the topics for discussion included the study of successes and failures in psychoanalysis, criteria for healing, attempts to draw up a typology of neuroses according to resistances and the question of prognosis. Freud felt that this research was not sufficient for the training of analytic practitioners. Moreover, Reich realised that his physiological insights into the function of the orgasm did not lend themselves directly to theoretical and practical applications. It was to overcome this difficulty that he developed character analysis. He started from the premise that characterological resistance always remained the same despite the diversity of materials. This permanence distinguished it from other forms of resistance. Characterological resistance was formed in childhood and had the same function as in the analytic situation. Reich presented his elaborations on character analysis at the 1927 IPA congress in Innsbruck. Three years later, he introduced the notion of ego armour, or character armour, which denoted a chronic modification of the ego. According to Reich, this armour served as a permanent protective mechanism against the drive demands and frustrations coming from the outside world. The constitution of a healthy body armour depended on the social order, morality, the satisfaction of needs and the economic structure of society. According to this perspective, the analyst was responsible for the therapeutic success of the cure, since the destruction of the character armour required an adaptation of the technique to each individual case. The logic underlying this technique of interpretation was not to be schematic – it could only be applied to particular cases. Reich believed that characterological attitudes could be understood spontaneously. The patient was no longer able to conceal a desire behind a word. This approach enabled him to treat difficult cases – the so-called narcissistic types – through psychoanalysis. He felt that he had succeeded in curing serious character disorders that were inaccessible to the Freudian method of free association.

For Reich, the economic point of view led to considerations concerning the political order. Since character armour exercised drive control, it was responsible for sexual dysfunction. The inhibition and rigidity resulting from this resistance prevented the full realisation of the sexual act and thus limited the energy released in the organism. In addition, the energy expended in preserving this armour led to a general impoverishment of the individual's life force. Modern man, diminished and reduced, resigned himself to performing thankless and tedious work that left him without the energy to rebel. It was as if the advent of the age of technology and the organisation of work in the capitalist system of production needed numbed individuals incapable of rebelling. Sexual repression was at the service of the functioning of an authoritarian society that enslaved its members. All forces of revolt were paralysed. Ultimately, character analysis showed that character was linked to the social position of the individual. Characterological structure perpetuated class society, and each social order created the forms necessary for its perpetuation. Reich conceived of two dimensions of character: one, the dimension that manifested itself in the permanence of resistances, and the other the character of the proletarian, the worker, the wealthy and the bourgeois. By means of this double usage, Reich felt that it would be possible to build a bridge between psychoanalysis and Marxist theory.

In spite of the friendly relations and intellectual collaboration that existed between the two men, Reich's position was not entirely shared by Fenichel, whose main criticism can definitely be dated to the period when a certain distance between them had already become evident. However, this criticism related to a disagreement whose origins dated back to earlier years. Fenichel could not admit that the resistances of the ego presented themselves in well-ordered layers, from the most recent to the oldest, in the course of the cure. He thought that Reich had been right to introduce a systematisation of the technique, in contrast to a handling of interpretation that aimed at direct contact with the unconscious, as was the case in the English school. He also had no doubt that there were older levels of repression than others, that there were successive layers of resistance. But he did not believe that they could appear in a systematic and organised way. Hence, the question under discussion – that of the systematisation of the technique – implied a structural-dynamic conception of the unconscious. By accentuating this rigorous principle of coherence, this position confused the successive identifications of the ego with the diachronic structure of the verbal chains unfolding in the course of the analysis. This barely left room for the unforeseen. Fenichel's perspective was more empirical. The experience that Reich acquired while working at the psychoanalytic community clinic in Vienna enabled him to study the neuroses of economically deprived individuals. He found that psychoanalysts rarely took patients' social conditions into account. At the Berlin Polyclinic, however, economic issues were at the forefront. After only two years of working there, he became convinced that the scope of individual psychotherapy was very limited. He realised that social action was often a priority, that only a small proportion of the patients were in a position to be helped by psychoanalysis. This experience led to his observation that there was a difference between private clients and those whose psychological difficulties, against a background of economic misery, made it difficult for them to adapt to society. Often regarded by psychiatry as psychopathies, moral follies or schizoid degeneration, the symptoms suffered by the poorest people did not, according to Reich, fall into any known category. These symptoms fell outside categorisation. Obsessive behaviour, hysterical twilight states, criminal impulses: none of these symptoms alone explained the impossibility of social integration.

'While these private manias were, in the case of the well-to-do, socially harmless, they had, in the case of the poor, a grotesque and dangerous character.'[31] Poverty was a factor that reduced inhibition. Under these conditions, antisocial, criminal and perverse impulses frequently prevailed.

Reich gave the example of a young and pretty working-class woman who had lost the use of speech shortly before meeting him and was tormented by the idea of killing her children. Starving and living in squalid housing, she had been abandoned by her husband. She was trying to survive and raise her three children as best she could by working as a seamstress. Her income proved insufficient, however, and the thought of drowning her offspring crossed her mind. Convinced that she had to protect her children from herself, she began to entertain the idea of going to the police and being hanged. This thought caused her throat to constrict. The spasms affecting her vocal cords were linked both to her need to keep quiet about her frightful plans for the children and to the location of the hangman's cord on her neck. Orphaned quite early in childhood, the young woman had been brought up in abject poverty. Adults had tried to sexually abuse her. She had had the fantasy of a protective mother whose breast she would have sucked. Oral satisfaction had always been in the foreground. Her children, in turn, shared her fate. After being abandoned by her husband, she transferred her hatred of him to them. Finally, her frigidity had not prevented her from indulging in sexual escapades. At times, the unfortunate woman would arrive in the middle of the night at Reich's home, terrified that she was going to kill her baby and herself. One day, Reich decided to visit her and went to the slum where she was living with her children: 'There I had to grapple not with the exalted question of the etiology of neuroses but with the question of how a human organism could put up with such conditions year in and year out.'[32]

Reich arranged to have her two eldest children placed in a boarding school and organised a collection to assist her. 'There was nothing,' he wrote, 'absolutely nothing, to bring light into this life. There was nothing but misery, loneliness, the gossip of the neighbours, worries about the next meal – and, on top of it all, there were the criminal chicaneries of her landlord and employer.'[33] The young woman was, in fact, being exploited to the extreme. She worked ten hours a day for a ridiculous salary. And yet, despite all this, she had a desire to read. So Reich lent her some books. Neurosis was generally considered a bourgeois disease by the Marxists, but Reich, who objected to that position, pointed out that cases like that of this young woman were not rare. The neuroses of the proletariat differed, he said, from those of the wealthy classes in that they embodied, even more tragically, the revolt of the human being against the unbearable. This is the style of case that Reich encountered in the psychoanalytic community clinic in Vienna in the 1920s.

From the institutional point of view, each analyst had agreed to work at the Vienna Psychoanalytic Institute for one hour a day without receiving any remuneration. Since the study of psychoanalytic theory also required at least one hour a day, it soon became clear to Reich that '*psychoanalysis is not a mass therapy*'.[34] It was better, he said, to focus on the prevention of neuroses.

Notes

1 Sigmund Freud, 'Preface to *Ten Years of the Berlin Psychoanalytic Institute*' (1930), *Standard Edition*, vol. 21, p. 257.
2 Simmel, 'Sur l'histoire...' (1930), in Colonomos, *On forme des psychanalystes*, p. 46.
3 The Frankfurt Psychoanalytic Institute's rapprochement with the Marxist orientation resulted in its closure by the Nazis in 1933.
4 Ernst Simmel, 'Sur l'histoire...' (1930), in Colonomos, *On forme des psychanalystes, op. cit.*, p. 53.
5 Letter of 13 October 1924 from Alix Strachey to James Strachey, in Meisel and Kendrick, *Bloomsbury/Freud, op. cit.*, p. 86.
6 Ernst Simmel, 'L'hôpital psychanalytique et le mouvement psychanalytique' (1937), in Jacqueline Poulain-Colombier and Philippe Christophe (eds.), *Le Patient de la psychanalyse* (Paris: L'Harmattan, 2007), p. 56. The article was originally published in the *Bulletin of the Menninger Clinic*, vol. 1 (1937).
7 *Ibid.*, p. 58.
8 Otto Fenichel, 'Rapport statistique sur l'activité thérapeutique entre 1920 et 1930' (1930), in Colonomos, *On forme des psychanalystes*, pp. 57–71.
9 Otto Fenichel, *The Psychoanalytic Theory of Neurosis* (New York: Norton, 1945).
10 Russell Jacoby, *Repression of Psychoanalysis, op. cit.*, pp. 33–34.
11 Wilhelm Reich, *The Function of the Orgasm* (London: Souvenir Press, 1983), p. 49.
12 Jacques Lacan, 'Variations on the Standard Treatment' (1955), *Écrits*, p. 270.
13 Jacques Lacan, *De la psychose paranoïaque dans ses rapports avec la personnalité* (Paris: Seuil, 1980), p. 51. See also the commentary in footnote 42, where the term 'resistance' appears.
14 Sigmund Freud, 'Character and Anal Erotism' (1908), *Standard Edition*, vol. 9, p. 170.
15 Sigmund Freud, 'The Disposition to Obsessional Neurosis' (1913), *Standard Edition*, vol. 12, pp. 323–324.
16 Sigmund Freud, 'Some Character-Types Met with in Psychoanalytic Work' (1916), *Standard Edition*, vol. 14, pp. 311, 315, 319.
17 Karl Abraham, 'The Influence of Oral Erotism on Character-Formation' (1925), *International Journal of Psychoanalysis,* vol. 6 (1925), 253.
18 Karl Abraham, 'Character-Formation on the Genital Level of Libido-Development' (1926), *International Journal of Psychoanalysis,* vol. 7 (1926), 217, 220.
19 Wilhelm Reich, *The Function of the Orgasm, op. cit.*, p. 73.
20 *Ibid.*; the emphasis is Reich's.
21 Jacques-Alain Miller (ed.), *Le Transfert négatif* (Paris: Seuil, 2005), p. 49.
22 Wilhelm Reich, 'Some Problems of Psychoanalytic Technique' (1933), *Character Analysis* (New York: Noonday Press, 1963), p. 4.
23 Sigmund Freud, 'On Beginning the Treatment' (1913), *Standard Edition*, vol. 12, p. 143.
24 Sigmund Freud, 'The Dynamics of Transference' (1912), *Standard Edition*, vol. 12, p. 102.
25 Wilhelm Reich, 'On the Technique of Interpretation and of Resistance Analysis' (1927), *Character Analysis*, p. 31.
26 Jacques Lacan, 'Variations on the Standard Treatment' (1955), *Écrits*, p. 275.

27 Wilhelm Reich, 'On the Technique of Interpretation and of Resistance Analysis' (1927), *Character Analysis, op. cit.*, p. 27. The emphasis is Reich's.
28 *Ibid.*, p. 36.
29 Jacques Lacan, 'Variations on the Standard Treatment', *Écrits*, p. 278.
30 Wilhelm Reich, *The Function of the Orgasm, op. cit.*, p. 167. The emphasis is Reich's.
31 Wilhelm Reich, *The Function of the Orgasm, op. cit.*, p. 76.
32 *Ibid.*, p. 77.
33 *Ibid.*, p. 78.
34 *Ibid.*, p. 75. The emphasis is Reich's.

Part II

The Institute and the rise of Nazism

Chapter 4

Institute, training and society

A Freudian objection to the prevention of neuroses

If the theory of character defence constituted, according to some, a valuable contribution to the metapsychology of interpretation, this contribution was nevertheless based on the natural rejection of the beyond of the pleasure principle. Reich had become convinced that negative transference was indeed the first phenomenon to manifest in the cure, but he did not come to the same conclusions as Freud regarding negative therapeutic resistance. Reich could not admit the existence of the death drive, which he interpreted as a calamity from which psychoanalysis was never to recover. But it was not just a whim, as his subsequent fanciful extrapolations on sexual energy would make explicit afterwards. In other words, Freud's death drive refuted Reich's idea that the misery of individuals was the effect of repressive sexual morality.

In his preface to the first edition of *Character Analysis*, written in Berlin in 1933, Reich evoked the characterological anchoring of the social order. This explained the oppressed classes' tolerance of, and submission to, the ruling classes. From then on, the scientific aim of character analysis was different from that of the therapeutic one. It was to highlight 'the means and mechanisms by way of which social existence is transformed into psychic structure and, with that, into ideology'.[1] If the patriarchal order prepared young people to accept the authoritarian order of society, 'the character structures of persons belonging to a certain epoch or a certain social order are not only the reflection of this order, but, much more importantly, they represent the anchoring of this order'. Civilised sexual morality is not reducible to the repression of the drives that civilisation demands and which Freud has described. The conservative element of the character structure of modern man is not to be confused with the superego. The first incidences of the frustrations related to sex education and the first identifications of the ego are prior to the formation of the superego, he believes. In fact, repression of the drives is always carried out for purposes of capitalist jouissance: 'Sexual suppression is one of the cardinal ideological means by which the ruling class subjugates the working population.'[2]

DOI: 10.4324/9781003215684-7

The possibility of a prophylaxis of the neuroses was based precisely on the observation that the psychic disorders from which the masses suffered had their origin in the repressive sexual morality of the authoritarian and patriarchal society in which they lived.

> The structuring of masses of people to be blindly obedient to authority is brought about not by natural parental love, but by the authoritarian family. The suppression of the sexuality of small children and adolescents is the chief means of producing this obedience.[3]

Reich was convinced that the theory of Marx and Engels undermined the conceptions developed in *Totem and Taboo* about the origin of morality. Freud described the social event that gave birth to the feeling of guilt and sexual repression. However, this event did not find its source in the conditions of existence – it was related to murderous jealousy of the primal father. Consequently, the problem was stated in this way: if Freud was right, if sexual repression and the limitation of drives were necessary for the development of civilisation and if this repression was also the cause of neuroses, then the prophylaxis of neuroses was impossible. On the other hand, if morality was a social product likely to change historically according to the interests of the ruling class, this prophylaxis was conceivable. The suppression of sexual misery of the masses could be combated by modifying the relation between the forbidden and satisfaction:

> The goal of a future prevention of the neuroses can only be that of creating character structures which allow of the sexual and social mobility necessary for psychic economy. For this reason, we must first try to understand the results of any denial of instinctive gratification in the child.[4]

Reich wanted to elaborate a history of sexual economy that would involve studying the foundations of psychopathology and neurotic character formation in their relation to sexuality. The father and the mother appeared to him as the executive organs of the influence of society on the child. In the working classes, the pedagogical influence of the mother was preponderant. If society offered no possibility of satisfaction to the sexual drive, if it offered only sublimation, which remained inaccessible to most individuals, substitute mechanisms would be put in place in order to find a replacement satisfaction. It resulted in neuroses, perversions, pathological character changes and disturbances in professional life. This is why the authoritarian patriarchal order led to the sexual distress of the masses.

In his study *The Invasion of Compulsory Sex-Morality*, published in 1932, Reich pointed out that the disintegration of the authoritarian family (*die Zwangsfamilie*) was one of the symptoms of the transformation of contemporary society. The active transformation of this process of disintegration could only come about by recognising the sociological role of sexual repression, both from the outside and from within: 'When practical preventive and educational measures [have been taken], the goal is prevention of armouring in man from birth onward.'[5] The origin of morality exposed in *Totem and Taboo* could, if necessary, be contradicted by drawing on Malinowski's ethnological researches on the sexual economy of the Trobriand Islanders. But the beyond of the pleasure principle was a more formidable obstacle since it was a metapsychological refutation of the social origin of neuroses. Reich tried to deny the existence of the death drive through the problem of the place of masochism in the psychic economy. The question of whether the latter was primary or secondary raised the question of the origin of the desire for unconscious punishment. By distinguishing between the fear of punishment and the desire for punishment, recalling that the fear of punishment – the fear of castration resulting from having experienced certain sexual desires – was the cornerstone of the clinic of neuroses, Reich came to the conclusion that masochistic desire could only be secondary, that it was only a way out of the complications that the inhibition of sexuality entailed. The analyst needed to eliminate this unconscious desire for punishment, which would only be a secondary neurotic formation. He had to release the patient's sexuality and not confirm his self-destructive tendencies based on hypothetical biological foundations. The negative therapeutic resistance of the patient reflected the theoretical and technical incapacity of the psychoanalyst who was unable to confer orgasmic power on his patient. The analyst could not help his patient overcome his fear of pleasure.[6] In such a case, the resistance came from the analyst. In reality, Reich considered the position that Freud adopted in the early 1920s to be hopeless. According to Reich, the inventor of psychoanalysis resigned after having fought for fifteen years for the recognition of psychoanalysis. Treated as a charlatan, betrayed by his colleagues, Freud the genius discovered that sexual repression led to mental disorders, but he feared mixing psychoanalytic science with the chaos of politics.[7] According to Reich, Freud was a man of science, and social pragmatics was totally foreign to him. His inability to change any neuroses suffered by the masses resulted in an attitude of resignation that led him to abandon the theory of the libido. Thus, Freud came to consider that happiness, pleasure, sexual fulfilment were objectives that were impossible to achieve at the collective level. According to Reich, in this movement of renunciation, Freud surrounded himself with colleagues who had only one goal: to make psychoanalysis socially acceptable. These colleagues transferred their conservative traditions into the psychoanalytic organisation itself, and Freud was dragged into the orbit of this bourgeois conservatism. He resigned, said Reich, because 'in the interest of self-preservation and the consolidation of the movement, he could not permit himself to say what, in a more honest world, he would certainly have stood up for all alone'.[8] His scientific mind took him beyond the intellectual horizon of his contemporaries, but the organisation he had created and needed for the sustainability and transmission of his work forced him to stay within the narrow limits of this conservative environment. According to Reich, because of his disillusionment, Freud came to think that the pathological character of the behaviour of individuals could not be changed. His pessimism vis-à-vis human nature led him to a wrong biological theory. Admittedly, the therapy of neuroses had been a fundamental step, but the eminent thinker could not find a sociological solution to the therapeutic applications of psychoanalysis. This was the crux of the matter: in order to preserve psychoanalysis from any connection with the political dimension, to isolate it, Freud advocated an ascetic ideal, a renunciation of sexual satisfaction based on a conservative doctrine of the cultural adaptation of psychoanalysis. It was to justify such an adaptation that the beyond of the pleasure principle was invented in 1920. Based on this reasoning, Reich envisioned the death drive as a theoretical justification that left the economic-sexual problem of the misery of the masses without a solution.

The publication of Freud's *The Ego and the Id* in 1923 had given rise to a new confusion in the analytic movement, said Reich. The analysts really did not know how to deal with the feeling of unconscious guilt, the superego. Psychoanalysts emphasised the ego at the expense of the theory of sexuality, which was then emptied of all substance. Reich said, ironically, 'The id was "wicked," the superego sat on a throne with a long beard, and was "strict" and the poor ego endeavoured to "mediate" between the two.'[9] The scientific level of the psychoanalytic communications of this period weakened; time and again, developments drew things from the side of ego psychology. Psychoanalysts spoke of sexuality without believing in it any more. And little by little, the organisation of the psychoanalytic movement took precedence over the task at hand. From 1924 to 1927, Reich continued to employ the term 'death instinct'. Nevertheless, in his clinical work, he denied its existence. In 1930, he felt that human sexuality had become the Cinderella of society.

Although Fenichel does not seem to have joined the KPD, as Reich did, he nonetheless supported his colleague's Marxist orientation and followed with great attention his research on the repression imposed by the authoritarian and patriarchal society. According to Fenichel, Reich's great merit was his courage – he dared to confront questions from which psychoanalysts usually fled for fear of encroaching on the realm of politics. Fenichel felt it necessary to develop the sociological dimension of psychoanalysis. The investigation of the resistance of bourgeois sexual morality to psychoanalysis was a priority. One must encourage both psychoanalytic practice among Marxists and Marxist dialectics among psychoanalysts. In an article published in *Imago* in 1931, Fenichel defended the future prospects that Reich had just outlined: the future tasks awaiting psychoanalysts, once the social revolution was accomplished, would go beyond the limits of the therapeutic application of the discipline. Psychoanalysts were to devote themselves to the study of the prehistory of humanity, the reform of teaching and the prophylaxis of neuroses. At the beginning of the 1930s, in

Berlin, it was noted that instances of the so-called classical forms of hysterical, obsessive and phobic neurosis dwindled and pathological variants of character took their place. Analytical practice could no longer be limited to the treatment of neuroses in the strict sense. The important thing, it was believed, was the possibility of modifying character by means of psychoanalysis well beyond the period of childhood. The emphasis on the education of the ego was already in play. It was necessary to teach the ego to support material derived from the drive. In 1935, Fenichel wrote an article on Reich's technical contributions.[10] The work that Anna Freud published in 1936 on *The Ego and the Mechanisms of Defence* leaned in part on his critical analysis. The statistical report that Fenichel had written six years earlier for the Berlin Institute had a place in this sequence.

The generation of psychoanalysts born around the year 1900 was marked by the decisive experiences of the European youth movement, World War I and the revolutions that followed. This generation did not engage in psychoanalysis for a quiet career. Before their twentieth birthdays, these future analysts were sometimes socialist or communist militants at the heart of the student youth movements in Germany and especially in Austria. Siegfried Bernfeld tried to propagate Zionism, socialism and psychoanalysis. The young Fenichel, who readily identified with Melchior's character in Wedekind's *Spring Awakening*, nearly got kicked out of high school for conducting an investigation into students' sexuality. To become a psychoanalyst, for them, was to continue their militancy, it was to defend new and subversive ideas vis-à-vis the established order. 'They never surrendered their youthful commitments; as they became analysts they changed only their vocabulary',[11] says Jacoby. But one question cannot be eluded: was their commitment to giving the socially oppressed classes access to psychoanalysis fully realised? In Berlin, the tension that existed between the desire for political and social renewal and the desire to be recognised and accepted in society was at the heart of a dilemma that needed to be explained.

The social extension in question

The Fenichel report of 1930 showed that there were substantial disparities in the social origins of patients received at the Berlin Institute. Most were from the middle classes. Eitingon had been noticing this tendency to embourgeoisement since 1922. Over time, this trend had only been further confirmed. Was the impoverishment of the middle classes under Weimar the only explanation? The economy had indeed improved in Germany in the mid-1920s. Catastrophic inflation was partly curbed. There was an improvement in living conditions and an intense cultural life, especially in Berlin. From the sociological point of view, a book published by Reich in the same year as *Character Analysis* provides data on the composition of German society during this period. His *Mass Psychology of Fascism* was, moreover, immediately banned by the Nazis and was not very well received, to say the least, by the socialist and communist organisations of the time. In 1932, the KPD had already prevented the publication in Berlin of books produced by Reich's Verlag für Sexualpolitik.[12]

According to Reich, fascism could not be explained solely by the data of political economy; the movement represented the nostalgia that resulted from the inhibition of natural sexuality. According to him, sex economy outweighed political economy and Marxist theory itself. The idea that the adherence of the masses to totalitarian ideologies was a phenomenon related to the repression of jouissance earned him the hostility of the Marxists. However, this book was a great success. The chapters devoted to the population's adherence to National Socialist propaganda are nevertheless quite impressive to read because they were written at the very moment when the events they were trying to interpret took place. The problem was thus addressed in the present tense by the author, who was wondering about the structure of the masses: 'What must be answered is: *Why do the masses allow themselves to be politically swindled*?'[13]

According to a 1925 census, data on the composition of the German population were as follows (Table 4.1):

Table 4.1 Census of German population in 1925

	Active population	*With families*
Workers	21.789 million	40.7 million
Middle classes	12.755 million	19.7 million

Let us now turn to the table (Table 4.2) relating to the composition of the urban middle classes in 1925, which appears in the section titled 'The economic and ideological structure of German society from 1928 to 1933':

Table 4.2 Composition of the urban middle classes in 1925

	Thousands
Smallholders	1,916
Small businesses (3 or more salaried employees)	1,403
Civil servants	1,763
Liberal professions and students	0,431
Small proprietors and rentiers	0,644
TOTAL	6,157

The 1925 census of the German working class is as follows (Table 4.3):

Table 4.3 Census of the German working class in 1925

	Thousands
Industrial, transportation and commercial workers, etc.	1,826
Agricultural workers	2,607
People working from home	0,138
Domestic workers	1,326
Social pensioners	1,717
Low-wage employees (up to 250 marks per month)	2,775
Junior officials (and pensioners)	1,400
TOTAL	21,789

In comparison, the statistics produced by the Berlin Institute in 1930 appear quite surprising. Of the 1,955 consultations carried out between 14 February 1920 and 1 January 1930, the distribution of the occupational categories of the patients accommodated was as follows (Table 4.4):

Table 4.4 Distribution of professional categories of patients of the Berlin Institute in 1930

	Consultations
Workers	69
Peasants	3
Artisans	157
Home employees	46
Office employees	173
Bank employees	25
Salesmen	42
Nurses	24
Other employees	54
Tradespeople	124
Primary school teachers	123
Civil servants	50
Doctors	28
Jurists	18
Technical professions	28
Artists	124
Other liberal professions	40
Students	160
Apprentices	30
Schoolchildren	75
Without indication of profession	313
Without profession	249
TOTAL	1,955

As a result, mainly craftsmen, clerks, shopkeepers, teachers, artists and students consulted the Berlin Polyclinic. These representatives of the middle class accounted for 44 percent of the consultations. The unemployed and those who did not report a profession, mainly women, accounted for 28.74 percent of the consultations. It should be noted that the liberal professions, doctors and lawyers accounted for only 4.3 percent of consultations. Compared with the number of workers in the German population as a whole and the total of 1,955 consultations over ten years, the figure of sixty-nine consultations for the category of workers is disproportionately small. If the poorest patients were undoubtedly the unemployed and those who did not provide information about a profession, it is certain that the Berlin working class as a whole had shunned the services offered by the polyclinic. The argument that the institutional project was to make psychoanalysis accessible to the middle classes ruined by the postwar crisis is not enough to explain this fact. Moreover, nothing prevented the working class from resorting to the free treatment offered at the polyclinic. Were there ideological barriers at work here? Did working-class prejudices operate as resistances to psychoanalysis?

Lacan taught us that resistance is primarily that of the analyst. Should we not look for the cause of the disaffection of the working class in the choices of the Berlin clinicians themselves – was it unconscious? Some psychoanalysts were saddened by the choice in favour of respectability, which had an impact on the entire institutional setup. They felt that like was attracting like; analysts who were doctors chose other doctors from the privileged social classes as pupils. The avant-garde ideas, the hopes placed in a possible alliance between the class struggle and psychoanalysis had been mastered and repressed by the institute's management. The tendency towards gentrification and respectability prevailed. The link, if any, between this trend and the rarity of patients from the most disadvantaged classes needs to be studied. For now, we must face the facts: the scarcity of working-class patients was a repudiation of the social openness and ideals defended by the creators of the polyclinic. This phenomenon was identified very early on, since the management of the polyclinic drew attention to it at the end of the first two years of operation.

In his article dedicated to the memory of Max Eitingon, the pioneer of psychoanalysis in Israel, Maurice-Moshe Krajzman comments on this point. He considers that the bourgeois intellectual had gradually become the only beneficiary of this enterprise and that it was therefore a partial failing of the Berlin Psychoanalytic Institute.[14] According to Krajzman, this should be attributed to the fact that the institute did not know how to transcend the social profiles of the time. If the social is indeed a form of organisation supported by a discourse, the involvement of Berlin psychoanalysts in the process of political and social renewal going on around them is open to question. Krajzman further contends that the functioning of the institute would have been perfectly consonant with that of respectable society at the time, hence the prevalence of bourgeois intellectuals, albeit impoverished or ruined by the crisis of the postwar period and the financial crash of 1929, among the patients.

However, such an explanation suggests that the desire to belong to respectable society was above all that of the analysts themselves. Although a Marxist-inspired psychoanalytic tendency existed in Berlin, it does not seem justified to try to unify the various temperaments and characters at work in the Berlin movement in order to merge them in a single aim. For their part, most Viennese psychoanalysts came from the Austrian liberal bourgeoisie. Like most Viennese intellectuals, they were sympathetic to the Social Democrats, who favoured the progressive establishment of socialism. Freud himself sided with the Social Democrats. His position was essentially pragmatic, not enthusiastic. He felt that nothing particularly good could come of politics, especially in Austria after the catastrophe of 1918. Moreover, being favourable to democracy, Freud had little admiration for the Bolshevik revolution. He affirmed this without hesitation in 1921: 'If another group tie takes the place of the religious one – and the socialistic tie seems to be succeeding in doing so – then there will be the same intolerance towards outsiders as in the age of the Wars of Religion.'[15] Freud reaffirmed his position more than ten years later in his correspondence with Albert Einstein. He wrote:

> Some people are inclined to prophesy that it will not be possible to make an end of war until Communist ways of thinking have found universal acceptance. But that aim is in any case a very remote one today, and perhaps it could only be reached after the most fearful civil wars. Thus the attempt to replace actual force by the force of ideas seems at present to be doomed to failure.[16]

For his part, in a short article dated 1922, Ferenczi pointed out that leaders of political tendencies based on historical materialism had the same resistance to psychoanalysis as other politicians. Proponents of social theory generally rejected the primacy of sexual life in the individual.[17]

In *Civilisation and Its Discontents,* Freud delivered his considered conception of the communist revolution by stating at the outset that economic criticism was not his business. What he questioned was the assumption that the suppression of private property would deliver humanity from evil. He described communism as an illusion without consistency because it entailed a conception of human nature that was completely erroneous. He opposed the idea that man was originally good, that jealousy and hatred of one's neighbour arose from the possession of goods, and that aggression and hostility would come to an end with the abolition of private property. Even if private property were to be abolished, sexual privilege – another kind of possession – would still exist. If it were decided to abolish sexual privilege, then the institution of the family would need to be abolished. Freud considered this hypothetical sexual liberation unimaginable. Basically, he said, communism rested on the principle of universal love, as in Christianity. In both cases, it was an illusion to the extent that the idea of universal love completely ignored man's tendency to satisfy his aggressiveness: 'It is always possible to bind together a considerable number of people in love, so long as there are other people left over to receive the manifestations of their aggressiveness.'[18] Freud gave historical examples of the effects of the narcissism of small differences, including fratricidal wars between neighbouring countries and the scapegoating role played by Jews throughout history. And, he asked, when the Russian bourgeoisie has been liquidated by the communist regime, who will be next? It is the very idea that happiness exists that leads men to believe in the most fatal utopias. The sacrifice of enjoyment imposed on us by civilisation makes the existence of happiness impossible. Freud's aversion to the Russian Revolution and communist ideology did not (as some have said) simply reflect the fact that he belonged to the Central European bourgeoisie, which had known the old empire. His reasoning was this: to believe in the happiness of universal love is to want it to exist, it is to want to impose it – and it leaves mass murder looming on the horizon. Let us not forget that this was written during the summer of 1929.

Most of the German-speaking analysts came from the liberal bourgeoisie and their ideal was not the intellectual engaged in the public debate, but the *gebildete Mensch*, the cultured man, whose culture implied the knowledge of several living languages, Latin, Greek, great writers of Western literature, history, the most illustrious works of art and their creators. This civilised man, of which Freud was an eminent example, had a form of education, a style of life, which could be schematically defined by his indifference to the accumulation of material goods and by his detachment from all things transcendental. The symbolic was, so to speak, his element. His function as an observer, interpreter, critic, exegete of the functioning of power or the state of the social order was not the most important thing to him. This distinguishes him, to some extent, from our customary definition of the intellectual. And even if one wanted to deny that a difference really existed between the *gebildete Mensch* inherited from the Enlightenment and the intellectual who, ever since the Dreyfus Affair, was more a man of knowledge addressing public opinion in order to awaken it, the evidence compiled by historians runs counter to the un-nuanced vision of leftwing intellectuals under Weimar. Not all of them were Social Democrats. In Germany, leftwing intellectuals often rejected the SPD's positions because they seemed too far from the dreams of their youth. The old bureaucracy was still in place and the judiciary was biased. Although weakened, the army still had a powerful influence on society. The implosion of traditional German political structures favoured, above all, the establishment of a democratic and bourgeois order. Widespread mistrust of the Social Democrats arose from their bloody repression of the workers' uprisings that took place at the beginning of 1919 and which had been aimed at establishing a communist regime in Germany. Fear that the Bolshevik revolution of 1917 would spread like an oil slick across Eastern Europe partly explains why the representatives of the German political class accepted the brutality of the repression. This abortive revolution of the German proletariat left deep scars. Committed leftwing intellectuals were deeply embittered.

Despite everything, if this desire for social renewal was not realised, it did not mean that nothing had changed. However, it would not be accurate to claim that all members of the German psychoanalytic movement had lined up as one behind the same ideals. As we have already indicated, the description of a group of enterprising psychoanalysts who all shared the same hope with regard to the coming socialist revolution is incorrect. Even though they undertook to participate actively in the transformation of a society that had been tested by total war, this proposition was unrealistic because social developments, the economic context and the prevailing political situation simply made it impossible. The analysts who worked in Berlin were not all engaged in the same way in the process of social renewal. They were not simply a group of personalities conquered by Marxist or socialist ideas. Max Eitingon, for example, belonged to the haute bourgeoisie. He came from a tradition that was not originally German and his penchant for Zionism penetrated his entire life. If he put his fortune at the disposal of the psychoanalytic movement, it was not so much due to any adherence to the ideals of the left but rather to his attachment to the Freudian cause, to which he decided to dedicate his life. His youth did not resemble that of his colleagues of Austrian origin who arrived in Berlin in the early 1920s. The institutional prototype set up by the German branch of the IPA was not solely in the hands of the Freudo-Marxists. Nor should we underestimate the influence of the privilege accorded to the medical professions at the level of candidate selection. This is an irrefutable fact. A good medical training, with its apprenticeship in relations with the sick and the knowledge of the possibilities and nature of somatic disorders, had been considered, despite all its defects, as the best preparation for the psychoanalytic profession by the institute's admissions committee. This preference weighed heavily in the selection of candidates who wished to undertake their training there. The number of people who attended Karl Abraham's introductory course on psychoanalysis in 1923 leaves no room for doubt. Fifty-four of the seventy-five attendees were doctors.

The ideal of making psychoanalysis accessible to the poorest classes was not accompanied by the desire for equivalent social openness with regard to the training of analysts. At the Berlin Institute, the preference for reputation and respectability, along with the concern to include psychoanalysis in medicine, rapidly won out over the transmission of psychoanalysis to new generations of lay analysts, to non-physicians whose consciences had been awakened by the recent social upheavals. Jacoby's conclusions concerning the fate of the Freudian left seems incomplete. He contends that revolutionary psychoanalysis would not have survived the Americanisation of the discipline, and also thinks that it would have traded its social and political outlook for something more comfortable and respectable. In the end, the didactic function of the institute prevailed over the social mission originally entrusted to the psychoanalytic polyclinic. This tendency had already begun before the disintegration of German psychoanalysis and the exodus of the political Freudians to the United States. The Marxist and revolutionary orientation of psychoanalysis was curbed and contained well before the advent of the National Socialist Party in Germany. The evolution that would lead to the medicalisation of psychoanalysis, whose spectre frightened Freud so much, did not depend solely on external circumstances. The transatlantic exile of the Central European analysts, the Americanisation of the discipline and the American rejection of lay analysis are not the only elements to be taken into account. The desire to make psychoanalysis acceptable by medicalising it came about via the strengthening of the therapeutic application, and also through the bias in favour of recruiting medical candidates. Should we be surprised at this movement when we know that the regulations relating to the training of psychoanalysts were developed by Max Eitingon, and that he was the president for life of the IPA's International Training Commission?

Uses of the initial consultation

Hans Lampl was charged with presenting the considerations concerning consultations at the polyclinic in the original 1930 report. He recalled at the outset that the initial goal of the Berlin Institute was to make the psychoanalytic method accessible to patients who lacked financial means. He stressed that initially, it was possible to take into treatment all those who wanted it. This remark is interesting in that Eitingon had not presented things this way in the 1922 Activity Report. According to Lampl, the very early years of the institute represented the golden age of the polyclinic.[19] At that time, in fact, the organisation still rested on the shoulders of just one man. Was this hierarchical pyramid structure perceived as being advantageous? Eitingon noted that at one point he himself was forced to take charge of selecting all the patients. He remarked that

> we very soon found it was far more advisable for the whole business to pass through the hands of one person and last year I took over the work of consultation entirely, so that it was easily possible to make a survey of all the material.[20]

Such a detail cannot be trivial – the desire for an overview wasn't just about convenience. This was an option whose purpose went beyond merely practical issues. Eitingon could select the cases that seemed the most appropriate for the training of students who were doing their practical training in the polyclinic. The director thus had an overview of the evolution of treatments carried out by novice practitioners. For Hans Lampl, this system of organisation was a huge advantage that nevertheless had not been able to maintain itself given the influx of patients.

After a few years, the function assumed by Eitingon was divided among several assistants. Lampl did not give their names. Each of the assistants had to devote half a day a week to it. According to Lampl, only those patients able to do an analysis were presented to Max Eitingon, with the result that Eitingon only met patients who had already been preselected by the assistants. This is a curious detail. Did this mean that these patients were received twice for the initial consultation, the first time by an assistant and the second time by the director, who either approved or rejected the assistant's opinion? Was the patient then referred to a third analyst for treatment? The process is surprising, but it is logically understandable in that it is unlikely that any but the most favourable cases for treatment had been sent directly to Eitingon. Consequently, it could only be a question of control exercised by the director vis-à-vis the selection made by his own assistants during the consultations. This implies that, despite the influx of patients over time, the indication of treatment still depended on the endorsement of the director. The consultation itself resembled that of other polyclinics. The medical model was prevalent, Lampl cautioned. Thus, there was no hesitation in performing a physical examination of patients who were seeking consultation for the first time. The most ordinary somatic pathologies – those related to ageing, among others – were side by side with neuroses and advanced psychoses. In some cases, patients were redirected to specialised medical consultations. This first evaluation had to be undertaken by a doctor. It should also be added that the consultation had a political use. The Berlin Polyclinic was meant to attract all those who practised psychoanalysis without having been analysed themselves, in order to persuade them to undergo training. It was necessary to try to convince them of the necessity of training at the institute. As Freud himself wrote in 1926, it was a requirement: no one should practice analysis without having acquired the right to do so through a specific training. From this point of view, the Berlin Institute was to serve as an instrument in the struggle against wild psychoanalysis. There is a remarkable example, dating from the end of 1924, showing how a whole network of psychoanalysts could mobilise to allow someone to do an analysis in the polyclinic. Eitingon's consultation appears to have been not only a filter but also a means of attracting interesting personalities to be analysed by members of the analytic society.

The case of Josephine Dellisch

In the autumn of 1924, Alix Strachey, a translator of Freud's works into English, travelled to Berlin to undertake her second tranche of analysis with Karl Abraham. Her husband, James Strachey, had gone back to England. Before that, the Stracheys had stayed in Vienna. The husband and wife had simultaneously carried out a first tranche of analysis with Freud. During

Alix's stay in Berlin between 1924 and 1925, the couple wrote to each other almost daily. This correspondence, mainly Alix's letters, is a wealth of information on the atmosphere and functioning of the Berlin-based analytical movement in the mid-1920s. The name of Alix Strachey is associated with that of Melanie Klein, who arrived in Berlin at the time of her divorce in 1921. Melanie Klein may even have begun to meet Abraham before that date to tell him about the difficulties she faced in analysing her own son, Erich. In January 1921 she moved with Erich to a boarding house near Abraham's home in the Grünwald district. Klein advocated the use of play and interpretation to initiate the transference with small children – how did the team react to this revolutionary thesis? Two trends emerged at the institute. Some, mostly doctors and Hungarians, were alarmed by her clinical practice with children, believing that Klein was misusing suggestion and causing a frightful weakening of the superego. Conversely, other analysts argued that it was beneficial to analyse early repression and the harmful effects of the infant superego.

Among Melanie Klein's Berlin supporters was Alix Strachey. She described to her husband the effects of Klein's presentation to the members of the institute in December 1924:

> The opposition consisted of Drs. Alexander & Radó, & was purely affective & 'theoretical' since, apparently, no one knows anything about the subject outside die Melanie & a Frl. Schott who is too retiring to speak, but who agrees with her. Abraham spoke sharply to Alexander, & Dr. Boehm (a faded, but possibly a very clever analyst, youngish & bird-like in manner) rushed in too to defend die Klein. In fact, everyone rallied to her & attacked the 2 swarthy Hungarians. She gave 2 specially brilliant examples. One, of an apparently utterly uninhibited boy, who exhibited & masturbated & wanted to assault everyone, i.e. a complete example of a so-called defective Überich, who turned out to be in a state of chronic latent Angst, forced to behave in this way as a compulsive act. This was to disprove the contention that what children need is to have their Überichs toned up. The second example disposed of Alexander's other objection, that it was useless & pernicious, to interpret the meaning of their symptoms to children, as (a) They couldn't understand & (b) They'ld faint with horror (!) She said that very often it was absolutely impossible to establish any contact with the child – any transference – until one had explained what it really wanted to do when it pushed a poker into its doll etc. [...] Well, it was most stimulating, & much more feeling was displayed than usual.[21]

These incredible allegations caused a break in Alix Strachey's analytical training. The meeting with Klein prompted Alix to organise Klein's first stay in England in the summer of 1925. As Walter Kendrick and Perry Meisel pointed out, Alix Strachey was lucky enough to be in Berlin at the moment when the study of psychoanalysis was at its peak. She arrived in Berlin in September 1924. As early as November, she went to the weekly meetings of the Kinderseminar organised by Fenichel for young Berlin analysts. When she began attending the institute, Alix Strachey wanted to perfect her German and wanted to take classes. More exactly, she began to converse with a 28-year-old Swiss primary school teacher named Josephine Dellisch. The Stracheys already knew her, having met her before in Vienna. The adventures relating to her symptoms were frequently mentioned in the letters they exchanged. Soon it was a question of getting her to consult an analyst again, but not just anyone. In fact, Josephine Dellisch had already met Heinrich Körber who was one of the founding members of the DPV. But the results of this analysis were not very conclusive, to say the least, since Josephine confided to Alix at the same time her distress but also her ambition to become a psychoanalyst by turning her back on Freudian theories. She felt, however, that she needed to undertake a new analysis. For her part, Alix went straight to the point when she noticed that her classmate was suffering from a castration complex doubled with a full-blown narcissism, which made it very difficult to maintain relations with her:

> Her desire to be superior to all, & hatred of being 'downed' is frightful. Added to all this, she's suffered for the last 8 years from a diseased hip which makes her lame & drives her mad with rage. – The net result is that the first 2 things she did today, when I called on her, were to thrust that wretched book of Adler's under my nose & tell me that *he* was the only man who could really understand her (or anything) & cure her; & to state that she wished to join the Berlin Psychoanalytic Society at once & drop in on the Poliklinik.[22]

Such was the stake: a young, cultured and lost woman proclaimed to anyone who would listen that she recognised herself in the traitor Adler's theory of the power of the will, all while asking to become a member of the DPV. One could make neither head nor tail of it! Alix Strachey thought this was a classic case of elation. A major mobilisation of several analysts on the Berlin-Vienna axis then took place.

Alix's first mission was to find things to keep this drifting young woman busy; she complained of it quite a lot in her correspondence. She first took Josephine to lunch, then the afternoon was devoted to touring museums. At this time, Alix noted that a crisis was shaking the educational community in Germany, which plunged the teacher into great distress. This was the disagreement between Gustav Wyneken and Martin Luserke, two famous pedagogues, about the function of boys' boarding schools in Germany. Wyneken had attracted a considerable audience within the youth movement. This reformer had founded the Wickersdorf Free School; he thought that young people would flourish on the basis of their own values. He wasn't a member of the SPD himself, but his ideas seduced the most leftwing supporters of the youth movement. Martin Luserke wanted to separate from Wyneken to found his own school on the island of Sylt. This context relating to the professional environment in which Josephine was evolving has to be taken into consideration. The subjective crisis that the teacher was going through during this period was linked to a specific circumstance: indeed, she had to choose sides. We could hypothesise that the conflict between the two pedagogues took the place, in her case, of the conflict between Freud and Adler. Dellisch was caught between a rock and a hard place. She wavered when making a choice. To put it this way, Josephine's subjective crisis was linked to the master signifiers of the time, and her identification reflected the upheavals and uncertainties among German youth. The youth movement, which had taken off before the war, was marked by romantic and nebulous idealism. When the crisis of the postwar period began, these groups began to express radical but disorganised and aimless social demands. These demands could 'just as well turn to the left as to the right, or even lead nowhere'.[23] The conclusion of the crisis navigated by the teacher shows that the genesis of her troubles was related to a crisis of institutions and, particularly, that of schooling.

At the end of October 1924, between two epistolary exchanges about the translation of Freud's study of the Wolf-Man, Alix pointed out that 'the Dellisch affair continues to get complicated'. Josephine, who thought her landlady wanted to rape her, had just rushed out of her apartment. This sketch of erotomania was noted by Alix in a rather ironic way: 'she was known to be mad, but not to be a saph'. This did not preclude her proposal that Josephine should come to Alix's boarding house in the Grünewald district. Alix felt compelled to do so in order to protect her comrade from the crazy project of going to live in a Christian hospice or a brothel. Suddenly, Josephine announced that she had made the decision to be analysed at the polyclinic for four weeks:

> She seemed frightfully anxious to find help somewhere, (Needless to say, this all came out at lunch at the Heidelberger Restaurant, & she was in tears) & at once, & it seemed as if she felt that she would be temporarily relieved by being able to vent herself on an analyst even for that short time. And I daresay there's truth in it. I ventured to suggest that nothing radical could be done under at least 4 months, & altho' she knew this perfectly well, she seemed quite bouleversée by it. People *are* queer.[24]

She also pointed out that when Josephine was in Vienna, Freud had offered to analyse her for free – '& the WOMAN REFUSED'. As a result, Josephine had tried to analyse her dreams by herself, an undertaking that provided her with such surprising insights that she had not recovered. Two days later, she had an appointment with Max Eitingon at the Berlin Polyclinic. Following the consultation, Eitingon advised her to meet Lou Andreas-Salomé, who had been based in Göttingen since 1903. It is quite likely that this advice came directly from Vienna and that Eitingon was the messenger. Indeed, it was the Freuds themselves who made Eitingon aware of Josephine's troubles. The Freuds also asked him to convince Lou Andreas-Salomé to agree to analyse this distressed young woman free of charge. At that time, Alix Strachey said, 'I imagine the Klinik is only too glad to foist (or hoist) some of its superfluous patients onto higher spheres. But no-one knows yet what will come of it' (letter of 28 October 1924). Alix was not entirely wrong – the Dellisch case was not yet over. On 3 December 1924, Eitingon wanted to speak urgently with Alix to announce that Lou Andreas-Salomé had refused to take her friend into analysis. The only alternative was to offer 'a *fraktionäre* treatment – a month at Xmas, 3 weeks at Easter, etc., to suit her schooltime'. But Josephine wouldn't hear of it, she changed her mind, she rebelled, she backtracked. Eitingon did not know what to do.

Anna Freud decided to intervene directly by persuading Eitingon to do everything in his power to bring the young woman back to her senses. One suspects that when a Freud decreed that it was necessary to try everything to allow someone to make an analysis, the director of the polyclinic obeyed. Moreover, we must not forget the bonds of friendship between Eitingon and Freud's daughter. On 6 December 1924, Eitingon showed Alix a letter from Josephine, in which Josephine made it clear that she would have to decline the offer of analysis because she was exhausted, she had no money, and was having no luck with finding accommodation in Berlin. It was therefore absolutely necessary that Alix take her back with her to the Pension Bismarck. Even better, for the moment Alix had to foot the bill. It was necessary for Dellisch to agree to meet another analyst very quickly, whatever the cost, without her suspecting for a moment what was going on around her.

> Anna Freud is to write to Eitingon (he's asked for a letter) telling him more about D.'s state of mind; & that I'm to see it, & write to D. pretending that Anna's been in communication with me (for of course Eitingon & the Poliklinik must not appear to be taking any special pains to catch her) & give her a good blowing up, in the hearty style, I think, & force her to take money & to be helped by me.
>
> (Letter of 6 December 1924)

Eitingon had said that finances were not a problem, because the money was there. The only problem was, as Alix pointed out to James, 'how to press it into that lunatic's hand'. She was worried about the idea of having to share the meagre resources that were forcing her to economise during her stay in Berlin. This adventure, however, allowed her to approach Eitingon and to get to know him better. Alix felt a deep respect for this man of taste whose house was furnished with thick carpets and valuable paintings, which evoked the

Victorian style familiar to this Englishwoman. In the end, a place was found in the polyclinic for Josephine and she begin an analysis with Franz Alexander.

Just before Christmas, Anna Freud managed to get a rich Viennese woman, Mrs Blumgart – who was none other than Ruth Mack Brunswick, the wife of Hermann Blumgart – to look after Dellisch during the first month of her fractional analysis at the polyclinic. This time, again, the thing was organised without the knowledge of Dellisch who ended up accepting financial assistance from this wealthy woman. Josephine, completely exhausted, felt that her mental state did not allow her, in any way, to remain isolated. She had to live a little while longer at the guesthouse with Alix. She felt absolutely unable to cope alone. Even though the analytic honeymoon with Alexander was short-lived, it still led to a result. The treatment at the clinic did not lead to the training expected at the institute, but it nevertheless allowed her to find a way out of her subjective crisis. Josephine Dellisch ended up returning to her teaching job. She left to join Wyneken in his free school in the mountainous region of Taunus. Alix Strachey went to visit her during the summer of 1926. She stayed in the quarters where her friend lived at this establishment.

Beyond the anecdotes that peppered the correspondence between Alix and James, this episode is quite instructive. First, it confirms that after only four years of operation, the polyclinic was working at full capacity. Moreover, we see how the consultations could be used to redirect certain urgent cases to analysts in private practice. The director of the institution also had to make sure that the external analyst agreed not to be paid. In this particular case, it is quite piquant to know that Freud had scolded Lou Andreas-Salomé about money the year before. In 1923 he had begged her to increase the price of her sessions. Freud had learned that his friend was exhausted working as an analyst for ten hours a day. According to him, it was a form of disguised suicide. Freud told her to increase her fees by at least a quarter or a half 'to correspond with the cascading collapse of the mark'.[25]

It is quite remarkable that a year later, despite the bonds of friendship that existed between the daughter-Anna (as Freud named her) and Lou Andreas-Salomé, the latter guarded her freedom of action and her clinical opinion concerning the situation in which Josephine Dellisch found herself as a result of Lou's refusal to take her into analysis. Anyway, let's keep in mind the fact that in 1924, free analysis was common and did not shock anyone. It was Lou Andreas-Salomé's refusal that forced Eitingon to see Dellisch again for a consultation. Moreover, if the idea of being analysed in four weeks seemed somewhat daring to Alix Strachey, the undertaking seemed at least conceivable over a period of four months. Were the combined efforts of Sigmund Freud, Anna Freud, Max Eitingon, Alix Strachey, Lou Andreas-Salomé, Ruth Mack Brunswick and Franz Alexander something exceptional? In October 1924, Alix Strachey commented on the working methods employed at the recent IPA congress in Würzburg. She explained to her husband that

'The idea of [these small working groups] is to rope in "wild" analysts & give them a chance of becoming orthodox ones by telling them about it & Poliklinik and persuading them to get analysed there themselves' (letter of 13 October 1924). Other testimonies also go in this direction; they confirm that the Berlin Institute was conceived as a special instrument in the fight against the spread of wild psychoanalysis.

This is not the least of the paradoxes. The Berlin Institute and the polyclinic attached to it were created to respond to the uncontrollable penetration of psychoanalysis into culture in the early twenties. Freudian theories faced considerable resistance throughout Germany for a long time. In the postwar period, things had changed. The psychoanalytic congresses of 1924 and 1925, which took place in Würzburg and Weimar, showed that psychoanalysis was beginning to find an audience beyond the boundaries of the capital. The extension of psychoanalysis could not be accomplished without guaranteeing the competence of its practitioners. In addition, deviances from within the movement were perceived as threats. The didactic training that was developed at the Berlin Institute was to serve these two interests of expansion and orthodoxy.

New guidelines for training

It was in Berlin that the standardisation of selection and training procedures for candidates was invented. A central body established at Eitingon's instigation in 1923 was responsible for ensuring managing admissions and teaching content. Before that date, these tasks had been shared between a few members of the institute in a rather unorganised way. The numerical increase of those who approached the institute for the purpose of training there was presented as the cause of an evolution that culminated in 1927, that is to say at the moment when Freud's fight in defence of lay analysis was in full swing. It was then that new measures were enacted by the teaching commission. These new Guidelines for the Training of Therapeutic Analysts were presented and commented on by Karen Horney in the 1930 report.

But before proceeding, we need to remind ourselves of the position publicly adopted by Freud concerning the training of psychoanalysts four years earlier. In 'The Question of Lay Analysis', he referred to the training provided by the new psychoanalytic institutes in Berlin and Vienna. The London Institute was about to open its doors. In all these places, an analysis was offered to students attending theoretical classes. The latter benefited from the supervision of experienced analysts from the moment their theoretical training was considered advanced enough to entrust them with fairly easy cases. It took two years for this training cycle to be completed, said Freud. At the end of this cycle, however, the analyst's training was not complete. The trainee analyst had to hone his skills in two ways: putting in the hours, and discussing with his seniors in psychoanalytic societies. Anyone who had followed the theoretical teaching and who had practised psychoanalysis was no longer a layman. Basically, whether or not the analyst in question was a doctor was beside the point. A more decisive criterion was the possession of what Freud called a keen ear for the repressed unconscious. Then again, too great an abnormality was likely to have a harmful effect on the psychic life of the patient. As the scientific definition of normality does not exist, such an estimate depends more on consensus: there is no test for psychological normality. The assessment of the qualities of the analytic candidate therefore depended on a subjective agreement. Referring to the need to train analysts in psychoanalytic institutes, Freud said that it was hardly possible to refer to any standard for assessing the qualities of the candidate. According to him, the future analyst must hear what is said behind what is heard. The 'keen ear' relates to the difference between utterance and enunciation.

Let's return to the *Guidelines for Training* at the Berlin Institute. These were based on a series of general principles. The training committee was composed of seven members and was responsible for teaching, properly speaking. This commission was responsible for the organisation and control of all the other courses taught by the institute. Courses were designed for social workers, lawyers, educators, pastors and doctors. The commission was also responsible for organising lectures for a cultured public. These guidelines were very clear on one point: medical studies were considered the most appropriate among the preparatory courses required for those applying to the teaching commission. An explanation of the criteria used for the selection of candidates was added to the presentation of the curriculum regulations that students had to complete. Before 1927,

> some much-needed regulations in practice were easily decided, such as the establishment of a curriculum or the provision that in future only the board, rather than one person, would be responsible for the admission of a candidate. But there was no clear agreement on admission criteria or curriculum details,

said Karen Horney.[26] According to her, the lack of agreement on these criteria made it necessary to adopt new guidelines.

The 1927 guidelines divided the curriculum into three parts: didactic analysis, theoretical training and polyclinic practice. The practical polyclinic experience was what the candidate had to perform after proving that his didactic analysis and theoretical training were sufficiently advanced to allow him to be entrusted with patients. The student carried out treatments under supervision. Karen Horney emphasised the evolution of the institute's position vis-à-vis didactic psychoanalysis. This evolution, which reflected the new guidelines, was linked to the candidate's aptitude. As Horney pointed out, analysis had a limit, it could not produce certain qualities in the future psychoanalyst. Certain character traits of the candidate were beyond the reach of his personal analysis, and would therefore persist. We find again at the didactic level this notion of 'character' which we already met with at the level of patient treatments at the polyclinic. Thus, they were not able to achieve a change as complete as they had hoped for through analysis. This was a finding from their experience. They had to admit that even with the same training, not all students had the qualities required to become analysts. It was not possible to transform just anyone into an 'ideal analyst or even moderately effective one' through their analysis, said Horney. The analysis would not modify two main stumbling blocks: an unreliable character and a lack of psychological skill. The future analyst had to be someone you could count on, but without a psychological knack, there could be no analyst. These two criteria would not be the result of analytical work – such was the reasoning.

Although it is hardly surprising to see the reference to character reappearing at the very moment when important developments were devoted to it in the technical seminars in Vienna and Berlin, another emphasis was placed on the psychological gift that didactic psychoanalysis could not produce. This implies that the analyst was not conceived of as a product of his own cure. The model chosen was rather that of development, maturation and prerequisite qualities. From that angle, it is quite logical that the members of the institute considered it inadvisable to entrust very neurotic patients to equally neurotic student analysts. Karen Horney put it this way: 'In other words, a serious neurotic always remained marked by an imbalance, a little less serious, no doubt, since he was analysed, but these antecedents were a contraindication to the practise of psychoanalysis.'

How was this vague concept of personal aptitude to be dealt with, especially since analysts likely to identify these initial qualities were often no better off in terms of having this 'intuitive gift' themselves? Only one solution to this dilemma had been found: trial didactic analysis. Nevertheless, this precaution was not enough to protect a profession haloed by a certain prestige from being entered into by unsavoury individuals. It was not uncommon for ageing women in need of adventure or unsuccessful men to be attracted to the institute's training programme. These people hoped that it would be easy to get work as an analyst and thereby enhance their social status. According to Karen Horney, all these bad prior dispositions were a set of contraindications to analytic training. On the other hand, it wasn't necessary to be too rigid. If medical training was considered at the time to be the best preparation for the profession of psychoanalyst, other professions should not be totally excluded from the training provided by the institute. Once again, it all depended on the personality and the aptitude of the non-medical candidate. A certain balance, a settled position marked by moderation and nuance, ideally guided the decisions of the teaching commission, which had to decide on the admission of candidates. It should be noted that this was an ideal because the guidelines introduced a disparity that was not in keeping with the Freudian position vis-à-vis lay analysis. It is clear enough from Karen Horney's account that personal aptitude was understood as a mixture of mental equilibrium and psychological aptitude. Obviously, this balance was difficult to detect in the candidate. The only accepted criterion was that the profession of analyst could not be performed by individuals who suffered from serious neuroses.

The training of medical candidates included didactic analysis, the theoretical course and the practical course. Didactic analysis was the first and most indispensable step according to Horney, who defended the official position established by Freud: didactic analysis took precedence over theoretical training. Eitingon had corrected his own point of view in order to make it consistent with Freud's. From that moment on, didactics was presented as a preliminary step to training at the Berlin Institute. The commission established a list of training analysts and the candidate had to choose a name from this list. The duration of the didactic analysis depended on the personality of the candidate; it had to last at least twelve months, at the rate of one hour of analysis per day. The teaching committee was responsible for evaluating the results. It could ask for an extension of the didactic analysis of the candidate or its suspension. The didactic analysis had to be almost completed before the practical training could begin. Medical candidates were advised to undertake their didactic analysis as soon as they obtained their state diploma. The theoretical curriculum itself consisted of compulsory courses and seminars. There were also optional and semi-annual courses and seminars. As these courses were held in the evening, this allowed doctors to continue their studies in specialities considered essential such as psychiatry, internal medicine or neurology. During the theoretical course, doctors had to acquire knowledge of psychology, sociology and the history of science and civilisations.

Thirdly, the practical course allowed students to gain the status of volunteer assistants at the polyclinic. It was specified that analytic treatment of patients was to be entrusted to those analysts who were in training and undergoing supervision. The compulsory technical seminar offered students the possibility of perfecting their theoretical and practical knowledge on the basis of the cases being treated. The training ended with the successful completion of this practical course. Only then was the candidate allowed to become a practising analyst. After a few more years of experience, he could ask to be admitted to the DPG, 'which serves him both to justify his training and to provide him with the possibility of continuous analytical improvement'.[27] On average, it took between three and four years to complete the entire curriculum. Each of these parts could be carried out outside the institute in places approved by the DPG. For their part, non-physicians had to acquire knowledge in biology, psychology, sexology, pathology and psychiatry. They had to attend courses at university or higher education institutions and had to experience contact with those who were suffering, especially the mentally ill. The institute was to provide them with this opportunity. At the end of their training, non-physicians had to commit to practice psychoanalysis within certain limits. For example, they could not make diagnoses or give indications without submitting them to a medical psychoanalyst. Neither could they analyse psychotics. Psychiatric borderline cases as well as psychoses with organic complications always had to be directed to their medically trained psychoanalytical colleagues. In her report, without giving any more precision, Horney added that a special status for candidates wishing to become child analysts was being prepared.

The candidate's training had to conform to a series of specific steps. We note that such a system bears some resemblance to university studies. Moreover, a certificate equivalent to a diploma was issued to students who had completed their studies at the institute. Richard Sterba, who was one of the first students at the Vienna Institute, completed his training course in 1927. He was appointed a member of the psychoanalytic society in 1925, when his training at the institute had just begun. After completing the course, he received a certificate signed by the director of the Vienna Institute – at that time Helene Deutsch – and from the president of the WPV, who was none other than Sigmund Freud. Grete Bibring and Richard Sterba were the only students to receive a certificate with Freud's signature. Institutes in other countries complained that the Vienna Institute had such a privilege. From then on, Freud stopped signing these certificates. When the Berliners realised that it was hardly possible for them to analyse each other, they called in an outside training analyst. Eitingon brought Hanns Sachs from Switzerland. The first training analyst of the Berlin Institute was, therefore, a layman at a time when they were not fully regarded as genuine therapists. Sachs embodied a counterweight to the considerable emphasis that the DPG had placed on medical practitioners.

The novitiate of the analyst

Hanns Sachs' brief report on didactic analysis, the shortest contribution to the 1930 report, is quite surprising. This is not unrelated to the long-standing strategy of silence adopted by the IPA regarding the organisation, results and purpose of the training analysis. To follow Sachs, the didactic training would be the equivalent of the priestly novitiate. The psychoanalyst, Sachs explained, cannot be considered a layman because he directs his gaze beyond the visible and onto what remains hidden. He must learn to see what escapes the secular vision of other men. Sachs emphasises the psychoanalyst's gaze:

> As we see, analysis needs something that corresponds to the novitiate of the Church. The acquisition of theoretical knowledge, a book knowledge, however complete it may be, is not enough. It demands from those who practice it a gaze constantly directed at things that they would rather turn aside from by internal necessity and moral requirement – things such as infantile sexuality, the Oedipus complex and ambivalence in human relations.[28]

The metaphor of the gaze insists on the formula according to which the analyst cannot immediately put on analytical glasses. It takes time to learn to endure the vision of this other reality, the unconscious, sustainably and without damage.

The training analysis set up for the first time at the Berlin Institute had two goals. The didactic goal allowed the future analyst to withstand the sight of unpleasantness without incurring any danger to himself, to get up close to the ugliness and suffering produced by human relations without harm. In a way, the didactic analysis would protect the soul of the analyst from the darkness of the drive life of the patients. The religious reference being very explicit in Sachs, it does not seem excessive to translate it in these terms. More classically, the other aim of the training analysis is to allow the future analyst to become familiar with the movements of his own unconscious in order to recognise them in others when they occur and to evaluate their importance correctly. Sachs insisted on the priority given to the didactic training in the spirit of the inventors of the Berlin training institution. This situation gave way to two problems that remained unresolved. It was a question of the choice of candidate and the preliminary training. Three years earlier, a shift had occurred via the new guidelines. Sachs made no comment on their soundness. The second problem, which remained unresolved, was the delicate question of the end of the training analysis, insofar as the usual criterion of removing symptoms was either lacking here or not sufficient. It should be emphasised that the training analysis was for the first time understood as an independent branch of analysis. Training was distinguished from therapeutic application. Once the candidate's training analysis had been judged sufficiently complete by the training committee, the student was allowed to undertake his theoretical training. The reference to religion will be taken up by Sachs later in an article on the prospects of psychoanalysis published in 1939 in the *International Journal*. He wrote about the shape that psychoanalysis should take in the future. Sachs pointed out that, as with the other sciences, psychoanalysis was not free from certain prejudices. The development of a science is always influenced by subjective factors, fantasies and opinions. This subjective element is responsible for errors that can be perpetuated over time and transmitted from generation to generation. In the scientific field, the truth is not written for all eternity.

> Every phase of every established science, no matter if it is one of splendid progress or miserable decay, will become, to a quite perceptible extent, a phenomenon of mass-psychology. Psychoanalysis has no right to assume that it forms an exception to this rule, although it started under conditions which were rather different from the usual ones.[29]

Sachs pointed out that at the beginning, psychoanalysis was the business of one man. However, it had quickly found shelter at the heart of an organisation to the extent where only a collective endeavour could face up to the exceptional resistance provoked in society by the Oedipus complex and infantile sexuality. Analysts were forced to stick together to stay strong. Psychoanalysis wasn't recognised by conventional research and teaching institutions. Analysts found themselves rejected from places where scientific knowledge was usually produced and transmitted. They needed a place where they could be together: a space of conversation and conservation. The organisation would thus provide a shelter, a refuge for the first psychoanalysts. Moreover, this collective allowed them to present their work and to test its validity in the company of their peers. It was a kind of scientific club made up of passionate people who also needed to counter the resistance that came from within the movement itself. We have seen that the fear of a weakening, of a transformation, of a betrayal of the ideas elaborated by Freud was a constant during the 1920s.

According to Sachs, the analytic organisation grew stronger as the success of analytic therapy attracted many physicians who had no prior analytical training. This is a new confirmation of the dangers that the diffusion and popularisation of psychoanalytic concepts has placed on the analytic community. The appropriation of analytic therapy by so-called wild analysts was perceived as a danger and one of the aims of the Berlin Institute was to thwart this uncontrollable expansion. So who could practice analysis and who could not? Someone had to decide. It was this function of guarantee that was taken up by the organisation.

> It became important that someone should have full authority to decide and declare who was entitled to describe himself as an analyst and who was not. The organisation, being already in existence, was, of course, invested with this authority. As a natural consequence the framing of rules concerning teaching and training and the supervision of their observance became a prerogative of the association.[30]

The question of the guarantee leads directly to that of the regulation of training, which had the effect of introducing a distortion insofar as the aims of science and those of the organisation are of a contradictory nature. Indeed, in research, science needs freedom, originality and invention. It cannot be deployed in the discursive regime of conformity, control and regulation. On the other hand, any organisation is supported by a practical perspective, its statutes provide stability over time, and its survival is its main objective. A division was established between regulation, which is essentially conservative, and progress, which is inherent to scientific advance. Sachs thus had the idea that the conservatism of the psychoanalytical organisation was structural. Like the figure of Moses, with which Sachs' article ended, Freud traced out a new path for civilisation, but his teaching had undergone so many transformations and distortions that it had become unrecognisable. It was to be hoped that the Freudian oeuvre could share the same fate as the Mosaic speech, that it would return to the light after having been forgotten and truncated. Sachs' criticism of the analytic organisation was rather subtle, it did not attack it directly. It pointed to a division that occurred when the aim of protecting analysts from a society that was hostile had overtaken the epistemological aims of psychoanalysis. Moreover, the establishment of professional regulation had focused on the survival of the organisation itself. Sachs' demonstration argues that early psychoanalysis was the business of one man and that its future, in its most optimistic version, would depend on returning to the teaching of Sigmund Freud:

> If we assume that every great man, every leader towards a new vision and a greater idea of humanity, has something in him of the personality and fate of Moses, then Freud has unintentionally given us a portrait of himself and his work.[31]

Notes

1 Wilhelm Reich, 'Preface to First Edition' (1933), *Character Analysis, op. cit.*, pp. xxii–xxiii.
2 Wilhelm Reich, *The Invasion of Compulsory Sex-Morality* (New York: Farrar, Straus and Giroux, 1971), p. xxvii.
3 Wilhelm Reich, *The Function of the Orgasm, op. cit.*, p. 8.
4 Wilhelm Reich, 'The Characterological Mastery of the Infantile Sexual Conflict' (1930), *Character Analysis, op. cit.*, p. 150.
5 Wilhelm Reich, *The Invasion of Compulsory Sex-Morality, op. cit.*, p. 158.
6 Wilhelm Reich, 'The Death Instinct', in *Reich Speaks of Freud* (Harmondsworth: Penguin Books, 1975), pp. 211–213.
7 Wilhelm Reich, *The Function of the Orgasm, op. cit.*, p. 214.
8 *Ibid.*, p. 215.
9 *Ibid.*, p. 124.
10 Otto Fenichel, 'Concerning the Theory of Psychoanalytic Technique', in Hanna Fenichel and David Rapaport (eds.), *The Collected Papers of Otto Fenichel: First Series* (London: Routledge & Kegan Paul, 1954), pp. 332–348.
11 Russell Jacoby, *The Repression of Psychoanalysis, op. cit.*, p. 46.
12 Wilhelm Reich, *The Mass Psychology of Fascism*, trans. Vincent R. Carfagno (Harmondsworth: Penguin Books, 1975), p. 23.
13 *Ibid.*, p. 70.
14 Maurice-Moshe Krajzman, 'Max Eitingon', *op. cit.*, p. 105.
15 Sigmund Freud, 'Group Psychology and the Analysis of the Ego' (1921), *Standard Edition*, vol. 18, p. 99.
16 Sigmund Freud, 'Why War?' (1932), *Standard Edition*, vol. 22, p. 208.
17 Sándor Ferenczi, 'Psychanalyse et politique sociale' (1922), *Psychanalyse 3, op. cit.*, p. 175.
18 Sigmund Freud, 'Civilization and Its Discontents' (1929), *Standard Edition*, vol. 21, p. 114.
19 Hans Lampl, 'La consultation à la policlinique', in Colonomos, *On forme des psychanalystes, op. cit.*, pp. 117–121. Lampl, a doctor, was born in Vienna in 1889 and began his psychoanalytic formation in Berlin in 1921.

20 Max Eitingon, 'Report', *op. cit.*, 261–262.
21 Perry Meisel and Walter Kendrick, *Bloomsbury/Freud, op. cit.*, pp. 145–146.
22 *Ibid.*, pp. 92–93.
23 Walter Laqueur, *Weimar, op. cit.*
24 Perry Meisel and Walter Kendrick, *Bloomsbury/Freud, op. cit.*, p. 96.
25 Ernst Pfeiffer (ed.), *Sigmund Freud and Lou Andreas-Salomé: Letters*, trans. William and Elaine Robson Scott (London: The Hogarth Press, 1972), p. 124.
26 Karen Horney, 'De l'organisation' (1930), in Colonomos, *On forme des psychanalystes, op. cit.*, pp. 125, 127.
27 *Ibid.*, p. 132.
28 Hanns Sachs, 'L'analyse didactique', in Colonomos, *On forme des psychanalystes, op. cit.*, p. 136.
29 Hanns Sachs, 'The Prospects of Psychoanalysis' (1939), *International Journal of Psychoanalysis*, vol. 20, 461.
30 *Ibid.*, p. 462.
31 *Ibid.*, p. 463.

Chapter 5

Psychoanalysis versus psychotherapy

The systematisation of the curriculum

The systematic organisation of the theoretical curriculum at the Berlin Institute had not been put in place until 1927. This organisation was based on a scheme that was modelled on the organisation of university studies. Systematisation was not only assumed, it also represented the culmination of a double process. It fell to Franz Alexander to explain the reasons for this development. On the one hand, the training offered by the institute attracted more and more students who had graduated in medicine. The organisation of the first year of studies was clearly intended for them. This was inspired, in fact, by the organisation of medical studies: anatomy and physiology of the psychic apparatus, psychoanalytic psychology of normality and elements of psychopathology. The theoretical curriculum required giving medical candidates the understanding of psychology that they often lacked, Alexander said.

Alexander also felt that psychoanalysis had accomplished its scientific mutation. At the outset, the concepts invented by Freud had to be flexible enough to adapt to the discoveries generated by clinical material, which was constantly being renewed. This first phase of psychoanalysis made it extremely complicated to set up a systematic teaching of fundamental psychoanalytic concepts. Little by little, however, the accumulated clinical experience confirmed the validity of the concepts. The era of empirical experimentation gave way to the properly scientific phase of psychoanalysis. From that moment, a systematic teaching of psychoanalysis could be envisaged. Only then was it possible to teach, in a systematic way, a discipline with the status of a science. Having acquired these credentials, psychoanalysis could be transmitted in the form of an organised curriculum. What became of the Freudian discovery in this transition? When psychoanalysis attempts to rival other scientific disciplines, such as biology or anatomy, all reference to the unconscious disappears:

> In parallel with the regrouping of isolated observations, the possibility of applying psychoanalysis is extended from the domain of pathology to

DOI: 10.4324/9781003215684-8

> other new domains of human psychic activity. The application of these was precisely the touchstone of the correctness of conceptual abstractions. Increasingly, psychoanalysis acquired the character of a general psychology.[1]

The establishment of the systematisation of the theoretical curriculum was linked to the idea that psychoanalysis had gone beyond the first stages of its development. Psychoanalysis had become scientific, and the previously slightly shady psychoanalyst had become a respectable scientist. This had an important consequence in that the teaching of psychoanalysis could now be modelled on the systematic organisation of conventional medical studies. One of the most surprising effects of the scientific development of psychoanalysis nevertheless heralded the decline of therapeutics. This is quite logical to the extent that the break with the clinical field reduced the therapeutic application of psychoanalysis to the status of simply being one application among others: 'The initial field, that of therapy, has become, while remaining predominant due to its importance, one possibility of application among many others.'[2]

At first, it seemed very difficult to develop a systematic curriculum with just a few teachers. Little by little, the growing number of qualified teachers made this organisation of studies possible. What did this last category correspond to? Alexander said nothing about it. In fact, the three founders of the institute were the first to teach the course. Abraham began to teach when the polyclinic opened in the spring of 1920. He continued up until June 1925, focusing his teaching on the presentation of the fundamental concepts of psychoanalysis. In 1923, he shared his course on neuroses with Hélène Deutsch, who came from Vienna as a guest. After this date, Abraham put the accent on the question of character development, on psychoanalysis of mental disorders, on the psychoanalytic theory of crime, and on the neuroses of the digestive system. Eitingon taught in Berlin continuously from 1921 to 1926; he also often shared his course with Simmel and Radó. His first course in 1921, on therapy and polyclinic practice, was intended solely for physicians with appropriate preparatory training. Subsequently, his courses did not deal with very specific topics, but they were nevertheless intended for candidates at a fairly advanced stage of training. Eitingon undertook work on therapeutic practice – analysis under supervision – until the spring of 1930. Simmel offered a course on war neuroses from October 1920. In 1921, he talked to general practitioners about the psychoanalytic perspective. He then dealt with analytical technique and therapeutic practice. In 1927 and 1928, his teaching focused on character defects, drug addiction, perversions, narcissistic neuroses and the psychoses. At the beginning of 1930, his teaching at Tegel was reserved for analysts already in practice.

Karen Horney taught in Berlin from 1920. She proposed using her medical training to spot cases from medical consultations that would be better approached through psychoanalytic treatment. In the spring of 1926, she dealt with feminine sexuality, particularly frigidity. This course was mainly intended for gynaecologists and female doctors. From 1928 until 1930, her teaching emphasised analytical technique and therapeutics; it was intended for candidates in training as well as practicing analysts. Hans Liebermann, another medical doctor, taught a course in obsessive neurosis from October 1920. From 1925 onward, he emphasised the importance of psychoanalysis in medical practice. Hanns Sachs joined the teaching team in the autumn of 1920. He focused mainly on the application of psychoanalysis to the humanities, but he also dealt with transference and resistance in January and March 1923. From 1928 until 1929, Sachs lectured on the theory of drives. Carl Müller-Braunschweig, a psychiatrist who also had a doctorate in philosophy, underwent an analysis with Abraham and Sachs. He was appointed to teach at the institute from 1922. He offered introductory courses in psychoanalysis and later specialised in studying the relationship between psychoanalysis and anthropology. In 1925, Müller-Braunschweig gave a course on the philosophy of psychoanalysis. In 1928, he dealt with the problem of standards and values inside and outside of science. It is striking to note that Müller-Braunschweig had moved away considerably from the Freudian corpus after he was admitted to the executive committee of the IPA in 1925. Subsequently, his credentials as a teacher at the Berlin Institute secured him a post as provisional director of the committee of the Aryanised DPG under the Nazi regime. His colleague Felix Boehm, who was in analysis with Abraham, started teaching in Berlin at the beginning of 1923. He lectured on perversions, on psychoanalytic practice and on case histories. Like other teachers, Boehm presented an introductory course in psychoanalysis for general practitioners in 1929. Although Freud considered him to be quite insignificant, Boehm wanted to offer himself as the saviour of psychoanalysis under the Nazi regime. Like his colleague Müller-Braunschweig, his credentials as a teacher at the Berlin Institute gave him a certain prestige that he would use without scruple when the time came.

The range of topics covered by Radó in seven years of teaching is quite impressive. From January 1923, his teaching successively focused on the concept of the unconscious, on the different types of neuroses, on therapeutic practice and on the question of transference. Likewise, Radó discussed what the doctor should know about psychoanalysis, the Freudian theory of anxiety and the symptom, love life, sexual function and technical propaedeutics. He also commented on new publications in psychoanalysis and related fields. In 1928–1929, he was responsible for a technical symposium with Karen Horney. He then led another technical seminar with Alexander, Horney and Sachs. A member of the BPV since 1921, Franz Alexander began teaching at the Berlin Institute in the autumn of 1924. His teaching embraced many themes, including dream interpretation, the place of psychoanalysis in culture, the presentation in several parts of the theory of neuroses, the study of recent publications, sublimation and its pathologies and the theory of, as well as therapy for, homosexuality. From the spring of 1929 to the beginning of 1930, Alexander collaborated in the technical seminar with Horney, Radó and Sachs. During this same period, he led a working group on criminology with

Hugo Staub, who was a lawyer by training.[3] In addition, Siegfried Bernfeld and Otto Fenichel, both of whom were doctors, taught from 1926 onwards. Bernfeld's past as a student activist encouraged him to base his teaching on the contributions of psychoanalysis to pedagogical psychology. At the end of 1928, Bernfeld led a working group on analytical child and adolescent psychology in collaboration with Jenö Hárnik. For his part, Fenichel devoted his first seminar to the work of Abraham, who had died six months earlier. His next three courses were centred on the psychology of the ego with, among other themes, the study of the structure and the genesis of the ego; the ideal of the ego; narcissism; the relations between the ego, the id and the superego; the ego and the drives; anxiety; and relations between the ego and the symptom. From 1927 until 1930, Fenichel emphasised the patient histories written by Freud as well as the Freudian theory of neuroses. Like Radó, Hárnik came from Hungary. He was a lecturer at the institute from 1926. His course titles show a certain originality: an early course, in 1927, focused on research into sexuality and sexual knowledge in childhood and puberty. Hárnik then offered a course on psychoanalysis as an art of interpretation in 1928 and another on the meaning of religious conflicts for analytical therapy. He collaborated with Bernfeld in a working group on child and adolescent psychology from the last quarter of 1928 until the first half of 1929. In 1930, Hárnik taught the psychology of 'love life', using examples from analytical practice. Dr Harald Schultz-Hencke, of whom Freud was very wary, joined the teaching staff in 1927. The names of his courses were not much different from those of his colleagues. He gave a seminar on the ego and the id in 1928 and other courses on the interpretation of dreams, on the stories of Freud's cases and on neurotic inhibitions. Finally, we must also note the interest in the psychology of religion that led Theodor Reik to offer teaching on this subject at the end of 1928. Reik then led a seminar on the application of psychoanalysis to literature and art and, at the beginning of 1930, devoted a lesson to the love affair between Goethe and Friederike Brion.

There were also teachers with guest status such as Geza Roheim, who came from Budapest and offered a cycle of eight lectures on psychoanalysis and ethnology in 1922. But there was, above all, Anna Freud, who led a seminar on psychoanalytic technique in work with children between September and October 1929. Some instructors endeavoured to present the most complete picture possible of their discipline to the students. Sachs, for instance, strung together thirty courses on different subjects in the space of nine years. Radó, for his part, presented forty-seven courses on distinct themes, including several seminars centred on therapeutic practice and analytical technique, between January 1923 and January 1930. Simmel, who had been one of the founders of the Berlin Institute and also the inspiration for the application of psychoanalysis to war neuroses, was also a pioneer in education. He dealt with twenty-nine different subjects over nine years. But when Schloss Tegel opened its doors in April 1927, Simmel began to present the applications of psychoanalysis to new indications: character defects, drug addiction, narcissistic neuroses and the psychoses. In 1930, the management of the institute initiated a project to create a psychoanalytic research institute that would be based in a closed psychiatric ward. Simmel's training efforts were a first step in this direction.

The two years of study at the institute were divided into six trimesters. Alexander said that in their first year the students should learn about the empirical foundations of analytical therapy. In the second year, they learned the principles of psychoanalytic technique. Freud's texts on dreams and the five psychoanalytic cases were studied. An important place was always reserved for the 'Three Essays on the Theory of Sexuality'. The systematisation of the curriculum resulted, in fact, in a pronounced division between compulsory and optional courses. In the middle of 1926, education was divided into five categories: general, introductory, private, seminar-based and practical work. The distinction between compulsory courses for beginners and advanced students on the one hand and optional courses with seminars on the other was established from the start of the school year in 1927.

Two stages should be distinguished in the development of the theoretical training provided by the institute. The first version of the study programme, which was developed in the autumn of 1927 by Alexander, Müller-Braunschweig and Radó, was compulsory for candidates in training who wanted to complete a full course that would include practice. This project was discussed by the teaching committee. This new programme of studies was added to the existing course programme at the beginning of 1928. The new programme subsequently evolved, and the emphasis was placed on practical work and seminars. The desire to systematise the theoretical curriculum was therefore introduced in Berlin following the debates on lay analysis in the summer of 1927. In its first version, 'The compulsory curriculum for complete training including practice' was divided into three parts: didactic analysis, compulsory theoretical courses and subsequent training. The subsequent training was divided into two subsections that corresponded to the therapeutic practical work, or analysis under supervision, and to the technical seminar. The new 1929 guidelines, presented by Karen Horney, were a modification of the first version of the systematic study programme developed two years earlier by Alexander and his colleagues. For example, during the first trimester of 1930, students in the first year of training at the institute had to attend the compulsory introductory courses in psychoanalysis by Radó, Boehm's seminar on Freud and Bernfeld's course on infantile sexuality. Students in the second year of training had to take Sachs' course on analytic technique as well as the seminar Fenichel devoted to Freud's theoretical writings. Further therapeutic development was reserved for candidates in training. It also fell under the category of compulsory courses and included the technical seminar led by Alexander, Horney and Radó, as well as the work on therapeutic practice organised by Eitingon and a few others. Eight optional courses were offered at Tegel, including Simmel's, which was devoted to psychoanalytic therapy, questions of indications, prognosis and changes in methodology. There was also Hárnik's optional course on the psychology of love life, Reik's course on Goethe and Friederike Brion and Karen Horney's course on sexual biology for doctors. Radó took care of the evenings of talks devoted to new publications. Finally, there were the optional working groups. One, on pedagogy, was moderated by Bernfeld. The other, on criminology, was the result of joint work by Alexander and Staub.

Systematic planning was seen as a necessity from the moment when psychoanalysis had to respond to new scientific requirements. 'In psychoanalysis, as in all science, the concepts drawn from observations have started to live their Golem's existence,'[4] Alexander pointed out. Psychoanalysis itself became systematised according to rules intrinsic to science. To this was added the fact that Freudian psychoanalysis had been the subject of various lootings: 'Isolated facts, tendentiously taken at random, were generalised and became the basis of a flattened psychoanalytic theory where analytical discoveries were violated by theory based on new ideological and philosophical criteria.' Psychoanalysis, having become scientific, would be able to measure itself against the parallel schools whose argument rested on the exploitation of a single concept. To overcome these rival schools, Freudian psychoanalysis had to present itself as a synthetic and coherent system. The requirement of scientificity should make it possible to combat these competing societies on their own terrain, that is to say at the level of affinity to the system that psychoanalysis could not have professed at the experimental stage.

The more psychoanalysis was drawn to the side of science, the more it became medicalised. In order to modulate the requirements introduced for a training mainly focused on therapeutics, compulsory courses on the applications of psychoanalysis to the human sciences were introduced in order to compensate for the candidate doctors' lack of humanist culture: 'He who had a literary or human-sciences training has more empathy with the psychic life of others than someone who, with current medical training, has learned almost nothing of the psychic life of the sick or of psychology in general.' The problem was to find a sufficient number of psychoanalysts duly trained and well versed in the human sciences. Such teachers could not be recruited from analysts with prior medical training. On the other hand, there was an additional step to take on the side of organic medicine. This path was, moreover, that of Simmel when he welcomed patients suffering from organic pathologies to his psychoanalytic hospital. In other words, the field of psychosomatics was a perspective that seemed to be in urgent need of development. It seemed logical to Alexander that research in psychoanalysis needed scientifically trained people. The therapist of the future must have received equivalent education in biology, medicine and psychoanalysis. The medically trained analyst embodied the ideal type of the analyst of the future: 'This imagined ideal type is one that we try to realise in our candidates as much as it seems practically possible for us to do today.' The circle was now complete. The systematic curriculum emphasised therapy; candidates were mainly recruited from among doctors, but medical training was considered insufficient. It was therefore necessary to introduce compulsory courses in order to broaden the humanist culture of candidate doctors. The problem was that there were not enough lay analysts specialising in the human sciences and able to teach. In line with the expansion of psychoanalysis in Germany and the choices that were made concerning training prior to the establishment of the institute, the era of the cultivated analyst, the *gebildete Psychoanalytiker*, was moving further away.

The practical training at the polyclinic

After having completed the whole cycle of theoretical training, the candidate was admitted to the practical stage. This last step led the student to receive his or her first patients under the supervision of an experienced analyst. From the point of view of psychoanalytic practice, in fact, the didactic analysis imagined by Freud was not considered sufficient for the training of the psychoanalyst. Supervision was presented as an answer to the central problem of the teaching of psychoanalysis. The function of practice under supervision clearly offset the difficulty raised by the difference between a doctor's training and that of the psychoanalyst. Sándor Radó stressed that it was not possible to offer the beginner a training through sitting in on the private conversation between a psychoanalyst and his patient. In medicine, on the other hand, the student attended the master's operations and the student subsequently operated under the supervision of his master. Analytical teaching could not be modelled on this medical training where the disciple and his master worked together. It was necessary to invent a new type of training which was adapted to the specifics of the psychoanalytic method. As Radó pointed out, this was the central problem of teaching, a problem that the institute had been trying to solve for a decade through its careful work.[5]

Freud had encouraged Eitingon to institute didactic analysis as the preliminary stage in the training of the analyst. In Berlin, it was conceived as a kind of way of improving the future analyst's psychic apparatus for future use. The didactic analysis also served to enrich the pupil's personality, strengthening it in its structure. It made it possible to transmit what was not taught in books. More astonishingly, it provided the student with the opportunity to steal his analyst's technique. Identification with the analyst was by no means unrecognised. On the contrary, the way the analyst worked was seen as a useful model for the future analyst. There were, however, two difficulties in holding on to this process. The student in training could only know his own case. He had to go to the analytic literature to get the clinical knowledge he lacked. As a result, the beginnings of his practice could be very problematic. How could the novice avoid coming across a situation that was way beyond his knowledge? Hence the need for practical training, which allowed the beginner to familiarise himself with a sufficient variety of situations. Supervision formed a natural counterpart to the candidate's didactic analysis; it was a protective measure because the management of the institute was already selecting suitable cases for the students. The important point was the emphasis placed on the learning of psychoanalysis as a technique, firstly through didactic analysis and then under supervision:

> The candidate acquires practical knowledge of the technique during the didactic analysis and must then apply it in a new situation that makes him pass from the passive role of the analysand to the active role of the analyst.[6]

As a result, supervision was introduced in Berlin as an indirect assistance and monitoring process. It was also a pedagogical supplement that made it possible to teach students technical elements that they had not acquired during their didactic analysis. Trainees were required to report regularly to the director of the institute on the treatments for which they were responsible. Reviews were organised between the director and the trainee. Sometimes it happened that the patient was invited. With the increase in the number of trainees, the director entrusted the function of supervisor to other teachers of the institute.

The technical seminar made up the second part of the practical course. The reference to medicine again appeared in Radó's writing: 'The analyst studies the individual case with a care that one cannot ordinarily imagine in medicine.' However, such study was so time-consuming that it only applied to a small number of cases. The presentations given by the students to the technical seminar each week allowed the students to familiarise themselves with a diverse series of clinical cases. The indication and structure of the case as well as the technical process used during the treatment were studied. Two modifications were introduced after a while. Indeed, given the influx of trainees, the technical seminar was divided into autonomous working groups. Similarly, participation in the technical seminar became limited; it was not to exceed the time of the actual training. Once the training course had been completed, the novice analyst was admitted to participate in the scientific sessions of the DPG.

Gregory Zilboorg, an American student who came to train in Berlin, was surprised by the modesty of the means initially used:

> It is disconcerting and it seems unbelievable that an institute which conducts more than a hundred analyses has only six consulting rooms, one of which belongs to the director and another to the doctor on duty. Is it not also very surprising that an old-fashioned, portable typewriter, such as one would not see in any decent office in America, and the work of a part-time secretary alone should be sufficient to carry out correspondence, registration, lists,

> etc.? Is it not also surprising that such an Institute continues to operate without an official budget or even a bank account? One wonders with amazement how it is possible to provide, quantitatively, so much work with such an imperfect device.[7]

If the Berliners managed to organise themselves so that they were able to treat and train a significant number of people during the first decade of the institute's existence, this testimony of an American introduces the nuance according to which the institution, such as it was, operated without much technical support. Zilboorg's list of an old typewriter, six consulting rooms, two of which were reserved for management, no specific budget, and minimal accounting suggests that the framework for analytic practice was supported far beyond its material means.

Despite the very positive impression that emerged from the original report, the Berlin Institute experienced a rapid decline in the early 1930s. This decline was linked to the fall from grace of its founder and to social and political upheavals. Everything happened fairly quickly. The Wall Street Crash caused the Eitingon companies to fail. Also, the management of the IPA, along with Freud himself, criticised Eitingon for his lack of skill in managing the Verlag. Eitingon complained, at the time, that the Berlin Institute was losing people. Between the time of the original report and 1932, four of the main members of the institute decided to settle abroad. Alexander, Radó, Sachs and Horney left Germany for America, where the new training institutes were beginning to operate. Radó's departure in particular shook Eitingon. Radó was a recognised and valued teacher at the institute, but he was also the editor of the *Zeitschrift* and *Imago*. Freud resolutely refused to replace Radó with Fenichel, who had been his assistant, as editor of the two journals because of his leftist political commitments. Eitingon attempted to force the issue, a move to which Freud responded by deciding to repatriate the offices of the two journals to Vienna. Eitingon then asked if he could drop the chairmanship of the IPA. Jones replaced him in this role from 1932 onwards.

Sigmund Freud's anxiety

By the beginning of the 1930s, Germany had been bled white. She had already experienced the humiliation of defeat, the fall of the imperial regime and the abortive Spartacist revolution in Berlin. The relative economic stabilisation that occurred in the mid-1920s was not enough to compensate for the effects of moral collapse. The possibility of an extension of the Bolshevik revolution to Central Europe had provoked violent reactions of fear and rejection; far-right groups were calling for a fight against the communists. The stock market crisis of 1929, the dramatic increase in unemployment and the rise of nationalist and anti-Semitic sentiments led to Field Marshal Paul von Hindenburg's politically irresponsible decision to invite Adolf Hitler, the leader of the National Socialist German Workers' Party (NSDAP), to take power. Hitler's accession to the post of Chancellor of the Reich on 30 January 1933 sounded the death knell for the great German intellectual enterprises. The programme of the Nazi Party, established on 24 February 1920, was declared the Basic Law of the German state.

Hitler did not even bother to modify or repeal the old Weimar constitution; instead, he organised power autocratically. The state had to submit to the will of its charismatic leader. According to Hitler's conception of the world, the state was nothing but a means of ensuring the dominant position of the Aryan race. The goal to be promoted was not the foundation of a monarchy or a republic; Hitler wanted to create a Germanic state that would favour a community of beings of the same species. To achieve this goal, the stain represented by the non-Aryan race had to be annihilated. 'The Reich as a state must include all Germans by giving them the task not only to collect and preserve the precious reserves of this people in its original racial elements, and must also lead them slowly and surely to a position of dominance,'[8] he wrote in *Mein Kampf.* In this vision of the world, no pact between Jews and Germans was possible. In 1924, he announced that the solution of the Jewish question would be the essential motif of his mission.

Is individual pathology likely to explain Hitler's anti-Jewish obsessions? One of the greatest authorities on Nazism believes that if there was a paranoid pathology involved, it was shared: it would relate not to an individual structure but to a social pathology of sects.[9] What is unfathomable is not Hitler's madness but the fact that a sect attained the status of a modern political party in such a dazzling fashion. How are we to understand the fact that a small Bavarian extremist party, all but written off after the failure of its attempted coup in 1923, managed to gain the favour of public opinion in record time? This would be the main puzzle for historians to solve. Historical works relating to Nazism fall into three broad categories of interpretation. The first category of interpretation makes Nazism a particular version of fascism. However, if one tries to draw comparisons between Hitler and Mussolini, nothing can explain the radicalism of the system spawned by Hitler, particularly the manifestations of racial theory that are specific to him. The second major category of interpretation – the Marxist one – holds that the Nazi state was the expression of a capitalism of exception. The ruling classes would have used Hitler to further their own interests. Here, too, materialist analysis comes up against the racial specificity of the National Socialist regime, which seems unjustifiable at the economic level. Since explanations geared to totalitarianism and economic organisation cannot account for the exceptional nature of the most appalling genocide of all time, the third major category of interpretation focuses on the personality of Hitler. Widely developed in those regions of the world committed to economic liberalism, this current has itself split into two opposing approaches. The Hitler-centric, or intentionalist, approach attributes all the evils concerned to Hitler's diabolical character. Developed primarily in the postwar years in the great Western democracies, the demonisation of Hitler absolved German society of any responsibility. The other path – referred to as structuralist or functionalist – is a reaction to the exaggeration of this intentionalist tendency. It follows the opposite path, trying to demonstrate that Hitler was merely an instrument of the system. In this case, the administrative apparatus is primarily responsible for the ideological drift. Hitler fades – he is only a minor actor in a tragic scenario. Currently, research is looking for a balance that would show that Hitler's exceptional position would not have been possible without the cult of personality that persuaded the masses to dedicate themselves to him. The déclassé individual, the failed artist who wandered the streets of Vienna before World War I, could not have experienced a meteoric rise without the veneration that the masses accorded to him because he presented himself as a saviour.[10] In January 1933, Hitler's accession to power was not seen as a change of cabinet but as the start of a new era. The Führer's will now became law. But, in turn, the subjugation of the masses to the will to destroy conveyed by the voice of the leader is an enigma that Freudian psychoanalysis is liable to shed light on through identification with the leader, the superego and the death drive.

The study that Wilhelm Reich published in 1933 on the mass psychology of fascism falls into the second category of interpretation. Indeed, Reich emphasised the reactionary aspirations of the classes that brought Hitler to the pinnacle of power. He focused on the sociological nature of National Socialist demagoguery. To understand how the masses were deceived, misled and subjected to psychotic influences by the Nazis, Reich identified the various levels of propaganda adapted to the social categories to which it was addressed. To gain the favour of industrial workers, the Nazis spoke to them of revolution. To seduce the petty bourgeoisie, which formed the basis of its electorate, they denounced the economic empire of the department stores that were competing with the small traders, the craftsmen and the small businesses. To attract the peasants, they defended small properties against large mechanised farms. To please employees and civil servants, the Nazis flattered them by declaring that they represented the pillar of the nation. Reich insisted that National Socialism was based above all on the disappointments and hopes of the petty bourgeoisie: the paternalist and capitalist model of domination represented, in his view, the petty bourgeois ideal.

German anti-Semitism was by no means a Nazi invention. Anti-Semitic legislation was developed by conservative officials in some ministries during the Weimar Republic. After World War I, the far-right conservatives continued relentlessly to demand the abolition of the emancipation achieved by German Jews in 1871. These officials later turned into zealous servants of the Third Reich. So the Nazis, when they came to power, drew their inspiration from previous legislative projects. However, the anti-Semitism that had spread since the end of the previous century was based on the premise of the biological inferiority of the Jewish race. Hitler's was different. His was a redemptive anti-Semitism that originated during the war and demanded warlike methods. As early as 1919, Hitler distinguished the emotive anti-Semitism of the pogroms from the 'reasoned' anti-Semitism that was to lead to a legal and methodical struggle to eliminate the Jews from the face of the earth. His conception of the world was apocalyptic, and his mission reconnected with that of Christ, who had had to fight against the Semites. For Hitler, the Jewish international was Marxist, and the ultimate danger came from the union of Jewish and Marxist elements. He wanted to purify the cradle of the German people immediately in order to protect them from the malevolent danger embodied by international Judaism. From then on, the Jews would be foreigners who could no longer claim German nationality. They simultaneously represented a monstrously powerful superhuman force and a subhuman factor that did not deserve to live.[11] By defending the German people against the Jews, Hitler was convinced that he was doing the Lord's work. And at that time, the Central European psychoanalytic elite was Jewish.

As early as the spring of 1933, Freud sensed that the Nazis would not spare the Jews of Europe and that they would attack freedom of thought: 'One cannot avoid seeing that persecution of the Jews and restriction of intellectual freedom are the only features of the Hitler programme that can be carried out. All the rest is weakness and utopianism.'[12] Like many of his contemporaries, however, Freud reasoned according to the first type of anti-Semitism, that of pogroms – which is to say the classical form. Like others at the time of National Socialism, Freud thought in terms of persecution, reduced activity, manifestations of hostility, emotive anti-Semitism. When Hitler became chancellor, who would have thought that 'reasoned' anti-Semitism would be realised in its ultimate form a few years later? The grip that the latter had on the masses was described in the mid-1930s by Brecht.

> Behold several million electors.
> One hundred per cent in all sectors
> Have asked to be led by the nose.
> They didn't get real bread and butter
> They didn't get warm coats or fodder
> They did get the leader they chose.[13]

But no one could have foreseen the radicalisation of Nazi politics that took place from 1938 onwards. As Friedländer points out, by the end of 1933 millions of people in Germany were perfectly aware that the new National Socialist regime had launched a policy of discrimination and exclusion against its Jewish citizens.

> It may have been impossible for most people, Jewish or otherwise, to clearly understand the goals and limits of this course of action. There was

> anxiety among the Jews in Germany, but no panic, no general feeling of imminent danger.[14]

Freud, who saw things unfolding from Austria, was anxious but did not panic. Not yet.

Like so many others, Freud initially assumed that Austrian Jews would be protected by the relevant provisions of the Treaty of Versailles. Like his fellow citizens, he also placed his hopes in Mussolini's Italy. At the time, in Austria, he thought that Catholicism would be the main bulwark against Nazism. Some speculated that the National Socialists would not stay in power for long, that it would only be a matter of months before the conservatives would take up the reins of power again by means of a coup d'état. The German Jewish philosopher Martin Buber calculated, for example, that the balance of forces would be overturned, that the Nazis would lose out to the conservatives, and that the conservatives would find it useful to have the Nazis fight the proletariat, and this in turn would divide the Nazi party and neutralise them. Or the Nazis might leave the government despite the fact that the balance of power in the Reichstag was favourable to them, as Martin Buber noted in February 1933:

> Anti-Semitic legislation would be possible only if the balance of power shifted in favour of the National Socialists, but, as I have said above, this is hardly to be expected. Jew-baiting is only possible during the interval between the National Socialists' leaving the government and the proclamation of a state of emergency.[15]

It occurred to Freud, though not to any great extent, to cling to the hopes aroused by the League of Nations, to the Treaty of Versailles, to the opinion that the Austrian Nazis would never be as brutal as their German counterparts, to the hope that they would be kept respectable by their enforced alliance with other rightwing parties. At that time, Freud decided to stay in Vienna and to keep the Berlin Institute open.

Up until the summer of 1933, Freud used the first person plural to reassure himself and to calm those who feared for his life:

> That will not be an agreeable state of affairs and will not make life pleasant for us Jews, but we all think that legal emergency declarations are impossible in Austria [...] Here legalised persecution of the Jews would immediately result in the intervention of the League of Nations [...] In such a way we lull ourselves into – relative – security.[16]

In the same letter, Freud used the first person singular to conclude: 'In any case, I am resolved not to budge an inch.' Therefore, the 'we' was referring to the Jews of Austria, to public opinion, to the information conveyed by the newspapers, while the 'I' allowed him to affirm his decision to stay put because the threat had not been proven. But also, conversely, it was in the first person that Freud confided his presentiment of the disaster to come:

> The world is turning into an enormous prison. Germany is the worst cell. What will happen in the Austrian cell is quite uncertain. I predict a paradoxical surprise in Germany. They began with Bolshevism as their deadly enemy, and they will end with something indistinguishable from it – except perhaps that Bolshevism, after all, adopted revolutionary ideals, whereas those of Hitlerism are purely mediaeval and reactionary. This world seems to me to have lost its vitality and to be doomed to perdition.[17]

When he wrote this, in June 1933, Freud was seventy-seven years old; he had endured five surgeries the previous year and no longer made much of his fears for his life. If he stayed in Vienna, it would not be only because he was old and sick. Freud told Ferenczi that even when he was young and in good health, he would have acted similarly for personal reasons. His body was worn out and sick, but his will was intact. Freud did not panic; he was someone who had great self-control, who was in full command of his emotions. In the first months after the Nazis came to power, it was not impossible that Freud would have toyed with the idea of dying as a martyr. However, he rejected this prospect, which was not in keeping with his more fervent desire to secure the posterity of psychoanalysis. In truth, Freud could not disappear as a martyr in Vienna. Politically speaking, it would have been a disaster and the negation of his lifelong struggle for the future of psychoanalysis. However, what worried him a lot was the future of his children and grandchildren. The only time he was ever seen crying was on the day he greeted his daughter shortly after her interrogation by the Gestapo. Her arrest prompted his decision to leave Austria.

As the weeks passed, Freud saw civilisation sinking into chaos. But as he sensed the worst and became anxious, Jones managed to distract him and reassure him. Jones explained that things weren't so grave, that there would be many solutions and that people were exaggerating what was going on in Germany. For example, when Freud learned of the appointment of a 'wild' psychoanalyst as a lecturer in psychotherapy at the University of Berlin in July 1933, the news alarmed him greatly. It was, for him, a bad omen. Hans von Hattingberg, a former member of the WPV, was commissioned by Dr Matthias Göring to develop a German 'soul medicine' (*Deutsche Seelenheilkunde*). According to Freud, von Hattingberg was 'an aristocrat, Aryan, fool, blockhead and a bad sort, in other words in every respect the right man for the post'.[18] For his part, Jung had offered himself as 'Führer of Souls' (*Seelenführer*), and he had caught the attention of the Nazis by making a distinction between Germanic psychology and Jewish psychology. At the beginning of the following year, as director of the *Zentralblatt für Psychotherapie*, Jung prevented the publication of the course programme of the Berlin Institute. 'According to this first announcement, the programme borders on the limits of the inadmissible,'[19] said Nazi neurologist Walter Cimbal. Matthias Göring therefore considered it urgent to send an envoy to monitor the lectures that were being given at the institute. Beginning in the summer of 1934, Göring would prevent Müller-Braunschweig from acting as he pleased with respect to the training of therapists. In November 1939, Jung opposed the publication of a portrait of Sigmund Freud in the *Zentralblatt*. Freud was right – von Hattingberg's promotion to professor of psychotherapy was a very bad omen. Von Hattingberg was one of those eclectic analysts who were favoured by the Nazis. The Nazis recognised them as the true representatives of psychoanalysis because they had succeeded in extracting it from the alleged ruts of its orthodoxy. The appointment of von Hattingberg to a position at the University of Berlin was one of the first signs of the crushing of Freudian psychoanalysis by a new form of psychotherapy. 'I could hardly believe my ears when I learned that, in Berlin, von Hattingberg was in charge of the PSA course at the university. I never trusted him. This was the post that should one day have belonged to Abraham,' Lou Andréas-Salomé lamented.[20]

Unlike Freud, Jones saw many advantages to the Nazi party's appointment of the buffoon, since von Hattingberg considered himself a psychoanalyst. If he had indeed worked with the Freudians in the early 1920s, he had distinguished himself by wanting to unify everything that claimed to be psychoanalysis. Von Hattingberg had opened his own psychotherapy clinic at St. Gertrude's Hospital in Berlin in 1932. Jones believed that his appointment as lecturer at the University of Berlin would prevent a ban on psychoanalysis in Germany. 'There will of course be a tendency to dilute it with other material, and it is there that we shall have to fight,' he warned.[21] At the same time, Felix Boehm, a non-Jewish analyst at the Berlin Institute, wrote to him that he wanted to get ahead of the 'synchronisation' (*Gleichschaltung*) desired by the authorities. Even if there were many reasons to be wary of Boehm, Jones still wanted to explore the situation. Consequently, in his capacity as president of the IPA, Jones agreed to meet Boehm in the autumn of 1933 in The Hague in the presence of the Dutchman Johan van Ophuijsen, who was the treasurer of the IPA. This episode demonstrates the way in which Jones sought to allay Freud's anxiety. The latter was, of course, greatly alarmed, but Jones saw the appointment of von Hattingberg as an event that was not entirely bad because it would allow psychoanalytic activities to continue. One wonders, however, if there really was any reason to rejoice in the fact that a 'blockhead and a bad sort' was to have power of life and death over psychoanalysis. When Jones reassured Freud about von Hattingberg's appointment, he was also trying to persuade him that the blow to the activities of the German psychoanalytic movement was greatly exaggerated.

The political context changed rapidly. Two laws in particular had immediate repercussions. The first law of 24 March 1933 – also known as the Full

Powers or Enabling Act (*Ermächtigungsgesetz*) – was intended to alleviate the plight of the people and the state. It gave Hitler the legal right to promulgate laws without reference to parliament and permitted the legal prosecution of all political opponents of the far right. After the Reichstag fire on 27 February 1933, nearly 10,000 members and sympathisers of the KPD were arrested and interned in concentration camps, including the camp at Dachau, which opened in March 1933. The second law of 7 April 1933 – relating to the restoration of the civil service (*Gesetz zur Wiederherstellung des Berufsbeamtentums*), concerned the reinstatement of the appointment of civil servants. It was a question of setting up a legal framework that would make it possible to eliminate communists, Social Democrats and Jews from the civil service in order to have a bureaucracy that would not object to the impending political programme. This law applied to two million civil servants and included an Aryan paragraph. Paragraph 3 stipulated that officials of non-Aryan descent should be dismissed. The implementing decree, which was promulgated on 11 April, indicated what was to be understood by 'non-Aryan': 'Anyone from non-Aryan parents or grandparents, especially Jews. It only takes one parent or non-Aryan grandparent.'[22] This was the first time since 1871, when the emancipation of Germany's Jews became law, that a decree had reintroduced the concept of officially stripping the nation's Jews of their rights.

One measure particularly affected Jewish analysts who were doctors. Since 1 September 1924, the Preussischen Gebührenordnung – the state body that fixed the prices of medical care – had given its consent for health insurance funds to cover analytic sessions billed by doctors. Competition had in fact been established between a small number of associations, each of which claimed to represent authentic psychoanalysis. The DPG's members contested this competition and wanted to distinguish themselves from other groups; the fight against wild analysts also had a financial component.[23] On 22 April 1933, the health insurance funds broke their contracts with Jewish doctors. This moment corresponded to a fracture because, in many cases, the analytical cures were indirectly financed by the state.[24] Two years later, the Nuremberg Laws would define Jews by blood, which would imply a strict separation between Aryan and non-Aryan practitioners. In 1938, the granting of the diploma of 'end of studies' to the Jewish doctors would be prohibited.

The propaganda that psychoanalysis was a Jewish science that glorified the vilest instincts was disseminated through the newspapers. Psychotherapy was understood differently because it could serve the interests of the German people. Martin Staemmler, referring doctor for the NSDAP's Office of Racial Policy, published an article on the subject of Judaism in medicine in the summer of 1933. This illustrious defender of Hitler's anti-smoking policy accepted the principle of the action of unconscious forces while vehemently denying their sexual origin:

> Freudian psychoanalysis constitutes a typical example of the internal disharmony of the life of the soul between Jews and Germans. That

> certain forms of suffering and certain disorders of the body are to be related to psychic disorders of which the patient himself most often has no idea, that processes in the subconscious are able to exert their harmful influence on the organic functions, that it is necessary to know these complexes and to endeavour to dismiss them – all of this must be fully approved. But that all these subconscious disorders are of a sexual nature, that everything inevitably arises from the sphere of sexuality, this is something foreign to the German and leads him down a path that brings him no healing. And when we go even further and bring into the sexual sphere each movement of the mind and each instance of misconduct by a child, and when, as the paediatrician of Chemnitz, Oxenius, recently wrote, the human being, for the psychoanalyst, is nothing more than a sexual organ around which the body vegetates, so we must have the courage to refuse these interpretations of the German soul and to say to these gentlemen of Freud's entourage that they must only undertake their psychological experimentation on human material belonging to their own race.[25]

According to Staemmler, the psychoanalysts were not the most harmful; the worst allies of the evil forces were the scientific defenders of homosexuality, sexologists and all those who attacked the values of female virginity and the monogamous family. A sexologist like Magnus Hirschfeld, who defended the idea of the innate nature of homosexuality and called for the repeal of the paragraph of the penal code that condemned homosexuals, would undoubtedly destroy the German family. These dangerous reformers were criticised for encouraging the Germans to limit their birth rate at a time when the Nazis were eager to combat its decline. For doctors like Staemmler, the advice centres set up by the World League for Sexual Reform would prevent the German people from multiplying. Hirschfeld, who in 1908 participated with Abraham in the creation of the first Berlin psychoanalytic association, had founded the Institute of Sex Research in Berlin in 1919. On 6 May 1933, it was closed by the Nazis. The books in the library were burned, along with those of Freud, in the Opernplatz (now Bebelplatz) four days later.

In 1929, having drawn practical conclusions from his research on the social origin of neuroses, Wilhelm Reich had undertaken to bring together doctors and nurses in Vienna. With his team, he had crisscrossed the city's poorer suburbs in a bus and created a free sexual hygiene clinic for information and prevention. After settling in Berlin a year later, he founded an association for proletarian sexual politics, known as Sexpol, which brought together sexologists and communists. This association, which claimed up to 40,000 members, inevitably antagonised the Nazis. Excluded from the Communist Party because of his ideas concerning sexual education, much disliked by Freud (who thought him mad) and viewed by the members of the institute as a threat at the heart of the psychoanalytic movement, Reich represented a digest of all the subversive ideas of the time. The publication in Berlin of his book on the mass psychology of fascism did not help. From the earliest days of the NSDAP's accession to power, Reich was in the Nazi regime's cross-hairs. For the Nazis, a Jewish doctor, a Communist and an advocate of sexual freedom was truly the devil incarnate. In the spring of 1933, Max Eitingon asked Reich not to go to the premises of the Berlin Institute because he risked being arrested there. He also advised Freud not to expel him. Unable to prevent this, Eitingon insisted, along with his colleagues, that Reich's expulsion should take place only after he himself left Germany in late 1933, but without effect. Boehm, who considered himself in possession of a mandate from Freud to represent psychoanalysis in Germany – but only on the condition that he would expel Reich – defended himself from having carried out this expulsion insofar as, at the time when the exclusion of Reich from the DPG was decided, in July 1933, Eitingon had not yet resigned from his post as director of the institute and of the society. Boehm always denied that he had been anything other than an administrator. He had had no responsibility at the time of the events concerned. After the war, at the Amsterdam Congress, he hinted that he had been a scapegoat. For a while, he played the part of the victim.

Freud sensed that the persecution of the Jews and that of knowledge would be linked. If the Nazis indeed considered psychoanalysis to be 'Judeo-Marxist junk', it was also a matter of erasing in the real the furrows traced by Freudianism because the latter was itself an eminent creation of thought. In order for identification with the totalitarian One to be realised, it was necessary to secure the rejection of thought. One no longer had to think about the internal division of man: one had to respond to the call of the superegoic imperative. The quest for unity, the exhilaration aroused by the German people's call for indivisibility behind their supreme leader – these were the slogans chanted by the far right. It was a question of harnessing the country's young people, who had been helpless since the dawn of the century and who, 'in [their] incompleteness [*Halbheit*] felt good and ardently desired a harmonious and total humanity'. And this was done to the tune of 'the song of the whole man, complete in itself [*in sich geschlossen*]'.[26] Faced with this unreasonable exaltation of the One, the conspicuously political significance of the Freudian discovery had to be eradicated at all costs. Besides, hadn't Freud discovered the wellspring capable of welding crowds together in the same ideal? Hadn't he written that the original father is the ideal of the crowd, which dominates the ego instead of the ego ideal, and that the masses seek their own submission to a dreaded and authoritarian father figure?[27] The breakdown into three psychic instances and the notion that the deepest motives for acts and thoughts have an origin that escapes us were ideas the Nazis found intolerable. More than the sexual origin of symptoms, the division of the subject introduced by the hypothesis of the unconscious was, in the eyes of the Nazis, an objection to the alleged unity of the new German man.

The guardianship of psychoanalysis

Freud later explained that the writing of *Moses and Monotheism* was undertaken during two distinct periods: the first in Vienna (from 30 September 1934), the second in England. He confessed that he was not comfortable with this process, which had forced him to make certain repetitions. The German annexation of Austria in 1938 – which he had not been expecting – had persuaded him to leave his homeland. These linked events at least had the merit of freeing him from the concern of provoking a ban on psychoanalysis in England, a place where it was still tolerated, by publishing his entire book. He questioned the reasons for anti-Semitism, showing that Christian dislike of the Jews was the result of displacement. Before Christianity had been forced upon them by decree of the Emperor Constantine, the people of the Roman Empire had been largely polytheistic, and hated monotheistic religion. This hatred was now directed at the Jews. Freud added that, from this point of view, the Christians were in fact 'ill-baptised'.[28]

Consequently, contrary to what Jacoby asserts, the political Freudians (by which Jacoby means the politically committed analysts on the left) were not the only ones concerned with social phenomena. Until the end of his life, Freud was interested in the psychology of the masses, starting from the question of the transmission of the murder of the primitive father down the centuries. The biologists of Freud's time refused to give this perspective any consideration, but Freud persisted with the hypothesis of the conservation of trace memory from the archaic heritage: humans have always known that they once possessed a primitive father and that they put him to death. The murder of Moses is only a repeat of the inaugural murder of this primitive father, and the killing of Christ is a later avatar.

> The poor Jewish people, who with their habitual stubbornness continued to disavow the father's murder, atoned heavily for it in the course of time. They were constantly met with the reproach "You killed our God!" And this reproach is true, if it is correctly translated,

Freud wrote.[29] This reproach was not the only explanation. Anti-Semitism was based on three motives: jealousy of the chosen people; circumcision, which referred to castration; and the fact that anti-Semitism was basically anti-Christian. So it was hardly surprising that the National Socialist revolution was hostile both to Judaism and to Christianity, given the intimacy of the connection between these two monotheisms. Contrary to what Freud himself had professed in the past, religion is not just an illusion; it is based on historical truth. He did not need the notion of the collective unconscious that was so dear to Jung because 'The content of the unconscious, indeed, is in any case a collective, universal property of mankind'.[30] Freud established a connection between this collective and hereditary patrimony and the existence of the symbol that arose from the time when language development in children took place without their having to be instructed. Original murder is written at the heart of the language – it is transmitted from generation to generation with the language and it constitutes the trauma or the central hole. Only a religious ecstasy is capable of reviving the intensity of what the child experienced with regard to the father – namely, the certainty of his irresistible power and the willingness to submit entirely to his will. This is the reason why the meeting with the long-awaited being is overwhelming, as evidenced by the story of the giving of the law on Mount Sinai. The return of the God-Father can only be experienced through ecstasy. For Freud, the ecstatic welcome, the abandonment of all judgement and the exhilaration of submission to a single being was no mystery. Nostalgia for the father justified contemporary anti-Semitism and the fanatical enthusiasm of the masses for the one who presented himself as the supreme guide of the German people.

For his part, Hitler had his own view of why the masses behaved as they did. He believed that they had a feminine mentality, that they were governed by the emotional dimension. The feminine mentality of crowds was already to be found in Le Bon, for whom the simplicity and exaggeration of crowds meant that they knew neither doubt nor uncertainty, which were supposedly feminine qualities: 'Like women, they immediately go to extremes,' he suggested.[31] Had Hitler read Le Bon's book? *The Psychology of Crowds*, to which Freud referred in his 1921 study, had been translated into German in 1912. If this book was not listed as having belonged to Hitler's personal library, Le Bon's description of exaggeration and simplicity of feelings was also found in the Führer. Hitler believed that the people needed simple and sketchy points of reference, such as positive and negative, love and hate, justice and injustice, truth and falsehood. No half-mixtures, no half-tone nuances, no subtle words.

In March 1933, Freud explained that the wave of panic provoked by the expansion of the Nazi movement into Austria was also being felt in Vienna, but he doubted that events like those unfolding in Berlin could be duplicated in his hometown:

> I have always explained that on no account would I leave Vienna – my age is the pretext. I would like to give you this principle: no provocation, but even less concessions. They will not be able to destroy psychoanalysis, and [we as individuals] are of less importance.[32]

Max Eitingon replied that, for his part, he would stay until the last moment to close the Berlin Institute. Besides, he would only be forced to do so. Concerning the closure of the Berlin Institute, Eitingon and Freud disagreed. Eitingon wanted to stay put in order to close the Institute, and he refused to countenance the possibility of temporarily handing over its management while waiting for better days. Freud wanted to stay in Vienna at any cost to end his days there. He refused to contemplate going into exile and had no intention of abandoning the language in which psychoanalysis was created. He felt that his departure from Vienna would be interpreted as signalling the collapse of the analytic movement. Similarly, the closure of the Berlin Institute seemed to him not to be in the general interest of psychoanalysis. At the time of the first anti-Semitic measures in Germany, Freud recommended staying put. His position was to hold on just until the last moment, just until the humanly acceptable limit. Heroism was not the only reason for his insistence. Freud speculated that if the ship were to be abandoned, his enemies would take it by storm. To leave Berlin would be to leave the field open to Adlerians, Jungians and psychotherapists of all stripes, whose standard profile corresponded to that – which he hated – of Harald Schultz-Hencke, whom Freud distrusted more than anyone. Schultz-Hencke had been in analysis with Radó and had taught at the Berlin Institute in 1927–1928. He was later banned from teaching because of his criticism of the libido theory and his attempt to synthesise Freudian psychoanalysis with the theories of Adler and Jung. Freud's fear of Schultz-Hencke was not entirely unfounded, except that the poison would actually be administered from the inside. It would come from the cravenness and opportunism of the current members of the Institute.

In the 1930s, Berlin and Vienna were the symbols of the creation of psychoanalysis and its insertion in the world. For this reason alone, Freud could not bring himself to abandon the two cities. Was he really convinced, as he wrote to Jones, that psychoanalysis could no longer be destroyed? The lesson of 1932 on the *Weltanschauung*[33] was particularly clear on one point: psychoanalysis does not need to create its vision of the world because it is part of science, because it is included in it. As a science, could psychoanalysis be safe from the destruction of democratic structures? This strategy, if it was that of Freud, could only cause disappointments insofar as the Nazis wanted to develop their pseudoscience of the German man. The National Socialist regime was bathed in a strange atmosphere of scientificity. Its ideology was based on a logic of exclusion stemming from the notion of race that scientific discourse had helped to produce, and we have often mentioned the social Darwinism of National Socialism insofar as hereditary biology made it possible to shore up the foundation of racial characteristics.

Since science cannot be reduced to biology, psychology, too, had to serve the recovery and expansion of the German people. Therapists were expected to use their skills to prepare people's spirits by strengthening them. Because the Nazis believed in technology, senior dignitaries became interested in the fields of corporate psychology and military skills. They allowed psychoanalysis to continue because they viewed it as one healing technique among others. They not only accepted its retention as a branch of psychotherapy; they also planned to get their hands on the primary instrument of its influence. The Berlin Polyclinic aroused jealousies. Once it had been Aryanised, what would prevent analytic therapy from participating in the national recovery effort? Couldn't such a project be part of a continuity given the fact that practitioners had been trying to unify the Freudian, Adlerian and Jungian currents in a single theory for several years? To achieve that, one would merely have to delete the name of Freud and not speak all the time about sexuality or the Oedipus complex!

In retrospect, such a calculation seems improbable and incoherent to us. However, in this moment of collective madness, the possibility was indeed envisaged – and, most confusingly, there were German analysts who were willing to take this route. Psychotherapy, far from experiencing a decline under National Socialism, experienced significant growth and even – according to some historians – unequalled development. Hitler wanted to campaign for the health of the people, and that required operational health services. From this perspective, the know-how of psychotherapists and psychologists was to help improve the efficiency and morale of the Germans. In his book devoted to psychotherapy during the Third Reich, Geoffrey Cocks notes that the advent of Hitler eliminated Berlin and Vienna as centres of psychoanalysis to the advantage of London and New York, but his research led him to relativise the official version, according to which German psychoanalysis would not have survived Nazism. This official version is believed to be related to the negligence of Freud's hagiographic psychoanalysts, who described a rejection of psychoanalysis on the part of medical circles before 1933 and the widespread oppression of its practitioners after that date. However, according to Cocks, the Nazis failed to destroy the practice of psychoanalysis in Germany; the discipline actually survived as a method within the medical profession: 'In a divided and cracked Reich that actually favoured the growth of psychotherapy in general, psychoanalysis presents us with a particularly spectacular example of survival.'[34]

Without going into both the complex history of the professionalisation of psychotherapy before, during and after the advent of Hitler and the profession's conflictual relationship with the representatives of academic psychiatry, we must bear in mind the fact that the survival of psychoanalysis took place at the cost of subjugation and submission. Without having been favoured by the Nazis, *psychoanalysis was tolerated on condition that it be placed under guardianship by psychotherapy.* In reality, it was the independence of psychoanalysis that was problematic – hence this desire of the representative of the psychotherapists who had rallied to National Socialism to reach out to the Aryan analysts of the Berlin Institute in order to break their irksome isolation. Even though he distrusted the Freudians, Matthias Göring did not want to discard anyone: 'We absolutely must give the old psychoanalysts the opportunity to say if they can bring something to the new state,'[35] he said in September 1933. In December of the same year, Fritz Künkel, a Berlin neurologist, sent Professor Göring a memo in which he indicated that the regrouping of the different schools was under way, that the Jungians, the School of Applied Characterology and Schultz's school of autogenous treatment would not pose any problem. 'The real problem child is and continues to be psychoanalysis. The regulations must aim to make the psychoanalysts renounce their splendid isolation. I would gladly say that this view is "softening the crust of schools",'[36] said Künkel.

If the psychoanalysts had to be persecuted because they were Jewish, Boehm related how he managed to convince the authorities that psychoanalysis was neither Jewish nor Marxist and that it could serve the objectives of the Third Reich. However, if the authorities agreed to keep psychoanalysis under guardianship, it was not only because of Boehm's activism. The threat of a ban was undoubtedly used to panic people and, therefore, to manoeuvre, spur and steer things in the direction desired. The spectre of a ban was used primarily to intimidate. It is not likely that Boehm, either alone or with the support of his other colleague, succeeded in changing the course of the Nazi administration's ban on psychoanalysis. To believe that would be to overestimate his influence. It would be fairer to suggest that the steps taken by Boehm with respect to the Ministry of the Interior and the Prefecture met with a favourable reception because a decision had already been made higher up. Boehm certainly struggled to find his way through the administrative labyrinth, but it was necessary that the wish to recover the know-how of the clinicians and the psychoanalytic polyclinic had to be present. The rescue argument is therefore not very convincing; it would be fairer to claim that Aryan analysts could count on a certain amount of protection in exchange for toeing the line. Moreover, this strategy was mentioned relatively early on – from September 1933, Müller-Braunschweig and Boehm indicated that instead of deciding to wait and see, they had approached the authorities in order to obtain the protection of psychoanalysis. Also, in the 1932–1934 activity report of the Berlin Institute, it was stated that the requests for treatment at the polyclinic remained constant; this was an encouraging sign of how deeply entrenched public confidence in the efficacy of therapy had become. During this same period, the number of Jewish teachers who had left Berlin had been more or less offset by the recruitment of Aryan members. Furthermore, while the drop in the number of patients and candidates in training had more or less stabilised, the number of people attending lectures had fallen considerably. But nothing was said about it. Müller-Braunschweig insisted, on the contrary, that the situation of psychoanalysis in Germany, apparently conducive to causing multiple tensions, had, on the contrary, had a beneficial effect. According to him, this resulted in closer ties – that is to say, solidarity – between the members of the DPG. It was then a question of getting closer to the psychotherapeutic movement. Thus, the participation of DPG analysts in the Nauheim psychotherapy congress in May 1934 was approved unanimously.

As early as April 1933, Kretschmer had resigned from the presidency of the General Society of Psychotherapeutic Medicine. Jung, its vice president since 1930, took over the presidency in June. The psychotherapists had chosen

Matthias Göring as Führer. He was the eldest member of the oldest branch of the Göring family in Westphalia, from which his cousin Hermann Göring was descended. Matthias's father had helped Hermann financially after World War I. Under the Third Reich, cousin Hermann's feelings for his family kept pace with his ever-increasing power; he watched and protected his loved ones a lot. As the eldest in the family's oldest branch, Matthias had occupied the place of honour at Hermann Göring's wedding banquet. These family ties opened the doors of the Bavarian Ministries of Culture, Education and the Interior to the psychotherapists around Matthias Göring. On 15 September 1933, this enabled them to create a new German section of their association under the name of the German General Medical Society for Psychotherapy (Deutsche Allgemeine Ärztliche Gesellschaft für Psychotherapie, or DAÄGP). In the autumn of 1933, there were, therefore, two German psychotherapy associations. Jung was the president of the international section, the General Society of Psychotherapeutic Medicine. Matthias Göring headed the German section, the German General Psychotherapy Society.

Matthias Göring was a neuropsychiatrist and a doctor of law. He had worked as an assistant at Kraepelin's clinic and converted to psychotherapy. His good nature and his white beard earned him the nickname of Papy Göring, or Santa Claus. Matthias Göring was not an imposing figure; he was a shy man who stuttered, 'a patriot of the old school, a member of the national veterans' organisation, the Stahlhelm, and a convinced Lutheran pietist'.[37] He always had his Bible with him. His main objection to psychoanalysis was the fact that the patient could not see the analyst, who was sitting behind him. This arrangement, he felt, was an obstacle to an honest, Christian symposium – an eye-to-eye encounter between the two protagonists. Despite his harmless appearance, the mere mention of his name was enough to silence the administration's doubts or threats. By pronouncing the magic name of Göring, the doubts faded, the doors opened and the psychotherapists placed under the protective wing of Papy Göring had access to significant material resources. As Cocks notes:

> Under Göring's guidance, psychotherapists could take an aggressive professional stance because they were assured of protection from their enemies, both among the Nazis and the doctors; they were also assured of the benefit of financial support for the development of their profession.[38]

As the psychotherapists around him sought ways to expand their actions, Matthias Göring was embarrassed about the prospect of taking over the leadership of the Berlin Institute. Boehm and Müller-Brauschweig, co-chair of the Berlin Institute since Eitingon's departure, met Matthias Göring in the presence of Herbert Linden, ministerial adviser for eugenics and race at the Ministry of the Interior.[39] It was Linden who suggested that they work together to create a new institute to accommodate the various branches of psychotherapy. Were Aryan analysts really backed into a corner by a Nazi doctor? Above all, they expressed the wish not to be ousted from the forthcoming training programme for psychotherapists. In August 1934, Müller-Braunschweig wrote to Jones that

> in view of the ongoing attempts by the Reich government to establish a college of Reich psychotherapists, we did not see fit to remain sidelined or inactive and let things develop without us. We did not want to give the impression that our activity had the least fear of daylight and we did not want to make a mystery of our conviction, which is that fourteen years of experience in the field of education and training, as well as our years – more numerous still – of scientific experiments, should allow us a say in my task of organising a Reich College of Psychotherapy and possibly founding an establishment of psychotherapists.[40]

Founded on 14 June 1936, the German Institute for Psychotherapy and Psychological Research, better known as the Göring Institute, was to fulfil three missions: research, training and education, and the management of polyclinics for people without resources. Representatives of three associations participated in its creation: the DPG, the C.G. Jung Society and the Applied Research Circle on Character. These three associations had the status of working groups. The analysts brought their library and their furniture as well as their skills. Until April 1937, the headquarters of the Göring Institute was located in the premises of the polyclinic, inaugurated in September 1928 by Eitingon and his team, at Wichmannstrasse 10. It then moved to Budapeststrasse 29. We must note that the programme of the Göring Institute was modelled on that drawn up by the founders of the Berlin Institute in 1920.

Matthias Göring's son Ernst Göring, who undertook a didactic analysis with Müller-Braunschweig without his father's agreement, remembered that his father was frightened by the prospect of taking over the management of the Berlin Institute. Matthias Göring related the reasons for his apprehension to his age (he was then fifty-seven years old), the distance of his medical office from the capital and the new house he had just built outside the city. However, he yielded to the insistence of his fellow psychotherapists. This indecisive and untouchable character was obviously chosen strategically by them to defend them and to promote psychotherapy under the Third Reich. Like other psychotherapists at the same time, Matthias Göring wanted to bring together the different trends in psychotherapy. He believed that the disputes between the different schools of psychotherapy and psychoanalysis were provoking unnecessary quarrels that were delaying or preventing the recognition of psychotherapy by the medical profession. From the mid-1920s, Germany's psychotherapists sought to reduce the differences between psychoanalysis and psychotherapy in order to present a united front against university psychiatry, which focused on diseases of the brain and the nervous system. As a result, unification and simplification had already been watchwords among these psychotherapists before the advent of National Socialism. When he became president of the General Society of Psychotherapeutic Medicine in 1930, Kretschmer campaigned for psychotherapy to remain the preserve of psychiatrists. Two years earlier, at the time of the society's creation, only doctors had been allowed to be members. The creation of the German branch led by Göring in 1933 was clearly in line with the opening up of psychotherapeutic practice to non-doctors. From 1936, the German Institute for Psychological Research and Psychotherapy (the Göring Institute) accentuated this trend, since it was permissible for any psychotherapist, whether a doctor or not, to become a member of the Psychotherapy Society if he had trained at that institute. During this whole period, except in 1938 and especially after 1941, the number of non-medical psychotherapists who worked at the Göring Institute exceeded that of doctors.

Jones's mission to Berlin

In March 1936, Anna Freud wrote to Jones that the existence of the institute and the Berlin group was no longer tenable under the same name and with the requisite conditions of independence. Indicating that the existence of an independent institute crystallised these oppositions, she referred to the two possibilities open to Felix Boehm. The first of these possibilities had to do with dissolving the DPG and the Berlin Institute and in stopping teaching, with each member being able to continue to practice analysis in private if he wished. According to Anna Freud, Boehm could not bring himself to dissolve the DPG and the institute because, despite the circumstances, both institutions were very active. She felt that such a decision was almost impossible to take because, strangely, work was in full swing: there were constant new requests for training, the institute's courses continued to be very well attended and the hospital services were referring many patients to the polyclinic. Anna Freud also pointed out that the therapeutic effectiveness of psychoanalysis was now recognised by the authorities. In these circumstances, putting an end to the activities of the institute was inconceivable.[41] So, despite its 'upgrade', it continued to function – and even to function well.

The second possibility for pursuing teaching activities was to ensure the sustainability of the courses while managing to federate the different branches of psychotherapy that felt threatened or that did not have an institute of their own. For this, Boehm would be forced to give up its independence. According to Anna Freud, Boehm's strategy involved him in making serious major compromises, which, in turn, forced him to leave the IPA. However, he could always, she said, ask to become a member of the IPA at a later time in recognition of the services he had rendered to psychoanalysis.[42] Nevertheless, it was not certain, according to Anna, that Boehm actually knew whether he was being of service to psychoanalysis rather than helping only the German analysts. Nor did he share the views of his colleague Müller-Braunschweig, who was already laying the groundwork for a German form of psychoanalysis adapted to the new ideology. Boehm had a dozen people around him who were ready to follow him. He expected to exercise influence over psychotherapists by successfully converting them to psychoanalysis.

Anna Freud also believed there was another story. She was not convinced by the one Boehm was telling himself. Boehm, she felt, would surely fail to convert the psychotherapists; he would end up isolated and would be very happy to be able to remain a member of the IPA. Boehm was someone who greatly feared criticism from others. Anna then asked Jones for advice, noting the fact that, in her opinion, it was understandable that Boehm wanted to try. If Boehm succeeded, it wouldn't be so bad. But if he failed, psychoanalysis would not lose much, since the group of practitioners around Boehm was not viable. Anna felt that she and Jones could do worse than let Boehm try, since there was nothing left to lose. Boehm was to send an official letter to Jones advising him of the DPG's withdrawal from the IPA. Anna Freud concluded by noting that Boehm seemed very honest to her. Basically, Boehm believed himself capable of bringing along the psychotherapists from the new German institute behind him – but Anna was not convinced. She felt that he lacked the qualities of a leader and that his attempt to preserve the autonomy of the DPG was doomed to failure. Besides, Boehm had not come to Vienna for advice; he had come to announce his decision to join Matthias Göring's team. In any event, Anna Freud perceived this approach as a gamble lost in advance. It was a badly handled effort undertaken by an anxious man who overestimated his own abilities. Her reasoning was that Boehm simply did not have the necessary qualities to lead this operation; he was, of course, well-intentioned, but he simply didn't have what it would take. Jones also looked at it from that angle. For him too, the Boehm option was the only option. Thus, Anna Freud and Ernest Jones had agreed on one point: since they had no one else on hand, it would have to be Boehm. The obstacle was human, not moral. Furthermore, Jones believed that, given Boehm's anxieties, he needed to prop Boehm up by assuming the role of the superego that spurs the failing self.

In her correspondence – kept at the London Institute – Anna Freud sometimes refers to '*mein Vater*'. At the end of April 1933, she reported to Jones her father's contention that if psychoanalysis were to be banned, it should be banned as psychoanalysis and not, as Reich argued, as a mixture of psychoanalysis and politics.[43] It is also very likely that Anna Freud's judgement – which was, to say the least, mixed – about Boehm's personality was a reflection of that of her father, who took a rather dim view of the man. The Freuds felt that the loss of what would remain of the DPG following the departure of Jewish analysts would hardly be tragic since this group was, in a way, already doomed. Boehm could try, of course, but nobody in Vienna believed he could succeed. For his part, did the current president of the IPA align himself with

Anna Freud's position? As he explained at the Lucerne congress, Jones helped Jewish analysts leave Germany to live elsewhere, which was not entirely unreasonable during those times. On the other hand, however, he both negotiated and enforced the resignation of the last Jewish members working in Berlin at the end of 1935. Jones was, moreover, criticised for this action, as well as for having suspended endeavours to help a psychoanalyst who had been arrested. Edith Jacobson, who was of Jewish origin, was a didactic analyst and a member of the teaching committee of the Berlin Institute. She had belonged to the Neu Beginnen resistance network since 1933. She had organised secret meetings in her apartment and was arrested on 24 October 1935. Jones learned of her arrest on 30 October and consulted Anna Freud in Vienna, along with Fenichel, who had taken refuge in Prague. In November, Boehm managed to convince Jones that any attempt to assist their incarcerated colleague posed a risk of the DPG's dissolution. A Norwegian member of the DPG, Nic Hoel, was in a position to make return trips between Berlin and London via Vienna and Prague. In Vienna, she met Anna Freud, who begged her to make Fenichel understand that Boehm was under enormous pressure in Berlin. Anna Freud also spoke of the guilt of Edith Jacobson, who had acted carelessly and betrayed Boehm.

Following a visit to Berlin, Nic Hoel wrote to Jones that the argument for the autonomy of science was not tenable in Hitler's Germany. The terms she used were precise and underlined the contradictions inherent in supporting the independence of psychoanalysis from a position of submission:

> My opinion, therefore, is that these analysts are not neutral, but the least one can say is that they are obliged, passively, to abandon the aspect of research, of investigation, which is analysis. I don't think they're doing this consciously, but in the end, their anxiety and their collaboration with German psychotherapists must have that influence.[44]

It was wrong to take into account only the negative aspect of the constraint. If it was felt that the Berlin colleagues were collaborating with the German psychotherapists because they were afraid and had little choice, any possibility of scientific independence was intrinsically denied. Hoel concluded her letter with a description of Boehm's anxiety about the Jacobson affair. Fenichel's presence in Prague was also a source of great concern to her. The mere mention of Fenichel's name represented an indictment of the Berliners; the Gestapo had come to pick him up at the institute and his sister-in-law had been arrested. Edith Jacobson was to be tried before an assize court in Berlin. Jones assumed that she would be released only to be returned to the Gestapo and re-educated in a concentration camp. He expected that the influence of the English would work in her favour and that they would succeed in getting her out of the camp in a few days. On 2 December 1935, he asked Anna Freud if steps should be taken while the case was still pending, and noted that it would be tried by judicial authorities who did not yet belong to the Gestapo. Wasn't it unwise to do too much, to attract attention? Jones noted that Boehm was extremely anxious and that he no longer trusted anyone. He believed that Boehm's anxious temperament required firm treatment, that there was no point in reassuring him. The right method with him was that of the decisive exhortation. In general, Jones considered that only external firmness would be able to reassure the Berlin group. He set out to embody this firmness, defining himself as the strong man whose presence would be necessary because everyone in Berlin was in a panic. According to Jones, Boehm had 'neither the personality necessary to manage the group nor the rapid knowledge of the strategy necessary' to act in this situation.

Jones arrived in Berlin on 30 November 1935 to deal with three pressing matters: the possibility of the dissolution of the DPG, the question of its affiliation to the IPA, the expulsion of the Jewish analysts. Jones's exact phrase here is 'expelling the Jews'. This latest affair caused him concern. When he arrived, the Jews of the Berlin Institute rebelled. They had accepted the idea of resigning the previous week but, in the presence of Jones, they pretended otherwise. The latter had to insist that they do so, which he deplored because theirs was already a lost cause. According to him, it was a 'hopeless cause'. He reported the episode to Anna Freud, explaining that the Jews had done a volte-face and had presented arguments against their resignation. Jones also believed that this action posed a danger to the DPG. It would suggest that the ideology of psychoanalysis was identical to the Jewish ideology, both of which were incompatible with the Nazi worldview.

Boehm reported on Jones's negotiations in Berlin. When he went to pick him up at the station on 30 November, he informed him of the shakiness of his official position following the arrest of Edith Jacobson and said that it was difficult for him to continue his activities with a group so constrained. Jones calmed him down by explaining that he was highly regarded at the IPA, that Anna Freud admired him and that his courage and tact were much appreciated. Only Eitingon did not share these enthusiastic opinions about him. Then Jones and Boehm went to meet their imprisoned colleague's lawyer. They learned there that any action undertaken in her favour could backfire, that only an intervention from abroad could perhaps help to get her out of the concentration camp. Jones then had a discussion with Boehm, Müller-Braunschweig and Kemper, which, he said, allowed him to address the most important issue of all, namely the dissolution of the DPG.[45] The evening continued with a dinner with the Boehm family where Jones had an opportunity to meet the new candidates in training at the institute. The issue of resignation from the IPA was discussed for hours. Jones agreed with Schultz-Hencke, also present at the dinner, for whom leaving the IPA would be an admission of guilt. The resignation of the Jews was not discussed, since this question had been settled for a long time.

> Jones claimed that he had always stood apart from any ideology, that, for him, a separation between psychoanalysis and any ideology was self-evident and he insisted that it was absolutely necessary to emphasise this attitude vis-à-vis the public. As president of the IPA, he promised to issue a certificate to us to that effect.[46]

The next day, 1 December, Jones met with members of the institute, and the Jewish members expressed concern. They were afraid of being identified with their arrested colleague and other people would think that they had been forced to resign. 'The fact that after the resignation of the Jewish members psychoanalysis could no longer be practiced as before has been hotly debated,' said Boehm. Again, Jones reiterated what he said to Schultz-Hencke, that resignation was tantamount to a confession that psychoanalysis was an ideology. This would hinder the continuation of the colleagues' activities in Germany. The Jews seemed reassured. A little later that same morning, Boehm organised a new discussion on three points: dissolving the DPG, taking the DPG out of the IPA and the departure of the Jewish members ('*Austritt der jüdischen Mitglieder*'[47]). The first point was quickly settled: the dissolution of the DPG was not necessary. The question of the resignation of the Jews from the IPA offered Jones the opportunity to reiterate his argument that the public should be emphatically persuaded that psychoanalysis was a medical specialty. The proposal to quit the IPA was rejected. 'In short, Jones seemed to view our situation in Germany much more optimistically than we did, perhaps he was influenced by some positive factors on our account,' said Boehm in disbelief. In fact, the Chief of Reich Doctors had just informed Boehm that he had been accepted into the Federation of Biological Doctors. Next came the volte-face by the Jewish members, which surprised everyone. The Aryan members demanded their immediate resignation, but the Jews stuck to the argument that their resignation would be interpreted as an admission of ideological affiliation. The atmosphere grew heated. Therese Benedeck spoke for the Jewish members. Embarrassed, Boehm adjourned the meeting, thanking Jones for attending. A lunch was then held, and Jones was assured that the previous week the Jews had agreed to resign. When Jones was about to leave the institute, Therese Benedeck approached him to inform him that the Jews would leave sooner or later. On the way back to the station, Jones begged Boehm and Müller-Braunschweig not to lose hope; he begged them to continue their courageous struggle.

Upon his return on 2 December, an exhausted Jones wrote to Anna Freud that the third point, relating to the resignation of the Jews, had been one of the failures of his mission to Berlin. On 4 December, Benedeck received a telegram from Jones advising Jewish members to resign immediately. The letter Jones wrote to Boehm on 6 December was intended to be reassuring. No, said Jones, the letter that the Jewish analysts were demanding from Boehm in order to resign could not be used against him at a congress of the

IPA. If it would help, it should be added that the issue had been discussed at length with Jones, who was president of the IPA. Jones believed that Benedeck was hatching a plot to discredit the DPG abroad. He believed that Benedeck was not like other Jews, that she was exerting a harmful influence on others. Jones wrote about her, distinguishing her from those other colleagues who seemed more sincere to him. He regretted her influence on them.[48] He also admitted to being relieved to learn that this particular colleague did not intend to come and settle in England. Two assemblies were held on 18 December 1935. The Jewish members discussed their resignation. In truth, they had interpreted Jones's haste to see them resign as depriving them of their free will. Their resignation was impossible since it was an order from the president of the IPA. For his part, Boehm went to great lengths to persuade them to the contrary. A new candidate from the Berlin Institute who was soon to be named a member of the IPA, Eva Rosenfeld, made him understand that she could only refuse this constraint. The Jews, she said, could not offer their voluntary resignation because it implied too high a degree of masochism, 'as if one had to execute oneself'.[49]

In their brutality and simplicity, these terrible words forever contradict the fiction of the voluntary resignation of the Jewish members at the end of 1935 with the aim of saving German psychoanalysis. It was not the Nuremberg Laws but the arrest of an analyst engaged in the resistance that had pushed Jones to drop everything and go to Berlin at all. Regarding Jacobson, Jones received written protests. Some expressed their solidarity with their imprisoned colleague. Jones duly 'called to order' Dr Anne Buchholtz, who had appealed to psychoanalysts in all countries regarding the imprisonment of their colleague. Buchholtz did not mince her words in evoking the heedlessness and bad advice of the Berlin group which, under the leadership of Boehm and Müller-Braunschweig, had taken the step of identifying with National Socialism. She asked if the fear that dominated the Berliners was reason enough to deprive an analyst of liberty in the long term: 'Let each analyst imagine for himself half an hour in a German prison,' she wrote.[50] Jones answered her dryly in June 1936, stating that she was malicious, that she should have warned him before launching her appeal and that she should have reminded herself that he had met Jacobson's lawyer as well as her friends and that he had acted in Jacobson's best interests during the time of her pre-trial detention. On 12 September 1936, the Fourth Criminal Division of the Berlin Court of Appeal sentenced psychiatrist and psychoanalyst Edith Jacobson to a two and a half years' imprisonment, accompanied by forfeiture of her civil rights.

Notes

1 Franz Alexander, 'Le cursus théorique' (1930), in Colonomos, *On forme des psychanalystes*, p. 142.
2 *Ibid.*

3 See Franz Alexander and Hugo Staub, *The Criminal, the Judge and the Public: A Psychological Analysis* (London: George Allen & Unwin, 1931).
4 Franz Alexander, 'Le cursus théorique' (1930), in Colonomos, *On forme des psychanalystes*, p. 142.
5 Sándor Radó, 'Le cursus pratique', in Colonomos, *On forme des psychanalystes*, p. 148.
6 *Ibid.*
7 Gregory Zilboorg, 'En Amérique' (1930), in Colonomos, *On forme des psychanalystes*, p. 166.
8 Cited in Eberhard Jäckel, *Hitler idéologue* (Paris: Calmann-Levy, 1973), p. 106.
9 Saul Friedländer, *Nazi Germany and the Jews, Volume I: The Years of Persecution, 1933–1939* (New York: HarperCollins, 1997).
10 Ian Kershaw, *Hitler* (London: Longman, 1991).
11 Friedländer, *Nazi Germany and the Jews, Volume 1*.
12 Sigmund Freud to Marie Bonaparte, letter of 26 March 1933, in Jones, *Sigmund Freud, vol. 3*, pp. 187–188.
13 Bertolt Brecht, *Fear and Misery of the Third Reich* (1938), trans. John Willett (London: Bloomsbury, 2002), p. 76.
14 Friedländer, *Nazi Germany and the Jews, Volume 1*.
15 Martin Buber, letter to Ernst Simon, 14 February 1933, cited in Friedländer, *Nazi Germany and the Jews, Volume 1*, p. 17. Buber had been teaching Jewish religious philosophy at the University of Frankfurt am Main since 1924. He resigned in 1933 and was banned from lecturing in October of that same year. In 1938 he moved to Jerusalem and took up a teaching position at Hebrew University.
16 Freud to Jones, Letter 606, 7 April 1933, in R. Andrew Paskauskas, *Complete Correspondence of Sigmund Freud and Ernest Jones, op. cit.*, p. 716.
17 Sigmund Freud to Marie Bonaparte, letter of 10 June 1933, in Jones, *Sigmund Freud*, vol. 3, p. 194.
18 Freud to Jones, letter 615, 25 July 1933, in R. Andrew Paskauskas, *Complete Correspondence of Sigmund Freud and Ernest Jones, op. cit.*, p. 725.
19 Walter Cimbal to Matthias Göring, letter of 21 January 1934, in Karen Brecht, *Ici, la vie continue*, p. 243.
20 Lou Andreas-Salomé to Anna Freud, letter 391 L, 25 February 1934, in Lou Andreas-Salomé and Anna Freud, *À l'ombre du père, op. cit.*, p. 558.
21 Jones to Freud, Letter 618, 18 September 1933, in R. Andrew Paskauskas, *Complete Correspondence of Sigmund Freud and Ernest Jones, op. cit.*, p. 728.
22 Friedländer, *Nazi Germany and the Jews, Volume 1*.
23 Régine Lockot, 'À propos des changements de nom de l'Association psychanalytique de Berlin', *La Revue Lacanienne*, no. 1 (2008), 23–34.
24 Klaus Dieter Rath, 'À propos de l'exercise de la psychanalyse en Allemagne', *Journal francais de Psychiatrie*, no. 12 (Paris: Érès, 2001), 43.
25 Martin Staemmler, 'Le judaïsme dans le médicine' (1933), in Karen Brecht, *Ici, la vie continue, op. cit.*, p. 240.
26 Werner Kindt (ed.), *Dokumentation der Jugendbewegung. Grundschriften der deutschen Jugendbewegung*, vol. 1 (Düsseldorf and Cologne: Eugen Diederichs Verlag, 1963). Cited in Peter Gay, *Weimar Culture, op. cit.*
27 Sigmund Freud, 'Group Psychology and the Analysis of the Ego' (1921), *Standard Edition*, vol. 18, pp. 69–143.
28 Sigmund Freud, 'Moses and Monotheism: Three Essays' (1939), *Standard Edition*, vol. 23, p. 91.
29 *Ibid.*, p. 90.
30 *Ibid.*, p. 132.
31 Gustave Le Bon, *The Crowd* (New York: Dover Publications, 2002).

32 Freud to Eitingon, Letter 755 F, 21 March 1933, in Michael Schröter, *Correspondance, op. cit.*, p. 774.
33 Sigmund Freud, 'The Question of a Weltanschauung' (1933), *Standard Edition*, vol. 22 (London: Vintage, 2001).
34 Geoffrey Cocks, *Psychotherapy in the Third Reich: The Göring Institute* (Oxford: Oxford University Press, 1985).
35 Matthias Göring to Walter Cimbal, letter of 6 September 1933, in Karen Brecht, *Ici, la vie continue*, p. 246.
36 Fritz Künkel to Matthias Göring, letter of 12 December 1933.
37 Geoffrey Cocks, *Psychotherapy in the Third Reich, op. cit.*
38 *Ibid.*
39 Psychiatrist Herbert Linden was uncompromising when it came to National Socialist legislation on the genetic transmission of health. He was an active participant in the T4 euthanasia programme for the mentally ill. There could have been as many as 70,273 victims during the first period of the programme, which lasted until 1941, and 30,000 during the second period of the programme, which went forward more discreetly and lasted until 1945. Linden committed suicide that same year.
40 Report by Carl Müller-Braunschweig, Secretary of the DPG, dated 13 August 1934 and addressed to Ernest Jones, in Karen Brecht, *Ici, la vie continue, op. cit.*, p. 244.
41 Anna Freud to Ernest Jones, letter of 10 March 1936, Archives of the London Institute of Psychoanalysis.
42 *Ibid.*
43 Anna Freud to Ernest Jones, letter of 27 April 1933, Archives of the London Institute of Psychoanalysis.
44 Nic Hoel to Ernest Jones, letter of 4 January 1936, in Karen Brecht, *Ici, la vie continue*, p. 251. This letter is dated 4 January 1935, which is clearly an error, since Edith Jacobson was arrested in October 1935.
45 Werner Kemper had been in didactic analysis with Müller-Braunschweig. He became a teacher at the Berlin Institute and was a very active member of the German Institute for Psychological Research and Psychotherapy.
46 Report by Felix Boehm, dated 4 December 1935, concerning the negotiations in Berlin. Cited in Karen Brecht, *Ici, la vie continue, op. cit.*, p. 255.
47 Boehm employed the term *Austritt* (departure, exit, defection), not *Rücktritt* (resignation).
48 Ernest Jones to Felix Boehm, letter of 6 December 1935, Archives of the London Institute of Psychoanalysis. Born in Hungary, Therese Benedeck was analysed by Ferenczi and completed her training in Berlin in 1920. She eventually left Germany for the United States and, together with Franz Alexander, joined the Chicago Institute.
49 Report by Felix Boehm, dated 4 December 1935, concerning the negotiations in Berlin. Cited in Karen Brecht, *Ici, la vie continue, op. cit.*, p. 255.
50 Anne Buchholtz, 'Appel à tous les psychanalystes de tous les pays', in Karen Brecht, *Ici, la vie continue*, p. 250.

Chapter 6

The end of an experiment

The refusal of the political

Some authors, including Russell Jacoby, believe that the psychoanalytic establishment's rejection of politics was reinforced under Nazism. A distinction should be made, however, between the rejection of politics and the rejection of politicisation – that is to say, the use of psychoanalysis for political purposes. According to Wilhelm Reich's second daughter, Lore Reich Rubin, it was Anna Freud who encouraged Jones to follow her on the path of apoliticalism. Rubin also contended that Anna considered herself number one and tolerated no rivals. Either you were loyal to her or you were not an analyst – and you were out. Reich, the polar opposite of a team player, thought himself an exception. At the end of the 1920s, the situation of these two personalities was physically and intellectually mirrored both in the programme and in the topography of the Vienna Institute. Anna's and Wilhelm's seminars ran concurrently on opposite sides of the same corridor. In a room at the end of the corridor, Anna was teaching defence mechanisms. On the other side of the corridor, Reich was teaching character analysis. As a result, it was impossible for students to attend both seminars during the same academic year.

Commenting on how Jones and Anna Freud went about ejecting Reich from the DPG, Rubin recalls that in 1933 the Freuds and Ernest Jones saw the communists as a bigger threat than the Nazis. For the executive committee of the IPA, the most urgent concern was to sever all ties with communism. After Reich's expulsion, the conservative tendency embodied by Jones and Anna prevailed, and the political Freudians duly felt it prudent to keep a low profile given the fact that their radicalism was no longer tolerated. From 1934 onwards, Fenichel and his circle began to correspond secretly by means of *Rundbriefe* (circular letters), endeavouring to find common ground with the positions defended by Reich before eventually distancing themselves from them. Rubin inherited a complete set of these circular letters from her mother, Annie Reich, who was herself in analysis with Anna Freud in 1927.[1] Rubin deduced that Anna Freud wanted to exclude Wilhelm purely because of personal rivalry. Jones, in accordance with the respect for freedom of thought

DOI: 10.4324/9781003215684-9

characteristic of the English, would have been instinctively inclined to respect everyone's personal choice in matters of political opinion, but he ended up agreeing with Anna and conspired with her to remove Reich from the DPG's membership list. Upon arriving in Lucerne, Reich was stupefied to learn that he was no longer a member of the IPA. From that moment on, he became completely enraged; he took his frustrations out on his wife and made terrible scenes for her. According to Rubin, the disloyal way in which Reich was expelled from the IPA tipped him into madness. In order to remain in Anna's good graces, all those who had been close to Reich quickly began falling over themselves to pretend that the opposite had been the case. Anna was subsequently nicknamed the Iron Maiden – a reference to a medieval instrument of torture in the form of a hollow metal figure of a woman whose interior was lined with iron spikes.

Concerning the Reich affair, Jones believed that psychoanalysis had to be protected from political entanglement. His one and only goal was the search for knowledge. He understood that an analyst could hold a political movement in high esteem, but, at the same time, he had to consider his responsibility towards his colleagues.[2] He conjectured that Reich was going to create a new movement that would unite psychoanalysis and Bolshevism. This new group, he felt, would be a threat to psychoanalysis – even outside the IPA – despite everything that had already been done to deny it.[3] Even if it is not the case that Jones aligned himself solely with Anna Freud's position regarding the links between psychoanalysis and politics, the fact remains that we can identify three distinct levels of relationship between psychoanalysis and politics in the early 1930s.

The first level had to do with circumstances and was linked to the regime of repression in Nazi Germany. In the earliest days of Hitler's dictatorship, terror was first unleashed against the German Communist Party (KPD) and the German Social Democrats (SPD) and only later against the Jews. The kind of tolerance previously shown in Berlin by Max Eitingon could no longer be sustained – all links with the revolutionary Marxist current had to be broken immediately. Reich was a radical who had come to Berlin in 1930 to fight the Nazis. Edith Jacobson belonged to a secret resistance organisation with connections to SPD circles. When the Nazis came to power and immediately began carrying out mass arrests of their opponents, some psychoanalysts demanded immediate separation from the dissidents in order to demonstrate that psychoanalysis was not a creation of Bolshevism. The political Freudians were also German, Austrian and Hungarian Jews. They had found asylum in Berlin during the 1920s and early 1930s. Now they were doubly threatened, since the Nazi government was hunting them down and the analytical movement was trying to separate from them because their ideas were becoming a liability. Reich's expulsion served as a warning to others that if they persevered in their dissent they would suffer the same fate. The clandestine correspondence between the dissident psychoanalysts commenced following their departure from Europe.

Without the phenomenon of Nazism, would the apolitical tendency nevertheless have gradually imposed itself within the IPA insofar as this orientation was very much in line with Freud's rejection of Bolshevism? A dividing line emerged when the alliance between Marxism and psychoanalysis was perceived, both in Vienna and in London, as a new heresy. Jones had hinted at the impending creation of a new and uncontrollable group, and Anna Freud's attitude wasn't purely a product of her personal aversions. Sigmund Freud found Reich's attacks on the notion of the death drive intolerable; he knew he was being criticised on the level of theory by the dissidents in Berlin. Reich, moreover, had posited a correlation between Freud's invention of the death drive and a melancholy phase in its author's life. In Reich's eyes, 'Beyond the Pleasure Principle' was the fruit of a theoretical stiffening that came about after the end of the war because death had prevailed over life and libido. In short, one had to choose between the position of the Marxist and the hypothesis of the death drive. In expressing their apoliticalism, psychoanalysts like Anna Freud and Ernest Jones sincerely believed that they were defending the scientific nature of psychoanalysis. Besides, it would be tempting to make the political Freudians the only authentic European representatives of the spirit of classical analysis before its mutation into ego psychology in America. This thesis, defended by Jacoby, emphasises the analytical interest in social phenomena in the classical and European period of psychoanalysis. It privileges the political commitment of psychoanalysts and suggests that those who had no time for leftist ideas were conservatives or reactionaries. In contrast, Jacoby adds, American psychoanalysis defended a politically neutral vision and was hostile to the political and Marxist orientation of dissident psychoanalysis. However, the apolitical trend had already been evident in Europe for quite some time before the Continent's analysts began going into exile in the United States. Furthermore, at the theoretical level, the division between political Freudians and apolitical psychoanalysts doesn't map neatly onto the divisions between progressives and conservatives. Indeed, character analysis, introduced by Reich in the 1920s, emphasised the ego's capacity for resistance. Reich also opposed the idea of regression, which, he felt, represented the introduction of the second topography. For her part, Anna Freud drew inspiration from Fenichel's reflections on character in order to write certain passages from her work on defence mechanisms. The division between politicised Freudians and reactionary conservatives is not always precisely where we think it is, and it is not obvious that the dissidents were entirely in agreement with one another.

It should also be remembered that Freud liked to provoke people. The atmosphere of scandal that his writings created did not displease him. Whenever his thought was on the verge of becoming a kind of orthodoxy, Freud turned it upside down by inventing concepts that no one else had ever imagined. His productivity was also a source of embarrassment for his students, who found it difficult to follow him. Even after the onset of his cancer in 1923, he continued to publish articles at an astonishing rate. The year 1930 saw the publication of *Civilisation and Its Discontents.* Three years later, Freud published his *New Introductory Lectures on Psychoanalysis.* From 1924 to 1931, there was an impressive succession of articles. In 1923, there came the publication of 'The Infantile Genital Organisation'. The following year, Freud published three articles: 'Neurosis and Psychosis', 'The Economic Problem of Masochism', and 'The Loss of Reality in Neurosis and Psychosis'. In 1925, he published 'A Note upon the "Mystic Writing-Pad"', 'Negation', 'Some Psychical Consequences of the Anatomical Distinction Between the Sexes', and 'An Autobiographical Study'. In 1926, he wrote 'The Question of Lay Analysis'. 'Fetishism' appeared in 1927, 'Humour' in 1928. 'Libidinal Types' and 'Female Sexuality' were published in 1931. As the Vienna Psychoanalytic Institute's Richard Sterba noted, analysts simply could not follow all this: 'One can easily imagine that we analysts felt we were being bombarded by the deluge of new ideas and rectified or developed ideas to which Freud's productivity subjected us during this period.'[4] The ground was constantly shifting, and nothing was certain. Freud's work could not, in fact, be understood as a system at the moment of its invention. No sooner had his students made great efforts to assimilate a new concept than their master had already invented something else. Things were going fast, almost too fast – analysts were having trouble walking in Freud's footsteps. This avalanche of ideas made schematisation and ready-made ideas impossible.

Freud was a very quick thinker. His remarkable memory allowed him to talk about a clinical case for several hours without reading from notes. He quickly assimilated everything he read. People saw him leafing through books, methodically turning the pages one after another – which was simply his way of reading. And what he had read, he never forgot. The speed of Freud's thought is rarely a subject of discussion, what with the emphasis usually being placed on his circumspection, his moderation and his intellectual power. Nevertheless, its singularity does not conform to the wax figure of the Viennese sage that tradition has tended to erect. In truth, Freud was someone who said and did quite unusual things. His practice was far from dogmatic. In any event, the evolution of his thinking baffled his contemporaries. Reich's stubborn attachment to the theory of the libido is a striking example of a lack of evolution. *Moses and Monotheism*, the last book Freud wrote, clearly demonstrates how he perceived himself: right up until the end, he would never cease to confuse, to scandalise, to attack the wisdom of the most reasonable. People begged him to stop, to publish nothing that could possibly harm the Jews who were being persecuted – yet he remained stubborn. Illness, intolerable physical pain, the advent of the Nazis, the prospect of the collapse of German-language psychoanalysis, forced exile – despite all this, he continued to work and write. His passion for truth and the risks he took in the name of intellectual adventure accompanied an unceasing tide of clinical and conceptual questioning.

A second level of explanation for the refusal of political involvement is linked to the desire to inscribe psychoanalysis in scientific discourse. The politically engaged psychoanalysts were ostracised in the name of the principle of the independence of science. The emphasis on the therapeutic application of psychoanalysis could all too easily serve to suggest that the discipline was not a vision of the world but something designed to cure people on the model of medical science. This orientation, which encouraged the definition of psychoanalysis as a science applied to therapeutics, had been much debated in the IPA during the 1920s. In the dark years of Hitler's Germany, might not the assertion of political neutrality have risked generating apathy of another kind? To allege that psychoanalysis had nothing to do with politics, that it could remain politically neutral and that one could continue to analyse and train analysts in the name of the independence of science led a character like Felix Boehm to completely ignore ethical considerations.

In 1933 and 1934, the condemnation of the subversive activities of the leftwing Freudians and the desire to separate from them as quickly as possible so as not to risk being compromised in the eyes of the authorities were, of course, driven by fear. There was, nevertheless, a third way, one that corresponded to the national policy of compromise adopted by the DPG. This position was not equivalent to an absolute refusal of political engagement. In his report to the IPA congress in Lucerne at the end of August 1934, Jones, as president of the organisation, wanted to counter the harsh criticism that had been levelled at Boehm and stated that people had the right to have different opinions regarding the appropriateness of the steps he had taken, but that it was also necessary to have a proper knowledge of the realities at stake. Jones added that Boehm had met with Freud in April 1933 in order 'to prevent the acute conflicts which actually occurred thereafter' and that Boehm had sent very precise accounts of the situation in Berlin back to the IPA leadership. 'I have reason to hope that Dr. Boehm's services to psychoanalysis will outlast any passing criticism to which he may be exposed,'[5] he concluded. This also had to do with a position of principle. Jones considered that it was in the interest of psychoanalysis to guard against any entanglement with politics and that its nature consisted in following a single tendency defined as the search for knowledge.

Saving psychoanalysis by proclaiming that it had nothing to do with politics because it was a medical technique would open the way to every kind of compromise. The reduction of psychoanalysis to mere therapy allowed certain analysts to engage in a policy of compromise with the Nazi administration in order to defend the interests of science. The Institute for Psychological Research and Psychotherapy (also known as the Göring Institute), of which Boehm became secretary, was a 'declared association' (*eingetragener Verein*), with the suffix 'e.v.' in its name. This signified that the institution's psychotherapists had been approved by the Ministry of the Interior. Its statutes had been written by Herbert Linden in person. Although the latter was a member of the commission responsible for studying the unification of the theories of the three schools of psychotherapy within the Institute for Psychological Research and Psychotherapy, the project was completely controlled by Matthias Göring. In this connection, Geoffrey Cocks explains that the involvement of the Ministry of the Interior was mainly confined to solving the problem posed by the psychoanalysts who remained at the Institute. However, the training of psychotherapists was carried out mainly under the guidance of psychoanalysts. This training included a didactic analysis in the form of three sessions per week on the couch. Even though they were restricted in their didactic activity following an incident that occurred in Vienna in 1938 and which implicated Müller-Braunschweig, the former members of the Berlin Psychoanalytic Institute retained control over the activity of the Berlin Polyclinic, which was attached to the new institute. Boehm was in charge of assessments, while Müller-Braunschweig remained responsible for lectures on the organisation of teaching. In 1942, he wrote a memorandum on the organisation of the theoretical curriculum, which reserved a place for the treatment of problems of heredity and race with lectures on the maintenance of the hereditary and racial heritage by individuals like Herbert Linden.[6]

During its first year of operation, the polyclinic of the Göring Institute received 412 patients; thirty-eight of them continued the treatment initiated at the Berlin Psychoanalytic Institute. An estimate by Werner Kemper indicates that half of the patients were treated with short-term therapy, as the method was already popular with most German psychotherapists. Geoffrey Cocks contends that the short-term orientation suited the Nazi conception of public health (*Volksgesundheit*). The short-term treatment was also favoured because it was in line with the steps taken to ensure that psychotherapy could benefit from the reimbursement plans offered by the social security system. Each patient was seen by a primary therapist to assess the most appropriate therapy method. Among the therapies offered were in-depth psychological treatment, where the patient lay on the couch and engaged in free association; face-to-face consultations with a psychologist; group or educational therapies for children and their parents; hypnotic and auto-hypnotic therapies; physical therapy (massage of nerve endings); gymnastics; respiratory exercises; and voice therapy. Hypnosis and auto-hypnosis were understood as the best guarantee of integration into the reimbursement plans offered by the health insurance funds. Psychotherapists also practised a form of therapy that was adapted to the requirements for reimbursement and allowed patients intervals between two phases of their treatment. With few exceptions, Jews could not be treated at the Göring Institute. The Nazi-controlled Deutsche Arbeitsfront (German Labour Front) became interested in the institute's activities and financed its operations from 1936 to 1945. From 1943 onwards, the racial origins of the patients appeared in the Göring Institute's files.

The policy of national compromise undertaken to protect the existence of psychoanalysis in Germany ended in disaster. It would be an understatement to say that in order to continue operating, Christian analysts of pure German stock abandoned the ethical principles at the heart of the Freudian experiment.

The argument for independence

The placing of psychoanalysis under supervision by Germany's new masters was based on the definition of the discipline and on its therapeutic use. From this point of view, it is edifying to note that the disintegration of psychoanalysis was orchestrated by the very people who felt that it should survive as a medical speciality. Freud's fierce fight for the defence of lay analysis in the mid-1920s had a premonitory value: reduced to therapy, psychoanalysis no longer exists. Undoubtedly, what continued to be practised under the name of psychoanalysis in Germany during the Nazi period had almost nothing to do with the practice developed by Freud.

What, then, is the actual status of psychoanalysis, given that it is neither a science nor a therapeutic method nor a vision of the world? And how does it relate to politics? What should first be understood is the factor of its independence and autonomy. Independence and autonomy from what? Is it from political systems, government bodies, bureaucracy, medicine, psychotherapy and institutional forms? Let's start with the principle that the desire for respectability in psychoanalysis is a dubious one, a desire that risks dragging the discipline down the slippery slope to a point where it tries to pose as a rival of medicine and as a technique that aims at healing. To secure their reputations at the heart of science and obtain an enviable social status, the German analysts who agreed to work under Göring's leadership presented themselves as sensible and reasonable individuals, as people who were amenable to adapting their discipline to the great movements of their time, to the ideals and needs of their fellow citizens, to the evolution of social mores and practices. The search for professional recognition pushed them to respond to the National Socialist project of absorbing psychoanalysis into psychotherapy. Trained in analysis, they consented to their profession's loss of independence by putting their know-how at the service of the state.

This is why the study of this dark period is instructive. It shows how, via a series of sacrifices and compromises and by agreeing to put themselves at the service of the master in the hope of obtaining official recognition accompanied by material rewards, German psychoanalysts sold their souls to the devil. The period under consideration allows the use of this expression without fear of exaggeration. We also learn that the process of self-destruction can be very fast. One could, perhaps, retort that the circumstances were exceptional and that such a unique event could never happen again. To which the response can only be that, yes, the example is extreme and that its value, when looked at through a magnifying glass, is only more enlightening. We can also understand better the reasons why psychoanalysts have accused certain historians of having confused psychoanalysis and psychotherapy under the Third Reich insofar as what happened during this period in Germany involved the former in the latter.[7] It should also be noted that this research is not finished. It would still be necessary to determine the extent to which Freud was betrayed by those who promised to fight to safeguard the autonomy of psychoanalysis. Eli Zaretsky, a professor at New York University's New School for Social Research, points out that everything that could be said on this subject remains suspect because the correspondence between Freud and Boehm is still under seal.[8] I recently consulted him on this subject, and he informed me that he does not know where this correspondence is to be found. Has it simply been forgotten? Or did he get his information from a source whose identity he would prefer not to disclose? It's a mystery.

I contacted the Library of Congress in Washington, DC, where the Sigmund Freud Archives are kept. My exchange with Leonard Bruno, Librarian of the Sigmund Freud Collection, revealed that the correspondence between Freud and Boehm was interrupted in 1929:

> No Boehm materials in our collections are now closed … The only Sigmund Freud-Felix Boehm correspondence we have is for the years 1919–1929. However, we do have Boehm's brief (one page) 'Recollection' which pertains to his relationship with Freud. It was written by Boehm in 1956 when he gave it to the Sigmund Freud Archives. It was closed until 2006 but is now available.[9]

The document referenced by Leonard Bruno reveals little information about the management of the Berlin Institute. Freud's correspondence with Boehm, which I was able to consult, was therefore interrupted in 1929, while Boehm, along with Müller-Braunschweig, was directing the Berlin Institute, an arrangement that lasted from the end of 1933 just up until the Berlin Institute's integration into the Reich Institute for Psychological Research and Psychotherapy, later referred to as the Göring Institute, in May 1936. Until we have proof to the contrary, the assertion that no exact understanding of the situation is possible, due to the inaccessibility of the letters exchanged by Freud and Boehm after 1933, seems unfounded. Let us also recall the existence of censorship, implemented very early on in Nazi Germany and alluded to by Freud in his correspondence with Jones: 'Among the striking symptoms of our time we must also put the reluctance to write, which spreads everywhere, although we know that letters to England are not likely to be opened like those to Germany.'[10]

Five years later, Müller-Braunschweig encountered serious difficulties when one of his letters to Anna Freud was intercepted. Commissioned by Matthias Göring to deal with affairs in Vienna, Müller-Braunschweig wanted to reassure her about the future of the international editions of the Verlag and the

Vienna Institute, stating that it would be possible to play a double game vis-à-vis the authorities. Müller-Braunschweig was immediately suspected of having sympathy for a Jewish woman. At a psychoanalytical congress held after the war, Boehm did not mention this episode. Their previous partnership was no longer valid and the two of them had a falling out. Boehm contented himself with pointing out that a prominent figure in the regime had suddenly become interested in the Jewish origins of psychoanalysis and that an unfortunate combination of circumstances had led to the dismissal of Müller-Braunschweig. The latter was no longer authorised to publish or teach. It is not entirely out of the question that the interception of his letter to Anna Freud was the deciding factor in the dissolution of the Vienna Psychoanalytic Society (WPV) by the Gestapo on 11 April 1938. Müller-Braunschweig's imprudent missive would also have resulted in the official dissolution of the DPG in Germany. Also interesting is the fact that in a letter dated May 1938, Jones wrote to Müller-Braunschweig, who was now banned from teaching, to tell him that he understood that the DPG could no longer continue to exist as an independent organisation in Berlin after the incident in Austria, despite the fact that the German authorities seemed to him to be definitively in favour of the connection between the local psychoanalytic society and the IPA.

At the end of his life, Freud left it to Anna and Jones to take care of the management of the psychoanalytic societies in order to devote all his energy to writing. What we do know is that at a meeting that took place in the Berggasse and to which Boehm had been invited to report on the activities of the new Institute for Psychological Research and Psychotherapy, Freud got carried away. He interrupted Boehm, telling him that after the Jews, it was now up to the Aryan analysts to suffer in defence of their convictions, and left the room. Sterba and Boehm, who had nothing in common, gave much the same account of Freud's outburst. This meeting took place in the first months of 1937, after the integration of the Berlin Psychoanalytic Institute into the Göring Institute. Boehm had not only made great sacrifices, but he had also made many concessions. Freud's position relative to the maintenance of psychoanalysis in Germany rested precisely on the difference between the terms 'sacrifice' and 'concession'. Sacrificing something is not the same as conceding it. The sacrifice highlights the gift and the loss – what one agrees to offer to the Other and the loss to which one resigns oneself. Among the Hebrews, these were offerings made to God at ceremonies. The concession belongs to a completely different register. It is a matter of law, contract, agreement. It refers to the abandonment of a grace, of a privilege, of a place. It connotes withdrawal.

Finally, the notion of the autonomy of psychoanalysis as a science obviously raises certain questions. One could first say that such a question makes little sense, not only because, according to the Rabelaisian motto, science has no conscience – a scientific advance with unfortunate consequences for humanity generally finds scientists to tackle the task – but also because, as

Lacan has shown, science does not want to know anything about the relation to truth as cause. This 'truth as cause' constitutes the most fundamental contribution of psychoanalysis. Lacan teaches us that the unequalled success of science unfolds on the basis of a fundamental rejection, a *Verwerfung*, of truth as cause. This cause is material; it is defined by the action of the signifier when separated from its meaning.[11] If Freud's trick was to pretend that psychoanalysis was a science in order to integrate it into civilisation, the same procedure was used to prevent its ban during the National Socialist period. The problem was that this ruse turned against psychoanalysis.

It will be recalled that in the spring of 1933 Eitingon's position vis-à-vis closing the Berlin Institute differed from Freud's. The former wanted to stay until the end but had also envisaged leaving in order to recreate elsewhere what he had established in Germany thirteen years earlier. For Eitingon, who was not a native German speaker and had already had to adapt to a culture other than the one into which he was born, the institution he had created was by no means inseparable from the German capital. It could be exported elsewhere. It is likely that the peace of mind and astonishing calm he displayed in 1933, when his colleagues were utterly panicked, was commensurate with his own adaptability. Also, Freud and Eitingon, while sharing the ideals of Zionism, had a different understanding of the creation of a Jewish state and the question of going into exile. Eitingon had contemplated the idea of going to live in Palestine before the war, at the end of his medical studies. Had Karl Abraham not proposed that he come to Berlin to work as a psychiatrist, Eitingon would probably have settled in Palestine before 1914. At the end of 1933, he spoke of his new life in Jerusalem as follows: 'One has an intense feeling – always easy to justify, but pleasant enough – that one belongs here. What is taking hold here seems very convincing to me.'[12] If Freud spoke of the joy that Eitingon felt on returning to the Holy Land, and if there are also many testimonies concerning his own relations with certain great Zionist leaders of the time, he was nevertheless wary of attachment to holy places. The creation of a Jewish home in Palestine was a political necessity, he felt, but the Zionist enterprise should not be based on religion. It was hardly to be expected that the man who had stated that religion was an illusion would publicly defend the right of Jews to pray at the Wailing Wall. In February 1930, Freud spoke to this effect in a letter to a member of the foundation for the resettlement of Jews in Palestine.[13]

Freud also knew that, were he to go into exile, the destiny of psychoanalysis would be changed forever. As will be recalled, he chose Berlin over London in the aftermath of the war. He preferred Eitingon over Jones. He wanted to defend the supremacy of German-language psychoanalytic publications over their English-language counterparts. Ever since the collapse of the Austro-Hungarian Empire in 1918, Freud had endeavoured to delay a process that was essentially inevitable. After 1933, the loss of many German readers would prove catastrophic for the Verlag. For all these reasons, Freud expressed his reservations about exile to Eitingon. No, he would never leave Vienna: his age, the requirements of his medical treatment, his habits, the objects to which he was attached – all these made him stay. He was convinced that the Hitler regime would annex Austria, but he believed that this eventuality would not result in the level of brutality evidenced in Germany. His life, he felt, would not be directly threatened, and even if life in Vienna was going to be terribly uncomfortable for its Jewish inhabitants, he believed that exile in Switzerland or England promised considerable inconvenience: 'Flight, I think, would be justified only in the case of lethal danger, and incidentally, if they kill you, it's one kind of death like any other.'[14] Exile, in fact, seemed almost suicidal to him – so much so that at the time of the bloody clashes that took place in the streets of Vienna between government troops and the Austrian Social Democratic Party's Republikaner Schutzbund (a paramilitary organisation) in February 1934, Freud also noted that he was having to fight against all the pressing proposals that were pushing him to go abroad.

> Well, we stayed – we refused to make a pre-emptive escape, and everything that is happening now suggests that we will be able to stay safe. Any relocation, under the conditions in which I find myself, probably relates as much to suicide as to attempted rescue.[15]

To refuse the preventive escape: that was the essence of the compass that Freud used to regulate his behaviour.

Obviously, looking beyond his attachment to a familiar place and to his habits – and also beyond the fact that his illness made it difficult for him to bear the idea of leaving – Vienna brought Freud something invaluable, something that he needed in order to be able to reflect, to work, to live. The hated and yet familiar city immersed him in a conflict that proved fantastically productive. It was in Vienna that he found his supporters and his opponents, his most loyal pupils and his most serious detractors. He needed the support of his friends and stimulating arguments with his enemies in order to lead his fight for psychoanalysis. Age and illness had little influence on his temperament in this regard.[16] The will to stay, whatever the cost, influenced the way Freud looked at the future of the Berlin Institute in 1933. He recommended that it be enabled to function for as long as possible, even if it meant living with danger, slowing down, waiting for the return of better days. Both for the institution and for himself, the same strategy applied. No preventive escape, no early closure. It was necessary to remain on the spot so that the original language of psychoanalysis, the language of Freud, could be sustained. If one relies on these statements, which repeatedly reference his refusal to leave early, his decision to continue with the activities of the Berlin Institute can be better understood. Freud recommended that the Nazis should not be given the slightest pretext for banning psychoanalysis in Germany, even if sooner or later a ban was inevitable. The emphasis, therefore, was on holding out: Freud applied to the psychoanalytic institution what he applied to himself. To exist for as long as possible was his way of fighting and resisting. Freud had been battling terrible pain since 1923, and he continued to do so until his death in 1939, putting up with appalling suffering that he faced with courage and dignity. It can be assumed that he opposed closing the Berlin Institute and ending the activities of the DPG in the same spirit of obstinacy and of fighting against the enemy, against the death drive. Freud's persistence had nothing to do with political blindness or unconscious anti-Semitic prejudice, as has sometimes been stated. Later in the decade, he became irate after reading a report by a foreign journalist who, in an attempt to boost the sales of the newspaper he worked for, had portrayed Freud as an exhausted old man who had been completely panicked by the events that followed the Anschluss. Freud, deeply offended, accused the journalist of having woven a tissue of lies. Tired and ill though he was during the last period of his life in Vienna, he was still Sigmund Freud: his determination was indisputable. When he chose to keep the Berlin Institute and the Berlin Polyclinic open at any cost, no one dared contradict him.

As will be remembered, in March 1933 Freud told Eitingon what the three options were for the Berlin Institute. In the first case, psychoanalysis would be banned in Germany and the Berlin Institute would be forced to close for administrative reasons. In which case, he said, 'This is the least there is to say or do – you will have held on until the very last moment before the boat sinks.'[17] In the second case, the institute would not be directly threatened, but its director would be dismissed because he was a foreigner. Freud pointed out here that the Berlin Institute was most definitely not Eitingon's personal property. 'In this case,' he said, 'it seems to me that you cannot close the institute. You certainly founded it and maintained it for a very long time, but you then entrusted it to the Berlin Psychoanalytic Society, to which it now belongs.' He added that closing the institute would certainly not be legal, and he also pointed out that the general interest of psychoanalysis required that the institute be preserved in order to survive until the return of better times. It was imperative to wait, to survive and hang on. The remark about ownership allows us to grasp the ambiguous status of the Berlin Institute. Did it belong to the man who had had both the desire and the will to create, finance and direct it for thirteen years? Or was it the property of the analytical movement, in which case its future would depend solely on a collegial decision made by the movement's members? Would the Berliners, for their part, accede to decisions made in Vienna? Could they decide to continue or to stop without the support of the IPA's steering committee? Was it a purely personal creation or an institution belonging solely to its primary patron? Or was it a collective enterprise and the heritage of everyone who belonged to the organisation? Could Eitingon have created anything without the support of Freud, Abraham, Simmel and a few others?

Eitingon, however, was utterly convinced that the Berlin Institute was his alone, that it was an instrument that he had simply put at the disposal of the

DPG. Should this instrument be threatened, should it risk falling into the enemy's hands, then it would be necessary to prevent this seizure. Closing the institute would, he said, be the wisest and most obvious precaution. This line of reasoning was greatly at odds with Freud's conviction that a decision to close the institute could not be made by Eitingon alone. If, said Freud, Eitingon was unable to continue as director of the institute due to an intervention by the Nazis, then 'someone indifferent, like Boehm, could continue to lead it'. In this event, the institute should restrict its activities and not receive too many visits. It should maintain as low a profile as possible. This second option was the one Freud preferred, but it was predicated on Eitingon's continued presence in Berlin. In this scenario, Boehm would figure merely as a man of straw – he would not be allowed take any initiatives on his own recognisance.

In the third scenario, the closure of the institute would not be imposed but Eitingon would have to leave voluntarily or be forced out. The situation would, therefore, be much the same as before, but the danger would be much greater because the room for manoeuvre would be reduced. The Freudian movement would no longer have a say in the direction of the institute, its enemies would be ready to pounce, and a psychotherapist like Schultz-Hencke would benefit. To avoid this catastrophe, there could be only one solution: the IPA would have to sever its links with the Berlin Institute. It would have to cancel the institute's accreditation and disqualify Schultz-Hencke until such time as he could be 'cleansed of his faults'.[18] Before proceeding with such an expulsion, it would first be necessary to start raising your voice and to issue a warning. With this last remark, Freud suggests that the threat of a break with the IPA would carry weight, that it would be a serious strategy, one that would make anybody think twice. Logically, the threat of cutting the DPG loose would only frighten those for whom belonging to the IPA counted for something. This suggests that Freud, perhaps unconsciously, had the idea that the break would be effected by those who wanted to maintain the connection and that the others would not care.

As we know, Freud favoured the second option – with the Berlin Institute remaining open and continuing its activities with a nonentity like Boehm at the helm – but he considered this discussion of future prospects a sad debate. *Disqualification* and *atonement*: these terms suggest that Freud had little hope of being able to save anything. He predicted that the danger of psychoanalysis being misused would come from the institute's being taken over by a psychotherapist. Harald Schultz-Hencke had taught at the Berlin Institute in 1927 and 1928 but was expelled for criticising Freud's theory of sexuality and for his connections with Adler and Jung. A founding member of the Society of General Physicians for Psychotherapy, in 1934 he played a part in the creation of the German Society of General Doctors for Psychotherapy, which wished to promote psychotherapy in accordance with National Socialist ideology. An editor of one of the ten articles in the book on German psychotherapy published by Matthias Göring, Schultz-Hencke viewed psychoanalysis as a 'science of the inhibited man' and believed that it should be renamed if one really wanted to categorise it as a purely speculative theory. By the time Freud admitted to being as wary of Schultz-Hencke as he was of the plague, the latter had already turned away from the fundamentals of Freudian psychoanalysis. Schultz-Henke's later evolution shows that he was not as harmless as he seemed, despite Eitingon's opinion to the contrary. Essentially, Freud was not so wide of the mark – he merely imputed to an individual who was hostile to his teaching the manoeuvres that would in fact be carried out by Boehm, the Berlin Institute's nonentity par excellence.

If the Freudians' enemies seized the Berlin Psychoanalytic Institute in order to put it at the service of their bad intentions, they would be punished; the IPA would be forced to disown it. As a punishment, it would be necessary to banish it and wait for the moment of atonement. *Entsühnung*, atonement – the word comes from religious terminology. When sin is material, one delivers oneself from it by means of ablution, fumigation, walking through fire. When sin is understood as demonic possession, the rites required aim at casting out demons. When it is a matter of a crime against the deity, atonement is effected by means of sacrifice, confession, or penance. Regine Lockot, who testified to having paid a personal price for bringing the demons of the DPG's Nazi past out into the open in the Germany of the 1980s, stresses that it is not easy to get an idea of what Freud had really meant to signify by *Entsühnung*. Indeed, in 1933 no one could have had an idea of the true extent of the crime.[19] Could Freud have imagined a crime that no one else could? That is the question.

'All kinds of things about Berlin that you should know and that frighten me'

In the event, Boehm was chosen to replace Eitingon. But instead of staying in Berlin, Eitingon quickly decided to leave Germany permanently, having refused to occupy the position of unofficial director. In addition, with regard to the matter of the institute's membership in the DPG, Eitingon felt that the DPG's juridical pretensions were based merely on the fact that the simple glass sign on the institute's door read: 'The Berlin Psychoanalytic Institute of the German Psychoanalytic Society'. In addition, the DPG had made little contribution to the institute's functioning. Eitingon also confided to Freud that the attitude of his three German colleagues – Boehm, Müller-Braunschweig and Simmel – had greatly impressed him insofar as they had assured him that he was really the only person who should be allowed to decide the fate of the institute. Eitingon had concluded that none of them really wanted to replace him as head of the institute. On this point, however, he was deluding himself. As a result, he preferred to leave things as they were and duly refused to resign. Nevertheless, he simply commented that his and

Freud's conceptions of exactly who owned the institute differed. He did not, however, confront Freud on this point. He also explained that the possible relocation of the institute in order to make his life easier was a completely secondary concern: 'The fact that I will not leave Berlin voluntarily and not a second before that moment when the pressure of events will force me to do so was, albeit tacitly, in the background of my remarks.'[20] The next day, Eitingon wrote a new letter to Freud, explaining that the activity of the Berlin analysts had not been disrupted and that everyone's nerves were more or less holding up. The only person whose nerves really were cracking, frankly, was Eitingon's wife, Mirra. Because of her, Eitingon had no intention of postponing the trip to the Côte d'Azur that he had planned for April 1933, during the Easter holidays. To calm his wife's nerves, Eitingon would be leaving Berlin at a decisive moment – but not without having planned everything in advance.

On 7 April, Eitingon asked Boehm and Müller-Braunschweig to meet him at the institute. He gave them a directive that detailed three options. Firstly, if, during his trip – which would last from 11 April until the end of the month – the authorities should demand the replacement of the DPG's steering committee by a new committee composed of Christian analysts of pure German stock, Boehm and Müller-Braunschweig should be appointed. A meeting of members should then be convened immediately to explain the nature of the measures thus taken under external compulsion. Secondly, if the Nazi authorities should merely demand that he resign from his post as director of the institute, the same should be done, with Boehm and Müller-Braunschweig replacing him. Thirdly, if the closure of the institute or the dissolution of the DPG should be required during his absence, it should either be simply noted or, should it not be possible to obtain a delay until his return to Berlin, Boehm and Müller-Braunschweig would have to decide everything that would be necessary during an administrative meeting. On the back of the directive it was stated that in the event of unexpected developments, the signatory authorised his two Christian colleagues of pure German stock to convene an extraordinary general meeting in his absence.[21] Eitingon had planned everything before he left Berlin. Everything, that is, except Boehm's willingness to replace him.

On 10 April, just one day before the Eitingons were scheduled to leave Berlin for Menton, Boehm caught his colleagues off guard by mentioning the publication of a certain decree prohibiting Jews from belonging to the executive committee of a medical association. He had, in fact, paid a visit to the authorities in order to enquire as to whether or not the decree also applied to psychoanalysis. He further explained that as a doctor – and after having read the decree, which had been published on 9 April in the *Medical Journal of Greater Berlin* and stipulated that all medical organisations should exclude Jews from their steering committee – he felt himself to be subject to the authority of the Reichsärztekammer (Reich Chamber of Physicians). On 10

April, he went to its offices to enquire as to whether or not the decree applied to psychoanalysts. When Boehm discovered that this was, in fact, the case, he objected, contending that psychoanalysis was a scientific discipline rather than a medical one. In essence, he addressed the Reichsärztekammer, whose authority he recognised, as a doctor while maintaining that psychoanalysis, as a nonmedical specialty, should not be subject to the decree! This is barely comprehensible unless he was being dishonest.

This first initiative on Boehm's part was immediately followed by another. As soon as Eitingon left Berlin, Boehm dashed to Vienna. He later explained that he had long been planning to go to Vienna and Budapest in the spring anyway. Again, a simple fact, nothing premeditated. A little trip to Austria at Easter, in 1933 – what could be more innocent? In Vienna, Boehm visited Federn and told him about the precarious situation in Berlin. Federn promptly called Freud, who invited both men to come to his house on 17 April. Freud asked Federn to stay and witness his interview with Boehm. (So much for trust!) Boehm explained to Freud that the reason for his visit was the publication of a decree by the Reichsärztekammer that prohibited Jews from serving on a medical association's executive committee. However, he went on, Max Eitingon did not want to resign from his office as president despite the information that Boehm had been given by the Reichsärztekammer. Boehm believed that Eitingon's attitude was putting the DPG in danger.

Freud immediately suspected Boehm's motives. According to the founder of psychoanalysis, the real reason for Boehm's eagerness was his opportunism. The decree had provided him with an alibi for replacing his eminent Jewish colleague. Freud replied that he did not believe that the early resignation of Max Eitingon could help in any way. If the Nazis wanted to ban analysis and shut down the Berlin Institute, they would do it anyway. Freud had no illusions about the Nazis: psychoanalysis, he felt, would, very soon, no longer have a place in Germany. His strategy would be to play for time, to delay a ban for as long as possible. To extend the deadline, a man of straw, meaning Boehm, could head the Berlin Institute. It must also be remembered that at the time when Boehm came to see him, Freud was in fact embarking on the path prescribed by the second option, which was predicated on Eitingon's continued presence in Berlin.

In fact, however, the Nazi administration did something quite different. Psychoanalysis was not prohibited – it was simply cleansed of Jews. This segregation would not produce the same effects as banning psychoanalysis, since it would allow Christian analysts of pure German stock to join the Aryan psychotherapists. The difference between the prohibition and the racial cleansing of psychoanalysis in Germany is a decisive factor here. Can it be said that Jewish psychoanalysts shared the same fate as Jewish doctors? The medical profession was Aryanised only gradually because the Nazis realised that public opinion would have to be prepared for such a move by information campaigns. If, during the summer of 1933, the press campaign focused on the relationship between medicine and Judaism, Hitler's circumspection played an essential role in the progressive implementation of the policy of eliminating Jewish doctors. At first, Hitler proceeded cautiously. The boycott of Jewish businesses, decreed at the beginning of April 1933, had not brought the results the Nazis were expecting. There had been national and international protests. In some cities in Germany, Jewish stores continued to be crowded. There had been difficulties in enforcing measures aimed at eliminating Jewish officials, which resulted in a considerable number of exemptions. What befell Germany's liberal professions is instructive in this context. Where lawyers were concerned, the exclusion measures were gradual. On 11 April, Jewish lawyers were expelled from the National Bar Association but were still allowed to practice. On 7 April, Hitler suggested that measures against Jewish doctors should not be applied indiscriminately. On 22 April, many Jewish doctors were ousted from clinics and hospitals run by health insurance funds, but some were allowed to continue working. In the middle of 1933, eleven percent of German Jewish doctors were still practicing throughout the profession. Historian Saül Friedländer has pointed out that this is a good example of Hitler's pragmatism: 'Thousands of Jewish doctors meant tens of thousands of German patients. Cutting ties between these doctors and this large clientele risked causing unnecessary dissatisfaction. Hitler preferred to wait.'[22] More than the ban on their practicing, what worked was the pervasive fear that resulted in boycotts, he adds.

In fact, though, the Reichsärztekammer document to which Boehm referred in April 1933 was not, strictly speaking, a decree. It actually consisted of four texts written by representatives of medical corporations. One such text was an instruction from the Führer's Commissioner for National Health, Gerhard Wagner, head of the Union of German National Socialists (NSDÄB), which had been founded in 1929. Wagner had authority over all organisations in the medical field. In 1934, he was appointed to the position of Reichsärzteführer (Reich Doctors' Leader); in 1935, he became head of the Reichsärztekammer. Until his death in 1939, Wagner ruled Nazi medicine. Boehm claimed that the Nazis would view Eitingon's continued presence at the Berlin Institute as a serious provocation. According to him, it would be seen as an act of noncompliance and as grounds for official retaliation – something that could only be avoided by obtaining Eitingon's resignation. Boehm made it clear that when he had visited the Reichsärztekammer to find out about the position of psychoanalysis in the context of the decree, he had done so not as a psychoanalyst but as a doctor who felt much constrained by the decisions of the professional association to which he belonged. In so doing, Boehm became yet another of the propaganda tools that the Nazis needed in order to spread their anti-Jewish ideology. In addition to his desire to oust his Jewish colleague – as Freud suggested – his interpretation of the medical status of psychoanalysis led him to throw himself directly into the lion's den. Freud explained to Boehm that the matter of Eitingon's early resignation was a problem of local tactics. He did not really believe in the risk posed by immediate disobedience: 'If they wanted to suppress analysis and the Institute, they would hardly be influenced by the date of resignation.'[23] He suggested that Boehm contact the authorities again to let them know that the director was temporarily absent and that a meeting of members would be called upon his return. Boehm was convinced that any such assembly would demand Eitingon's resignation. If that were the case, Eitingon would resign only if it was absolutely necessary – which it would be if the assembly actually voted to oust him. He would have no choice but to abide by their decision.

It must also be remembered that Freud had almost lost the Verlag the previous year. We know of the value he accorded to the dissemination of his thought in the German language. One of his main concerns had always been to provide an increasingly wide public with written support for his work. In order to mobilise his colleagues in different countries and to encourage them to come to the assistance of international psychoanalytic publishing, Freud explained to them that the effects of the destruction of the German psychoanalytic movement would be felt at the international level. Eitingon, directly linked to the Verlag crisis in the spring of 1932, was blamed by the IPA leadership – and particularly by Jones – for having left Storfer (who, after the defection of Rank, had managed the Verlag absolutely disastrously) in place for far too long. Freud also took responsibility for this mismanagement by blaming himself for letting Storfer accumulate errors and debts. Freud's son Martin had then taken over from Storfer and had succeeded in obtaining a moratorium with the creditors. The British, American and German psychoanalytic associations provided liquidity. In order to actively contribute to saving the Verlag, Freud began to write the 'New Introductory Lectures on Psychoanalysis' in the summer of 1932. In addition, the manner in which Eitingon had dealt with the increasing power of the leftwing faction in Berlin had displeased Freud. This coterie, led by Fenichel and Reich, had grown considerably since 1931. The publication, the following year, in the *Zeitschrift* of Reich's famous article on the masochistic character – an article that Fenichel, the editor of the review at that time, had agreed to publish – had greatly annoyed Freud, who had wanted to add an editor's note to the piece. In a subsequent reprint, it was mentioned that Reich was a member of a German political party and that he had adopted the methods and objectives of Bolshevism. Reich's article had originally been published without this warning. In the same year, the Verlag refused to publish his work on character analysis.

Bernfeld was commissioned to write a response to Reich's article. In his refutation, he pointed out that the neuroses neither originated from capitalism nor dated from the age of bourgeois sexual morality. He also asserted that it was just as wrong to claim that the neuroses had only come into existence in the nineteenth century. Once considered signs of demonic possession or proofs of fate, they were later believed to be diseases until Freud succeeded in overcoming the prudishness of the 1890s. According to Bernfeld, the sociological analysis undertaken by Reich, who held that capitalism extracted profit from the sexual repression of the masses, was above all an attempt to justify psychoanalysis in the eyes of the communists. It was an argument designed to convince the Russians that psychoanalysis could work in concert with the revolution in order to free the people from capitalist exploitation. What Reich's analysis left out was the break introduced by Freud's discovery. The important thing, said Bernfeld, was that Freud was right – and that that was something that no sociology could explain. Reich, he continued, believed it was possible to eliminate the communists' distrust of the Freudian approach to sexuality, but on this point he was still mistaken because it was based on his own subjectivity. 'If Reich takes on the task of bringing psychoanalysis closer to the Comintern, he would do well not to determine the meaning of psychoanalysis according to his personal sexual ideals,' Bernfeld remarked, not without irony.[24] Reich held that psychoanalysis was likely to establish itself in communist territory on the condition of ridding itself of certain errors in order to become an authentic empirical science. He distinguished two types of psychoanalysis. The first, the original, was based on the theory of the libido. The most recent was based on the hypothesis of the death drive. Bernfeld was not exaggerating: Reich believed that the concept of the death drive represented a genuine split with psychoanalytic theory, a rupture from which psychoanalysis could never recover.

And so, at the beginning of 1932, Freud was complaining to Eitingon about the existence of certain uncontrollable and unusable personalities. First, he cited Ferenczi's obstinacy and his dubious analytic technique. Then there was the matter of Rank's desertion. And now there was Reich's and Fenichel's attempt to hijack the psychoanalytical reviews for purposes of Bolshevik propaganda – 'all kinds of things concerning Berlin that you need to know about and that make me fearful'.[25] Freud believed that the corrosive influence of the times was to blame and that people's characters were starting to fall apart. His criticism of Bolshevism placed it in the category of illusions, along with religion. Towards the end of the lecture titled 'The Question of a *Weltanschauung*', one of Freud's definitions of illusion is that it is something that aspires to achieving a metamorphosis of the fundamental human drive. To the extent that Bolshevism wanted to institute a new order in which aggressive inclinations would be neutralised by the abolition of private property, it was, said Freud, an illusion, one that aspired to change human nature in a matter of decades. Bolshevism was a religion, except for the fact that its paradise was to be inaugurated here on earth and in the near future. This much-hoped-for transformation of human nature being as yet unaccomplished, it seemed justified to inflict on all men the relentless pressure of an education of consciences coupled with a prohibition on thinking. Such use of force, Freud thought, might go as far as murder. In Russia, he noted, human nature had not improved and the aggressive drive had not disappeared.

Hatred was now directed outwards, targeting the revolution's enemies. The main lesson of this text was, he said, that the material misery of the masses could not be relieved by a radical transformation of the social order: 'Even then, to be sure, we shall still have to struggle for an incalculable time with the difficulties which the untameable character of human nature presents to every kind of social community.'[26]

These considerations should be understood as a warning, as Freud's response to the analytical movement's infatuation with communism. Indeed, the controversy triggered by Reich's article in the *Zeitschrift* had led Fenichel to organise an opposition group of leftwing psychoanalysts in Berlin and thus to antagonise Freud even further. For his part, Reich became 'a nuisance' for Freud.[27] The Reich affair was still preoccupying Freud at the time of Boehm's visit on 17 April 1933. Measures taken in Germany against the communists raised fears that Reich might be arrested at the premises of the institute. Reich was presenting himself both as a psychoanalyst and as a communist. Freud asked Boehm to arrange for Reich's expulsion from the DPG as quickly as possible. The following summer, the board of directors of the DPG held several meetings that included discussions on the subject of Reich's ejection. Eitingon wanted no action to be taken before he himself resigned from office at the general meeting scheduled for the autumn. Reich was, nevertheless, struck off the list of members. His expulsion from the DPG resulted in the cancellation of his IPA membership, which was announced in Lucerne.

A simple replacement of people?

Ernest Jones's version of Boehm's visit to Vienna was not entirely neutral. Jones, who was not present during the interview, relied on the letter that Freud wrote to Eitingon later that same day. At certain points in his narrative, Jones delivered an interpretation of the facts. If we base ourselves solely on his narrative, what emerges from it differs appreciably from Freud's description of the proceedings, with particular regard to a point that does not have the character of a detail. In fact, Jones attributed to Freud a judgement relating to the alleged harmlessness of the replacement of Jewish analysts by analysts of German origin. Let us compare the two versions we have at our disposal.

In his biography of Freud, Jones reported on Boehm's visit to Freud's house as follows:

> On April 17, 1933, Boehm visited Freud in Vienna to ask his advice about the situation. The immediate question was the new order that no Jews were to serve on any scientific council. Freud was of the opinion that merely to change the personnel in this way would not prevent the government from forbidding psychoanalysis in Germany. Yet it would be wise not to give them that pretext by refraining from making the change, and he agreed that Boehm replace Eitingon on the council.[28]

In this passage, Jones essentially portrays Freud as saying that the replacement of the Jewish members was an act of no importance.

Fanny Colonomos and Elisabeth Marsault, two authors who have written about psychoanalysis at the time of the rise of Nazism, have commented on this, emphasising the formulation's segregative nature. Establishing a link between the resignation of the Jewish members of the Berlin Institute's steering committee and the admission of three Jewish analysts – Therese Benedeck, Edith Jacobson and Edith Weigert-Vowinckel – to the teaching committee, they deduce that this had to do with balancing a segregative measure with a compensatory measure: 'Freud and the Berlin psychoanalysts seem to have believed in the possible autonomy of institutional analytical practice under a dictatorship, [a form of] political blindness that cost analytical theory dearly and led to bastardised practices.'[29] But this replacement of people is an 'error of judgement that neglects the culturally destructive dimension of anti-Semitism – not because the men of culture are predominantly Jews, as in the DPG, but because of the totalitarian essence of the phenomenon'.[30] They added that this error was shared by the Jews themselves. These assertions need be examined. Did Freud really neglect the culturally destructive dimension of anti-Semitism, as these two authors maintain?

It should be remembered at this point that National Socialist policy can be divided into three periods. Before the war, the civil rights of the Jews were rescinded and many were forced to emigrate. The early days of the war saw a period of expulsion, including a plan – which was never realised – to deport the Jews to Madagascar. In 1942, addressing the Reichstag, Hitler recalled the prophecy he had made on 30 September 1939, according to which the war would result in the annihilation of Judaism:

> Formerly, in Germany, the Jews laughed at my prophecy. I don't know if they're laughing today, or if they've had the urge to laugh. But now I can assure you of this: everywhere, the urge to laugh will pass away. And it is I who will, with this prophecy, have the last word.[31]

Following the invasion of the USSR in June 1941, German mobile killing units conducted a campaign of mass murder that affected entire Jewish families on Soviet territory. At the end of July 1941, Hermann Göring authorised Reinhard Heydrich, director of the Reichssicherheitshauptamt (Reich Main Security Office), to begin preparations for the implementation of the 'complete solution to the Jewish question'. The third period witnessed the implementation of the General Government's plan for the systematic liquidation of the Jews in three extermination camps in Poland.

As Germany's prospects of winning the war became increasingly uncertain, the messianic tenor of Hitler's anti-Semitism increased. After the failure of his campaign against the USSR and the setback of the American landings in North Africa, he spoke of the gift that National Socialism would give to the world by eradicating the Jews of Germany and Central Europe. In November 1942, Hitler declared that people always mocked his prophetic pronouncements but that soon they would have nothing to laugh about:

> Innumerable numbers of all those who laughed back then are no longer laughing today, and those who are still laughing will stop doing so before much longer. We will know it in Europe and it will spread all over the world. People will acknowledge the demonic danger represented by international Judaism – and we, the National Socialists, will watch over it.[32]

For Hitler, the notions of Judaism and internationalism were so tightly connected that he put forward – on at least two occasions – the absurd idea of international world war. This division of Nazi policy into three distinct periods is not gratuitous; it shows the progression of a programme based on the messianic conviction that the wicked Supreme Other and his sarcastic laughter would be eliminated.

Freud and Eitingon's discussions concerning the future of the Berlin Institute took place during the first period of National Socialism, which largely entailed stripping the Jews of their civil rights and giving them strong incentives to emigrate. Freud knew perfectly well that Germany would descend into barbarism and that among the many insane proposals put forward by Hitler the only two that could actually be achieved were the persecution of the Jews and the abolition of freedom of thought. Jewish thought would soon have no place in the Reich. Yet Freud felt that ultimately his personal decision to leave Vienna and go into exile could only be predicated on the existence of a direct threat to his life. We need to be clear that it was the lives of others that concerned him. At that time, his own life was no longer particularly dear to him. If it were 'only' a matter of persecution and restrictions on his activities, he felt duty bound to stay. Dying in Vienna was not a prospect Freud found unthinkable. In the last letter he addressed to Ferenczi, he soberly indicated that it was a possibility that needed to be considered:

> There is certainly no personal danger for me, and if you assume life in oppression to be amply uncomfortable for us Jews, then don't forget how little contentment life promises refugees in a foreign country, be it Switzerland or England. Flight, I think, would be justified only in the case of lethal danger, and incidentally, if they kill you, it's one kind of death like any other.[33]

It was only after the events of March 1938, when Freud realised that the Austrians were in no way inferior to the Germans where barbarism was concerned, and, above all, when two of his children, Anna and Martin, had serious trouble with the authorities, that he reconsidered his position and agreed to leave his homeland.

Colonomos and Marsault suggest that, ultimately, Freud and his entourage believed above all in the scientific nature of psychoanalysis. This illusion, they contend, would have led the Freudians to believe that the successful integration of psychoanalysis into society as a science could make it independent of political circumstances. Indeed, German analysts, like Freud himself, seem to have believed, at least at the outset, in the extraterritoriality of psychoanalysis in relation to history, and to have adjusted their strategy towards the Nazis in line with this conviction.[34] They conclude that by not wanting to offer a pretext to the Nazis, Freud would have ceased to be an analyst by virtue of having yielded to the illusion of the independence of science. Blindness, illusion and apoliticalism are therefore the main complaints made against Freud and his followers for agreeing to let the two German organisations continue their work rather than dissolving them.

What of blindness, then? Freud and the Berliners would not have grasped the fundamentally destructive scope of anti-Semitism. It has been said that they were blind to the seriousness of the situation – that they would, in some way, have consented to anti-Semitic measures by reshuffling and substituting people in order to make the institution last as pure form, as an empty shell. By privileging psychoanalysis as a therapeutic practice, the psychoanalysts would have behaved like any professional class seeking to protect itself, just as doctors, lawyers and solicitors fight to safeguard their professions by deciding to adapt to difficult conditions. The crucial signifier in this case is that of adaptation. That of Freud, we recall, was sacrifice. To put it another way, the analysts would have sacrificed their ethics in order to enable the institution to survive and continue functioning. As has been noted, Freud said he was ready to sacrifice his own name in order to ensure the survival of German-language psychoanalysis. It is fundamentally important to grasp the fact that, for Freud, what was at stake was much more than rescuing the institutions themselves. His entire life's work had taken shape and developed in a single language – German. Following his departure from Austria and the confiscation of all the books that had been stored in the Verlag, Freud endeavoured to publish, without delay, an original German edition of his works in England. He told Arnold Zweig that it was impossible for him to abandon his mother tongue. One's mother tongue, he explained, is like skin: one can't change it.

And what about illusion? That would relate to a belief in the extraterritoriality of psychoanalysis as a science and as a practice. This also implies that Freud overlooked the widely recognised fact that science is not independent of politics. Obviously, this is a judgement that Freud's actions after 1918 utterly refute. Relating to the question of the extraterritoriality of psychoanalysis in 1932's 'The Question of a *Weltanschauung*', his reaffirmation that psychoanalysis belonged to the discourse of science led to the original argument according to which psychoanalysis depended on no ideology and could not serve the interests of a political party. The call to revolution, to the belief in the possibility of rapidly effecting a change in the ways in which human beings function, was not only politically questionable – it was foolishness, an aberration, an illusion that ignored the drive demands. In his exchange with Albert Einstein, which took place that same year, Freud again explained that the Bolsheviks, for the moment, had above all been carefully armed and that before they could overcome the aggressiveness inherent in human nature they would have to fight terrible civil wars.[35] This questioning of illusion in politics objects to the image of the scientist sheltered in his ivory tower and looking at the landscape from his window. Conversely, Freud continually interpreted the world around him. Withdrawal was completely foreign to the position he had adopted with regard to civilisation. Freud was not detached – he was angry, which is very different. During the 1930s, Paula Fichtl, the family servant, pointed out that sculptor Oscar Nemon's bust of Freud represented him in a state of anger. Freud retorted: 'But I am angry, I am angry with humanity.'

Commentary on contemporary political events was part of the very substance of Freud's work. There was a profound reason for this, one related to the very progress of his theory. Based on his research into the origins of the moral conscience (*das Gewissen*), Freud had posited that, like individuals, civilisation also possesses a superego that governs its cultural evolution. Freud did not contest historical materialism's value as truth, but he showed that there was another explanation, that there was another truth that he had brought to light:

> It seems likely that what are known as materialistic views of history sin in under-estimating this factor. They brush it aside with the remark that human 'ideologies' are nothing other than the product and superstructure of their contemporary economic conditions. That is true, but very probably not the whole truth. Mankind never lives entirely in the present. The past, the traditions of the race and of the people, lives on in the ideologies of the super-ego, and yields only slowly to the influences of the present and to new changes; and so long as it operates through the super-ego it plays a powerful part in human life, independently of economic conditions.[36]

Through its individual and collective double face, the superego was thus a pivot point between the subject and the social. Freud's 1921 study of group psychology was, according to its author, only the beginning. In relation to the strain of the civilising process, both that of the superego in its singular expressions and that of the ideologies of the superego in their collective forms, psychoanalysis had something to say.

There remains the subject of the 'apolitical'. Freud's lecture on the *Weltanschauung* concluded with the need to take into account the fact that man is a fundamentally asocial being because instinctual satisfactions cannot be fully sublimated. It is impossible to transform them in their entirety into cultural requirements. There is always a remainder, which corresponds to the way in which everyone is satisfied at the level of the drive. In this sense, would it be more justified to posit a gap between concept and action? In the spring of 1933, Freud was aware that the Nazis were establishing a regime that would make life unbearable for all Jews in Germany. It seems a matter of some delicacy to reproach him for his lack of clairvoyance concerning the intrinsically destructive component of anti-Semitism insofar as it cannot be considered separately from the fact that the extermination of the Jews of Central Europe had a before and an after. A threshold had been crossed, and from that moment onwards anti-Semitism could no longer be synonymous merely with deprivation of liberty, with restrictions on activities in the professional, academic and political fields and with prejudice, exclusion and rejection. There is no doubt that the reality of the concentration camps changed the meaning of anti-Semitism. Neither the policy of compromise championed by Jones in Lucerne nor the duplicity of German analysts like Boehm and Müller-Braunschweig are justifiable. However, the judgement relating to the blindness of Freud and his entourage vis-à-vis the intrinsically destructive dimension of anti-Semitism represents a road that, for different reasons, need not be taken. The first of these considerations is that it is always easy to think things through in retrospect and to cite the Jews' blindness to the fate that awaited them. This question goes beyond the limits of the psychoanalytic movement to touch on the problem – by far the most crucial of all – of the failure of speech and language faced with the reality of the extermination of the Jews of Europe on an industrial scale.

The second consideration requiring attention is that the reproach made by Colonomos and Marsault results from their interest in an entirely separate controversy. They believe the error of judgement according to which psychoanalysts opted for the survival of the institution at the expense of ethics requires reflection on the relationship that psychoanalysts have with the psychoanalytic institution. Through their study of psychoanalysis at the time of the rise of Nazism, these two authors make no secret of the fact that, for them, it is a question of illustrating the contradiction that exists between the clinical and scientific autonomy of psychoanalysis with regard to outside interference. It is, in fact, an example of 'multiple institutional storms',[37] splits and counter-splits having led to the incessant recasting of psychoanalytic institutions. They compare the situation of psychoanalysis in France after the dissolution of the École Freudienne de Paris (EFP) and the creation of multiple analytical groups laying claim to Lacan's teaching to that of psychoanalysis in West Germany after 1945, when that country's two psychoanalytic societies were claiming direct descent from the Berlin Institute and the DPG. According to these authors, the question of origins and legitimacy comes up every time. To analyse the situation from the perspective of fantasy, it would be necessary to show how psychoanalytic institutions create for themselves – as does the patient in treatment – a foundation myth, a story of origins that allows them to privilege their prestige and their power at the expense of an assumed parentage. The situation of the Berlin Institute at the time of the rise of Nazism and the faulty thinking they impute to the Freudians who preferred to maintain, rather than dissolve, the institution to which they belonged allow the two authors to undertake a barely veiled criticism both of what happened when Lacan dissolved his own school at the end of his life and of the consequences of his action. This interpretative bias therefore functions as a filter colouring the image by giving it an anachronistic aspect. In addition, shedding light on the particularities of the last period of Freud's life by bringing it closer to the events that followed Lacan's demise is far from convincing. Thus, the imputation to Freud of an unconscious anti-Semitism accompanied by the drawing of parallels between the collaborationism of analysts from the IPA's German branch with the situation of the EFP after Lacan's death is not just anachronistic – it also makes for uncomfortable reading. Finally, and even though the matter was not addressed by these two authors whose insights are nothing if not simplistic, we will temporarily set aside the question of the choice of object made by Jones, who found in a Jewish woman (Anna Freud) the partner who suited him. Things are not remotely clear-cut here; they are located in a grey area of ambition, cowardice and neurosis.

The National Socialist danger was already present before 1933. Someone who said he wanted to destroy international Judaism had to be taken seriously. Hitler's *Mein Kampf*, published in two volumes (one in 1925, the other in 1926), lays bare the radicalisation of his thinking. His programme had three elements: the struggle against international Judaism, the elimination of Marxism and the need to conquer the USSR in order to extend the *Lebensraum* (living space) of the Germanic peoples. The former agitator in Bavarian beer halls who had previously contented himself with parroting hate slogans drawn from the far right had changed his thinking in the aftermath of the Russian Revolution. It seemed to him that the Jews now dominated Russia and that Judeo-Bolshevism had wiped out the old ruling class of the German race. It was necessary to take back from Russia what the Jews had taken from it – and, for that, Germany needed a leader who was capable of raising up the German people and giving them the strength to launch a titanic battle. After his failed coup and his subsequent imprisonment in Landsberg Castle, Hitler came to believe that he was the great man Germany was waiting for to initiate the confrontation. The first signs of a cult of personality appeared as early as 1922–1923 among members of the Nazi Party; however, many people still believed that Hitler was simply someone with decidedly cranky ideas. The collapse of the German state and its economic structures provoked by the financial crash of 1929 turned everything upside down. It allowed him to attain the status of someone sent by providence to save the desperate German people. The Weimar Republic seemed completely powerless to stem the country's dizzying descent into crisis. In addition, after his release from prison Hitler gradually managed to curb the internal strife within NSDAP. His simple ideas, which he hammered home relentlessly – the aspiration for national unity, the grandiose vision of Germany rising phoenix-like from the ashes and the mission of liberating humanity from Judeo-Bolshevism – won hearts and minds at a time when the crisis of the German state, provoked by the Great Depression, was undermining everything. As Ian Kershaw notes:

> In the building of mass support, it was less an intrinsic Nazi doctrine than the style of articulation and presentation of fears, phobias and nebulous expectations far more generally prevalent than among the traditional core support for the *völkisch* Right that was decisive. And when it came to presentation, Hitler was peerless.[38]

This union of racial and foreign policy was the essence of Hitlerism. When it reached its peak, however, its components came into conflict. In 1942, as the Battle of Stalingrad raged, the leading Nazis quarrelled among themselves concerning whether to favour the transportation of military equipment to the Eastern Front over the transportation of Jews to the extermination camps in Poland – and vice versa.

Freud, of course, knew none of this. He died in London on 23 September 1939, at three o'clock in the morning, after receiving a fatal dose of morphine from his doctor. His suffering was at an end. He had lived just long enough to learn of Hitler's triumph in Vienna on 14 March 1938 and the German invasion of Poland on 1 September 1939. It was on that day that Hitler addressed the Reichstag, promising that the war would result in the obliteration of Judaism. In this regard, it is important to remember that Freud's questioning of anti-Semitism had never ceased and that it continued right up until the end of his life and the stubborn writing of *Moses and Monotheism*. Freud conjectured that psychoanalysis had provoked opposition because its inventor was Jewish. According to him, only a Jew could have invented psychoanalysis because he was prepared to endure this position of rejection and exclusion. In the case of the Berlin Institute's non-closure, Freud did not underestimate the persecution that the new government would be capable of in Germany. It was his high conception of the capacity of psychoanalysis to resist, aligned with his own ability to fight on, that had led to his demand to keep both the institute and the DPG going following Hitler's appointment as chancellor. Underestimation of the meteoric speed with which the Hitlerian regime would shatter Germany's democratic structures, already damaged by the financial crisis of 1929 and its aftermath, was not unique to Freud. All political opposition to the Nazis was quashed in less than six months. In April 1933, in Prussia alone, there were 25,000 prisoners in pre-trial detention with no judicial oversight. The destruction of democracy and the establishment of despotism could not have happened without the backing of the ruling elites and the support of the masses who favoured the recovery policies initiated by the Third Reich. The destruction of parliamentarianism and Marxism in political life was consecrated by the promulgation of the one-party state on 14 July 1933. By that date, any challenge to the authority of the Führer was already over. Professional organisations and associations, along with other interest groups, purged their leaderships and Nazified their statutes very quickly: falling into line was the rule in many of the professions. More often than not, the Nazis did not even need to terrorise these organisations' representatives. The conservative right, which had set up the new regime, believed it had the country's new chancellor under its thumb and rallied to the Nazis, completely convinced that Hitler and his henchmen would serve its interests while the country waited for the crisis to be resolved.

However, in the spring of 1933, Freud's mood was fluctuating between despondency and hope. His idea that people should endeavour to resist until the crisis ended is quite logical. Although he had a hunch that civilisation was falling off a cliff, he was shaken when he learned of Eitingon's decision to leave for Palestine, and he asked the acting president of the IPA to organise the resistance. This choice can all too easily seem absurd, unfortunate and wrong. We can interpret it in many ways, and yet nothing helps. As simple and strange as it sounds, Freud wanted to preserve the Berlin Institute for the same reasons that he refused to leave Vienna. Convinced that psychoanalysis would, sooner or later, be prohibited in Germany, and that nothing in the world would be able to make the authorities back down as soon as such a decision had been taken, Freud argued that, in order to delay the deadline, the Nazis should not be given a pretext for rushing such a decision. It was necessary, he felt, to play for time, to wait until the Nazis fell from power. However, in light of the fact that Boehm was claiming to have succeeded in convincing the Nazi administration of the merits of psychoanalysis during the summer of 1933, this version of the story seems untenable, especially because Matthias Göring and his entourage had admitted to wanting to put an end to the intolerable isolation of the psychoanalysts of the DPG ever since Hitler's accession to power. Our assumption is that the Nazis were pretending that they needed persuading. Their intention, as an episode from 1936 involving Herbert Linden will show, was to take advantage of the expertise of therapists of all stripes and to make use of the experience and the prestigious premises of the most famous among them.

With regard to the matter of simply replacing people, one could say that what was unfortunate – the bad choice – was not so much the resignations as the substitutions, the replacement, in order to reassure the authorities, of Jewish analysts by Christian analysts of pure German stock. The idea was not to provoke, not to challenge, not to give a pretext to those who could, overnight, declare psychoanalysis to be just as *unerwünscht* (undesirable) as the Jews. Freud felt that the Berlin Institute should remain in place while awaiting better days, and one cannot help but think that this 'waiting until the last minute' approach was the expression of a subjective position rather than an instance of blindness. As long as one's life was not directly threatened, Freud felt, one had to resist – one had to stay the course and keep working even if the fight seemed lost. It was this character trait – his obstinacy, his stubbornness – that had been foundational, from the beginning, to his fight against the enemies of psychoanalysis, which he kept up despite his sickness and suffering. His overall attitude, which can seem disconcerting, was all of a piece with his singular obstinacy. It was the expression of the most prominent feature of his personality: his stoical resistance to pain and misfortune. Freud's iron control of his emotions astonished everyone who met him. Do not abandon the two centres of German-language psychoanalysis: this demand was a projection of Freud's mental attitude in the face of adversity. Freud was aware that the dictatorship of the right would certainly mean the quashing of social democracy in Germany. But the possibility of discriminatory and legal measures being taken against the Jews in Austria still seemed inconceivable to him.

Compared to the Germans, the Austrians appeared to be amateurs where brutality was concerned: 'In such a way we lull ourselves into – relative – security. In any case, I am resolved not to budge an inch,'[39] Freud wrote to Jones just ten days before Boehm's visit. If one wishes to maintain the thesis of blindness, this statement obviously concerns the idea – which was entirely incorrect, as the aftermath of the Anschluss was to demonstrate – that the Austrians were more civilised than their German neighbours. On this point, it is possible to reply that in 1933 Freud shared the illusions of those among his associates who refused to believe that Austria would sink into chaos. How could they have anticipated the outburst of insanity that followed the resignation of the Austrian chancellor, Kurt von Schuschnigg, on 11 March 1938, when Vienna turned into a nightmare straight out of Hieronymus Bosch? The Austrian capital's inhabitants wrecked Jewish businesses and assaulted their owners. The Wehrmacht's battalions were greeted with cries of joy. A torrent of envy, jealousy, bitterness and malice swept over civilised Austria. Even Nazi officers were stunned by this surge of hatred.

Now let us study the other version. In a letter to Eitingon penned just hours after Boehm's visit, Freud wrote:

> Here, the story of a visit by Boehm. He told me about the decree stating that no Jew can be president of an association; he told me that he had gone to the Reichsärztekammer to ask if this also applied to our psychoanalytic association, that he had given you a positive answer before your departure, but that you had announced that you would not resign on your own and that you would only yield to a direct order. He then asked to hear my point of view, but he probably wanted me to urge you to resign immediately; he believes that, when one has shown oneself to be ineffective, one risks the kinds of measures that, as a rule, cause more fuss than a purely formal change of personnel intended for the authorities. I was completely satisfied to have Federn in attendance during the

> interview, it being understood that he could testify to any distortions that might be made later. *I replied that it was a matter of local tactics that I was in no position to judge from a distance.* I didn't really believe in the risks of immediate disobedience; if [the Nazis] wanted to suppress analysis and the Institute, they would hardly be influenced by the date of resignation. I then advised him to tell the authorities that the president [of the Berlin Institute] was simply absent and that we would settle the matter during a general meeting following his return. Boehm takes it for granted that the majority of this meeting will invite you to resign. That would be the force that you demand and to which you could yield. [Boehm] was quite clear in assuring me that this step would change nothing relating to the interior life of the [DPG], and that he and [Müller-Braunschweig] would refuse to make any essential concessions concerning the functioning of analysis. I made him understand that in such a case we would ask for, and impose, the exclusion of the Berlin Institute from the IPA. He told me that this was not going to happen, that they themselves – the new bureau – would bring about the dissolution of the [DPG] before then. It all sounded very loyal, but it was still clear that these gentlemen are in a hurry to enter the bureau, and I have great doubts about their reliability.[40]

Note that the purely formal change of personnel was something expressed by Boehm that Freud transcribed. The expression 'He spoke to me' refers to the speech made by Boehm, while Freud's words are introduced by 'I answered'. The particular care taken by Freud when transcribing his interview with Boehm was completely overlooked by Jones, who attributed to Freud the words of the person who was actually speaking to him. Ultimately, Freud emphasised external constraint, differentiating it from subjective decision. This goes in the direction of the difference, as previously noted, between sacrifice and concession. You had to be forced to leave, you had to wait for the moment when you would have no choice. Until that limit was reached, you had to resist.

Eitingon sent his reply to Freud's letter of 17 April 1933 from the Widjers Grand Hôtel in Menton. He could not understand why Boehm had gone to Vienna if all he wanted to do was obtain Freud's approval to request his resignation. In fact, Eitingon had organised everything before leaving for France. Six days before his departure, he had discussed his plans with Müller-Braunschweig and Boehm. During his absence from Berlin for the Easter holidays, his resignation – should the authorities demand it – ought to be understood as a fait accompli, he said. The two Aryans were expected to divide the functions of president of the DPG and director of the Institute between them. Eitingon followed the course of events without anticipating anything; it had not been his intention to call an early general meeting. At that time, Fenichel had already left for Oslo to prepare for his emigration, which took place in the autumn. Simmel, afraid of being arrested, had moved to Zurich in March 1933. When Fenichel returned to Berlin, he noted the great concern of his younger colleagues. Eitingon's quiet wait-and-see attitude was no longer enough to reassure them. The day before his departure, Eitingon finally decided that, in his absence, the convening of a general meeting for the purpose of obtaining his resignation would be possible, but only in the case of absolute necessity. He would therefore comply with the decisions of this meeting. Moreover, only out of necessity and for the good of the analytic cause would he bow to something so degrading. Any further evolution of discriminatory measures against the Jews could only be the result of an external constraint. Like Freud, Eitingon firmly rejected the position of voluntary submission. He had no intention of precipitating a crisis – he was simply taking precautions before embarking on his trip. In 1933, Eitingon was already entertaining thoughts of moving to Palestine, whereas Freud only considered departing for England when he began to fear for his own life and for the lives of his family. Things came to a head on 22 March 1938, when Anna Freud was arrested and taken to Gestapo headquarters in a black sedan. For Freud, psychoanalysis was an ideal for which his own name was well worth sacrificing. For his part, Eitingon did not want to leave it to anyone to ensure that the Berlin Institute would continue to operate once he himself had been forced to leave. On the one hand, a sacrifice can be made in the name of the ideal. On the other hand, mere substitution of personnel is not desirable. The analytical cause cannot come into conflict with its Jewish origins. The emphasis on sacrifice was, in Freud's case, more marked.

On 21 April 1933, Eitingon indicated that he was not completely opposed to preventive measures, but he insisted that these should be implemented slowly and steadily. During the meeting that took place at the institute before his departure, Boehm had indeed mentioned the famous decree that was actually nothing more than a set of instructions intended for medical societies. Fenichel, Eitingon and Müller-Braunschweig were of the opinion that the decree did not pertain to psychoanalysis because psychoanalysis was not a corporate medical association. Boehm's decision to enquire into the matter on his own initiative struck them, in retrospect, as having been both useless and dangerous. His hastiness, they felt, did not bode well. Eitingon believed that Boehm had gone to Vienna to seek Freud's blessing. He concluded that having Boehm as president of the DPG and the Berlin Institute would be the greatest misfortune imaginable at that time. In the event, the general assembly was not convened in Eitingon's absence. Originally scheduled for 2 May, it was postponed to 6 May, which was also Freud's birthday – something Eitingon always marked with a greeting. 'The fact that I'll be there makes me very happy,'[41] he wrote to Freud at the end of April, when he was still on the Riviera. On this occasion, he alluded to his wife's fear of returning to Berlin. This confirms that Mirra's anxiety was one of his reasons for going to Menton. At the DPG's extraordinary general meeting on 6 May 1933, Müller-Braunschweig and Boehm demanded the removal of Jewish colleagues from the association's board of directors. This request was rejected. Anna Freud and Ernest Jones lauded Eitingon's capacity for resistance. It must also be noted that, in his biography of Freud, Jones conflated the general assembly with the occasion of Eitingon's resignation, giving the impression that Eitingon handed in his resignation during the meeting of the assembly. Jones's precise language is as follows: 'On Eitingon's return to Berlin, a general meeting was held and he had to resign.' In fact, however, Eitingon remained in post until the end of the year. It was also in May that the proposal to unite the Berlin and Vienna institutes was rejected – Eitingon, unlike Anna Freud, did not believe that Austria could provide more certain refuge than Germany.

On 10 May 1933, four days after the assembly had refused to accept Eitingon's resignation, Freud's books were burned in Berlin's Opera Square (now known as Bebelplatz). He responded by commenting that civilisation had indeed progressed: in the Middle Ages, it was the authors who were burned. Then, on 22 May, Ferenczi died. Freud said that in the last weeks before his death, Ferenczi could no longer stand or walk and that his madness had become apparent. Ferenczi's obituary was presented in June at a ceremony organised by the DPG. Anna Freud asked Eitingon to delete a passage where he described how the steering committee had reacted to Freud's announcement that he had cancer in 1923. The passage concerned reads as follows: 'Deeply distressed by the knowledge of the danger and the need for an invasive and mutilating operation, we were all looking at the older brother, Ferenczi.' The reference to the fact that Freud's predicament was understood by the steering committee as signalling the imminence of the DPG's demise was deleted. Freud greatly appreciated Eitingon's tribute to Ferenczi.[42]

Another cause for disillusionment presented itself in May. Freud was under the impression that Jung could not leave Switzerland. However, the latter immediately accepted the office of president of the General Medical Society for Psychotherapy following Kretschmer's resignation. In-depth reading of *Mein Kampf* was placed on that organisation's teaching programme by Matthias Göring with a view to making it the basis for future work in psychotherapy. In mid-July 1933, a newspaper announced the lessons that Hans von Hattingberg, a member of the IPA until 1925, was in charge of teaching psychotherapy at the University of Berlin. Did Freud speak in private differently than in his writings? Did he not try to reassure his colleagues about the future of psychoanalysis in his books? If he had become discouraged, what example would he have set for the analytical community as a whole? In his private correspondence, Freud indeed gave free rein to his pessimism – as he did when he stated that the early resignation of the director of the Berlin Institute was going to be useless because the authorities would ban psychoanalysis anyway. Such an opinion was certainly not naive. Freud foresaw that psychoanalysis would soon have no future in Germany. In August 1933, he wrote to Jones that Berlin was lost and that Budapest, in the wake of Ferenczi's death, was nothing.

The tribulations of a nonentity

Nazi policy vis-à-vis psychoanalysis was not to destroy it but to reduce its influence by mixing it with other therapeutic methods. Boehm, along with his colleague Müller-Braunschweig, went a considerable distance in bringing psychoanalysis into line with the Nazi project. The de-Judaised version of psychoanalysis would no longer be allowed to mention Freud's name. It was to be aligned with the new therapy of the German man, designed to ensure the disappearance of conflicts and the recovery of the life forces of individuals. It was necessary to cure those beaten down by fate and to give them the courage to contribute to the recovery of the nation. The new therapy would participate in the general mission of Hitlerian politics: the material and psychological preparation of the people for war with a view to building the Germany of the future.

As early as October 1933, in order to reassure the authorities, Carl Müller-Braunschweig published an article in a journal of the European Racial Alliance, under the title of 'Psychoanalysis and *Weltanschauung*'. In it, he defended the idea that psychoanalysis had been diverted from its goals. The discipline, he said, had sometimes been discredited because it had been practised by untrained clinicians. It was, he contended, by no means as anti-German as might be imagined:

> Psychoanalysis strives to transform the dispirited and incompetent into capable and strong beings; to transform the instinctually inhibited into assertive beings; to turn those fantasists who are strangers to life into human beings capable of looking reality in the face; to change those who are subject to their impulses into people who can control them; to turn egotists incapable of love into human beings capable of love and sacrifice; to turn those who care for nothing into people capable of serving a common cause. Thus it does a wonderful job of education and can do valuable service for a heroic conception of life turned towards constructive reality, the lines of which have been newly established.[43]

Müller-Braunschweig emphasised the ego's capacity for synthesis – the dramatic battle between the drive forces, on the one hand, and, on the other, the spiritual forces that flowed from the demands of the superego. The vision of the world conveyed by this highly distorted presentation of analytic treatment was very much aligned with the ideology of the Third Reich.

In a report he wrote after the war for presentation at the IPA congress in Amsterdam in 1951, Boehm stated that he had merely based his attitude on Freud's own wish not to give the authorities a pretext to ban the activities of the DPG during the Nazi period. He had, he said, always acted with Jones's full agreement and with Anna Freud's blessing. It was during the general assembly held on 18 November 1933 that Max Eitingon would have suggested restricting the members of the management committee to himself and Müller-Braunschweig. This restriction was, however, offset by the inclusion of Edith Jacobson and Therese Benedeck as members of the Berlin Institute's training committee. The scientific and teaching activities of the polyclinic then continued as usual until November 1935, when, according to Boehm, two Berlin psychotherapists and several members of the Nazi Party suddenly became interested in the fate of psychoanalysis. He and Müller-Braunschweig duly met with them. During this meeting, it was explained to them that psychoanalysis might be allowed to remain in existence with an entirely Aryan membership. Boehm then pointed out that most of the Jewish members had been gone since 1931. Under the influence of this threat and moved by the desire to protect psychoanalysis, Müller-Braunschweig and Boehm then contacted Jones. Without providing details, Boehm then indicated that the DPG's few remaining Jewish members had decided to resign.

Thus we see how the supposedly voluntary resignation of Jewish analysts was carried out in Berlin and how they interpreted it. It was clearly a degrading act of submission for them. In March 1936, Boehm met Anna Freud for six hours in Brünn. It was no longer possible for a German citizen to travel to Austria, which prevented him from travelling to Vienna himself. At the end of this long conversation, Anna Freud supposedly told him that her father approved of his new orientation. Boehm emphasised that it was only after having this discussion that he informed the representative of the medical department that he would accept the new proposals. Boehm argued that he had acted with the Freuds' consent. The medical representative immediately wrote to Matthias Göring to put forward the idea of creating a new institute that would bring together different therapeutic orientations. The proposed organisation's practitioners would all enjoy the same rights and privileges. In April, Boehm met with the head of the Nazi Party's University Affairs Department. In June, Matthias Göring took over the new institution with Boehm as his secretary. In November 1936, Göring moved to the premises of the Berlin Institute. Furniture and books from the library were made available.

In other words: in the spring of 1936, an official of the Medical Department of the Ministry of the Interior – Dr Herbert Linden – had given his assurance that psychoanalysis would not be banned as a therapeutic method. However, for ideological reasons linked to the philosophy of the Nazi Party, Freud's work would no longer be tolerated. Göring, who was now president of the German General Medical Society for Psychotherapy, wanted to establish a therapeutic institute (*Poliklinik*) in Berlin. In fact, as soon as the Göring Institute was created in May 1936, influential members of the Nazi Party demanded that the DPG separate from the IPA, which prompted Boehm to meet with Anna Freud in order to proceed to the official split. From now on, neither the term 'psychoanalysis' nor the existence of an independent institute would be tolerated by the authorities. When Boehm met Anna Freud for six hours in Brünn, the issue of the split between the DPG and the IPA was on the agenda. But despite the fact that a note relating to the split had already been prepared for the next congress, which was scheduled to be held in Marienbad, Jones opposed the split because he intended to have the DPG's silent adherence to the IPA continue until the situation in Germany improved.[44]

Boehm continued his Amsterdam address by specifying that in January 1937 he had met Sigmund Freud for more than an hour and told him that it was no longer possible to avoid teaching elements of Jungian theory to students at the new institute. According to Boehm, Freud would have replied that this posed no particular difficulty. Shortly afterwards, however, Freud held a meeting at his home at which – according to Boehm – Anna Freud, Jeanne Lampl-De Groot and Martin Freud were present. Boehm no longer remembered the names of the other participants. For three quarters of an hour, Boehm delivered his report. This was the point when, suddenly, Freud interrupted him by saying that the Jews had been persecuted for centuries for their beliefs and that it was now up to the Christian colleagues to suffer in order to defend their own convictions. Freud added that he attached no importance to the fact that his name would no longer be mentioned in Germany, provided that his work would still be presented correctly. With that, he got up and left the room. Since the same episode was reported by others, it is not beyond the bounds of possibility that Boehm was forced to share it at the congress without, however, explaining more on the subject.

This report by Boehm relating to the situation of the DPG from 1933 onwards requires comment. Despite all the efforts made by Jones, Müller-Braunschweig and Boehm to comply with the various requests made by the authorities, the official dissolution of the DPG was announced on 19 November 1938. The DPG then changed its name, becoming a simple working group (Arbeitsgruppe A) within the Göring Institute. Boehm also failed to mention the fact that after the arrest and execution – on 13 May 1943 – of the psychoanalyst John Rittmeister, who was the director of the polyclinic at the Göring Institute, Arbeitsgruppe A was forced to change its name to that of the College of Casuistry and Therapy (Referatenabende für Kasuistik und Therapie), which operated until the spring of 1945.

In trying to justify his active involvement with the Göring Institute, Boehm not only portrayed himself as a simple executive who had decided nothing on his own but also claimed to have been both a victim and a scapegoat. At a meeting in Zurich in 1949, Anna Freud reproached him for his past attitude by mentioning the way in which the Dutch psychoanalytic association had secretly continued to work following its dissolution. Boehm considered this comment unjustified, claiming, in response, that he had always acted in accordance with the advice that Freud and Jones had given him. In any case, he alleged in 1951, how could a psychoanalytic association's scientific life have developed within an institute directed by Matthias Göring? This was a judicious question, but wasn't it a little too late to ask it? At the time, teaching activities, training analyses and all meetings were under the supervision of

Göring and his wife, he added. It was no longer even possible to refer to the Oedipus complex. The line of defence presented by Boehm at the Amsterdam congress was therefore as follows: he had only followed the instructions of others; he had undertaken to keep a promise made to Freud; he had taken no initiatives of his own; and he had consulted on all important decisions with the president of the IPA. In addition, the last of the DPG's Jewish members had offered their resignation in 1935. In this report, which was intended to justify his activities under Nazism in the hope of reintegrating the DPG into the IPA after the war, Boehm therefore stressed the support he had received from Jones throughout the latter's 'rescue' mission. Which is hardly disputable.

For understandable reasons, the version of events developed by the IPA leadership emphasised the aid given to German exiles rather than the compliance of the DPG and the Berlin Institute with Nazi demands. In his biography of Freud, Jones mentioned the irreversible destruction of German psychoanalysis rather than the participation of psychoanalysts in the activities of the Göring Institute. Be that as it may, a certain number of elements relating to the fate of the Berlin Institute in the early days of the Nazi regime appear in the correspondence exchanged by Ernest Jones, Anna Freud, Boehm and Müller-Braunschweig, which is kept at the Institute of Psychoanalysis in London. In early October 1933, Jones informed Anna Freud that he had full confidence in Boehm and Müller-Braunschweig. He considered it necessary to support them in their efforts to save the situation.[45] What is also known for certain is that Boehm and Müller-Braunschweig gave Jones detailed accounts of the situation in which they explained the merits of their policy of preventive action.

There are other testimonies to be considered, however. Richard Sterba, the only non-Jewish member of the Vienna Psychoanalytic Institute in 1938, mentions Boehm's boast to the effect that he was proud to have worked for the incorporation of the Berlin Institute into the Göring Institute. He also painted an unflattering portrait of Jones at that time. Sterba recalled that in November 1936 the bureau of the Vienna Institute met on a Sunday afternoon at Freud's house. 'The discussion which took place there showed what Freud's attitude was towards those members of the Berlin society who had remained in place after the Nazis had taken over,'[46] he said. Sterba, the Vienna Institute's librarian at the time, was summoned, along with several colleagues, in order to learn about the report that Boehm, who had come from Berlin, was to present concerning the evolution of the Berlin group's activities.

Sterba climbed the steps of the Berggasse 19 staircase with Boehm. Freud welcomed them with his customary kindness. Boehm then presented his report, which was designed to justify what he had done 'with (or to) analysis under the Nazi regime'. He began to recount, with a measure of self-aggrandisement, how the Berlin Institute had been absorbed by the Institute of Psychotherapy directed by Reichsmarschall Göring's cousin. Sterba points out that, according to Boehm, it was a feat to have succeeded in ensuring that psychoanalysis could still be taught at the institute alongside Adlerian and Jungian psychology. Freud asked for explanations. He wanted to know how long this teaching lasted. Boehm explained that each of the courses concerned would take two years. Freud replied that that was understandable in the case of psychoanalysis but that two weeks was more than enough time in which to teach Adler's psychology. Boehm was embarrassed by this remark, which directly targeted that levelling of psychoanalysis in which he himself was involved. Boehm then suggested that someone from the Vienna Institute should go to Berlin to see the situation for themselves. Freud then asked Boehm to specify exactly who he had in mind. Boehm immediately picked Sterba, who wasn't Jewish. Sterba then said that he would gladly accept the invitation – but only after one of his Jewish colleagues in Vienna had been invited to speak at the Berlin Institute. At which point Freud smiled and Boehm was left tongue-tied. Sterba adds that Boehm's attitude made a bad impression on everyone insofar as he had arranged for psychoanalysis to exist in principle but not in fact. Boehm had achieved this result by chicanery, disingenuousness and yielding to political pressure. The meeting ended with an exhortation from Freud: 'You can make all kinds of sacrifices, but you must not make any concessions.' It was obvious that Boehm had already made many concessions. 'We left sad and worried about our future,' Sterba writes.

Speaking of Jones this time, Sterba relied on the testimony of Helene Deutsch, who described the secret plan that Jones, the president of the IPA at the time, had devised in order to save psychoanalysis in Austria. This plan concerned him directly, since Jones foresaw that two Aryan analysts would have to stay in Vienna in order to work with the Austrian branch of the Göring Institute. When Sterba asked Jones to help him obtain an emigration visa for the United States, the latter replied curtly that he would do absolutely nothing to allow him to obtain such authorisation. Sterba, Jones said, would be the last to be able to receive aid from the association of which he was president (the IPA) because he, Sterba, would have to stay in Vienna with August Aichhorn to keep the memory of psychoanalysis alive and await better days. Sterba then hastened to check that the Freuds had approved his departure from Austria, which was indeed the case.

When Jones came to Vienna to rescue Freud, he was greatly upset by Sterba's absence. At that time, he had planned to transfer the Vienna Psychoanalytic Society to England, but his efforts to rescue Austrian psychoanalysis failed because many of the Austrian analysts preferred to go to the United States rather than to England. Sterba was never made aware of this plan to move the Viennese group to England. According to Sterba, Jones had put his plan together without actually speaking to the people it concerned. The plan to leave a non-Jewish analyst in Vienna to wait for better days bears certain similarities to the way in which the so-called rescue of German psychoanalysis was organised. Was this strategy premeditated? Sterba and

Deutsch were of the opinion that such a plan did exist in the case of Austria. In any event, Sterba's testimony stood out by a mile from the concert of praise that generally greeted Jones's actions in Central Europe. Jones is best known for having set up, in 1938, with the help of his secretary, Miss Taylor, a rehabilitation fund to help psychoanalysts and their families to leave Austria following the Anschluss.[47] It is striking to find, under the very pen of his biographer, Brenda Maddox, the remark that the rescue of German psychoanalysis, which Jones believed to have been achieved, was not worth it.[48]

Berlin is lost

Another important question is that of the motives of German analysts under the Third Reich. Were they simply officials in the service of the regime or opportunists who tried to take advantage of the situation? Freud felt that these gentlemen seemed to be in a great hurry to occupy the best positions. Once again, if the decision to leave them in control was dictated by the desire to be able to survive the situation while waiting for better days, did the opinion that nothing could be saved actually have a measure of credibility at the time when these untoward events were taking place? A possible ban on psychoanalysis was the overarching threat. In the spring of 1936, however, this threat was lifted at the cost of a loss of autonomy and the ceding of the Berlin Institute to a new breed of therapists focused on the treatment of the soul.

In Berlin, the Nazis tolerated the Aryan analysts who chose to continue their activities when their Jewish colleagues could no longer do so. Some did not resist this deadly call; they saw it as an opportunity for career advancement, as something that offered the possibility of professional promotion following the departure of their Jewish colleagues. By adapting psychoanalysis to the constraints of the moment in order, they claimed, to save it, they ended up working for the disintegration of the analytic movement in Germany. Jones eventually admitted that Müller-Braunschweig was a dangerous anti-Semite who was flirting with National Socialist ideals. He also recognised that his Jewish colleagues' doubts about Boehm's dedication were well founded. On one occasion, Jones himself actually complained about the resistance put up by a number of what he called 'ultra-Jewish' psychoanalysts. However, it was his fight for the medicalisation of psychoanalysis that carried him along this path.

Freud's reaction in the spring of 1933 has often either been misunderstood or has been commented on only with reference to the concise formula according to which Freud did not commit himself too much. This is incorrect. Freud strongly opposed Eitingon on the issue of closing the Berlin Institute, challenging the latter's right to make the decision alone. It was also said that Freud had made the wrong enemy, that he had failed to appreciate the true severity of the anti-Semitic threat. He would, some contend, have overlooked that danger because he was obsessed with the threat represented by certain practitioners who were mixing his doctrine with Adler's. It was also suggested that his great age, his illness, his apoliticalism, even his ambivalence towards Judaism – he was now in the process of writing *Moses and Monotheism* – had led him astray. Some still believe that Freud was blind to the true nature of the Nazi phenomenon and that but for this blindness he would have accepted Jones's attempt at rescue and would also have endorsed the resignation of the Jewish members of the Berlin Insitute's steering committee. In short, some say, Freud failed to properly perceive the danger of Hitlerian anti-Semitism. This, they believe, was his greatest fault. It is also necessary to mention – in order not to have to return to the subject – the suspicions of a faction militantly opposed to psychoanalysis that has fought to portray Freud as a supporter of the Italian, Austrian and German fascist movements. As for the preposterous idea that Freud himself would have worked with Matthias Göring in Berlin, it would seem to be the product of a fantasist. We will confine ourselves to quoting something Matthias Göring said at a psychotherapy congress in 1934:

> I say today that we must see in *Mein Kampf* a scientific book; it lacks only the scientific expressions to which many publications owe their veneer of scientificity when they are not scientific. I go further – anyone who reads the Führer's book … and studies its essential nature will notice that it has something specific that most of them lack: this is what Jung calls intuition. It is more important than science.[49]

In August 1933, Freud spoke of the dark misery of the times as having wiped out any inclination on his part to take action. He also complained about his isolation. He saw from a distance that the IPA was heading for disaster and said he was quite prepared to see it disappear in the global crisis. At the end of the summer, he said: 'Berlin is lost, Budapest devalued by the loss of Ferenczi, and one cannot tell in which direction they are drifting in America.'[50] At that time, Freud already knew of Eitingon's decision to leave Berlin for Palestine. According to Lou Andreas-Salomé, the departure of the director of the Berlin Institute was a cruel disappointment to Freud, who felt abandoned. Far from Europe, Eitingon was now in the background. Jones, as president of the IPA, was expected to organise the resistance. We have pointed out that Freud foresaw that the danger would come from those who boasted of knowing psychoanalysis and who claimed to have gone beyond it and corrected it. According to him, the enemies of psychoanalysis would have the features of old friends. Freud knew all the compromisers, the men of ambition, the courteous practitioners, the therapists who had been welcomed at international congresses and who had published their works in journals of psychoanalysis. But Jones continued to reassure him – as if whispering in his ear – that the movement had friends in Berlin and that the appointment of von Hattingberg should be interpreted as offering psychoanalysis a chance to survive. When Jones met Matthias Göring in 1936, he found him very likeable.[51] He also saw Boehm as being proud but easy to handle. Exhibiting his customary narcissism and self-assurance, Jones managed to lull Freud to sleep. His plan was to shift the centre of gravity of the psychoanalytic movement to London, leaving two outposts in Berlin and Vienna. Strategically speaking, it was not just a rescue plan.

Psychoanalysis itself was not prohibited in Hitler's Germany – it was simply off limits for analysts who were Jewish. If fear of the ban was not unfounded, we saw that very early on, from the spring of 1933, many practitioners wanted to take control of psychoanalysis and adapt it to the requirements of the ideology of the Third Reich. The presence of Göring, ever the protector of psychotherapists, was a factor that Freud did not mention in his letters. Unless one had had unusual powers of divination, it would have been hard to imagine in advance that there could be such close ties between German psychotherapists and the Ministry of the Interior. Like other scholars in their speciality, the German analysts who set out to collaborate with the Nazis imagined that they had ideas to offer. On the other hand, the Nazis appreciated science as long as it was the kind of pseudo-science that could serve their propaganda purposes. Scholars offered their services to the Nazis, but the Nazis had no real need of their discoveries. The Nazis had their own conceptions and felt no need to consult great scholars. What interested them was not *Wissenschaft* – science as such. What they wanted was technology plus technicians with no ideas. In any case, only so-called racial science had any worth in their eyes. To presume that scholars inspired the Nazis would be to give the Nazis too much credit, according to Hannah Arendt. A number of truly exceptional figures did adhere to the Nazi ideology – men like the jurist Carl Schmitt, the historian Walter Frank, the theologian Gerhard Kittel and the philosopher Martin Heidegger – but they were drowned in the mass of insignificant personalities who replaced them. Since the Nazis did not need old-fashioned thinkers, anti-Semitic intellectuals or nationalists to plead their cause, they substituted second-rate personalities for the most gifted scholars.[52] On the other hand, the attitude of scientists during the National Socialist period was largely characterised by their constant docility. Subsequently, this voluntary submission gave way to the incredible ease with which the Allies convinced the scholars who had contributed to the German war effort to come and work with them in what had once been enemy territory. Could this comment by Arendt on the collaboration of German scholars also apply to the psychoanalysts who practised under the Nazi regime? The big difference, no doubt, is that the brightest of them were no longer there or were about to leave. After Abraham's death in 1925, the Berlin group had experienced difficulties. There were, to Freud's annoyance, disagreements between the various members, and Eitingon seem incapable of fixing the problem. The worsening of the situation in Berlin also saw the departure of Alexander, Sachs, Horney and Radó, all of whom had decided to join the new American psychoanalytic institutes. In the months following the establishment of the Hitler regime, Wilhelm Reich – the communist – fled to Denmark. Simmel, who represented the socialist doctors, took refuge in Zurich. Eitingon was making preparations to move to Jerusalem. Fenichel left for Copenhagen and later went to Prague. The management of the Berlin Institute and the DPG was now in the hands of people who were not recognised by their peers as being particularly brilliant.

There were two ways to approach the promotion of someone who was indifferent. There was that of Jones, who considered Boehm to be an ordinary person who was anxious to shake things up but easily handled. And there was that of Eitingon, who greatly distrusted Boehm and, unlike Freud, found an Adlerian like Schultz-Hencke much less frightening: 'The one I fear is not [Schultz-Henke], whom you quote, but the brave nobodies, not very shrewd but possessing very slow, subordinate ways of thinking,'[53] he wrote to Freud in March 1933. A month later, Eitingon added that the presidency of Boehm was the greatest misfortune of the present time, one that could only be mitigated by the presence of 'one of us'[54] in Berlin. He felt that someone had to stay in Berlin to deal with the stupidity of the nonentities; he himself, however, was in no position to resolve the situation. In other words, Eitingon established a link between stupidity and dishonesty. He said there were two categories. There were 'them' – that is, Boehm, Müller-Braunschweig, Schultz-Hencke and Werner Kemper. And there was 'us', meaning himself, Simmel and Fenichel, even if the latter wasn't much appreciated by Freud. One after the other, they were going to have to leave Germany in order to flee the mounting terror. Eitingon soon realised that the problem with the nonentities was their inability to see their own deficiencies. Despite their slow and subordinate thinking, they often exhibited quirky thinking, senseless lusts and chimerical intuitions. The worldview developed by Müller-Braunschweig bore witness to this. In the wake of Abraham's work on the oral incorporation phase, Boehm's ethnological investigations into cannibalism also resonate curiously: 'The idea of ritual murder is based on superstition with regard to blood, as well as with regard to the concept as well as the practices stemming from the belief in the virtue of freshly spilled blood, especially human blood.'[55]

Edith Ludowyk Gyömröi knew Boehm fairly well, since the Berlin Institute's teaching committee had selected her, much against her will, to be one of his student analysts in the 1920s.[56] Gyömröi, who described Boehm as a man of disgusting habits, eventually became his assistant. When Boehm first referred patients to her, he demanded that she pay him back half of the fees she received. At the time, Gyömröi was barely getting enough to eat. Her first meal of the day was often the cake that accompanied the coffee her colleagues offered her in the evening, after the seminars. In her memoirs, Gyömröi twice mentions the moment when an elated Boehm explained to her that he had found a way to adapt Freudian psychoanalysis to the ideology of Adolf

Hitler. He had just come from delivering a talk to the Führer in which he proved, with citations from Freud, that psychoanalysis could be used for the education of heroic individuals. Gyömröi mischievously replied that they shouldn't have to say this. Having said that, she left without further ado.[57]

A little later on, Gyömröi informed Boehm that she had to leave Berlin. Boehm, who was sitting at his desk, abruptly grabbed some flowers from a vase and handed them to her. At the end of April 1933, eager to know what the analysts in Vienna thought of him, Boehm asked Gyömröi to put in a good word for him when she met Freud. Boehm then proposed that, during the discussion she was going to have with Freud, she might want to express her gratitude to him in order to counterbalance the fact that Freud might have heard less flattering things about him.[58] In other words, Boehm instructed an analyst of Jewish origin to tell Freud good things about him, which suggests that Boehm was perfectly aware that Freud did not support him – all of which flies in the face of his claim to have been commissioned by Freud to manage the DPG's affairs in exchange for expelling Reich. Boehm explained that he was simply carrying out his assigned tasks and that he never took an initiative without first referring the matter to Vienna. Obviously, Boehm was manoeuvring. In the spring of 1933, when the Nazi terror took hold, this nonentity risked everything. A grand idea had taken hold of his mediocre mind – if he succeeded in getting the Jewish analysts to leave the Berlin Institute, their positions would be up for grabs and he, the man of no talent, could become the leader of psychoanalysis in Germany. For that, however, he needed Freud's approval, which is precisely what he was after when he visited Freud in Vienna on 17 April. As he was not entirely sure that he would succeed, he asked Gyömröi to talk him up in conversation with Freud. Why would he have chosen a Jewish woman as his emissary? It seems that nonentities of Boehm's ilk often consider themselves to be unusually cunning.

With the departure of Jewish analysts, Berlin psychoanalysis lost its elites. The people who now headed the Berlin Institute and managed the DPG had none of the prestige of Simmel, Fenichel and Eitingon. After the war, the Aryan analysts presented themselves as victims of the National Socialist regime who had secretly fought for the preservation of Freudian psychoanalysis by means of cunning and dissimulation. From this angle, Arendt's comments on the scholars and technicians who offered their services to the National Socialist state can also be said to apply to the second-rate psychoanalysts who were tolerated, integrated and overseen by the Nazi dictatorship. Their scientific contributions turned out to be relatively useless. As early as 1936, the Ministry of the Interior decided that there was no longer any reason to give the Aryan analysts privileged status. From the authorities' point of view, once their training methods had been assimilated and their premises confiscated, the old psychoanalysts of the Berlin Institute were no longer of any interest. Why, the authorities asked, was it necessary to allow them their own offices and special facilities? Ultimately, it was only Boehm's work on homosexuality that would be used to treat 'inverts' in the military. At the end of 1944, Boehm gave his approval to treating homosexual soldiers as criminals. Many were sterilised, imprisoned or sentenced to death.

Here, as in other areas, the Nazis first cleaned up the vocabulary. 'Now that Freud's books have been burned, we must delete, for example, the word "psychoanalysis", as well as the term "individual psychology", which could be replaced by "applied character science"',[59] Göring told neurologist Walter Cimbal in the summer of 1933. At that time, Göring already held the title of Reichstherapeutenführer (Head of Reich Therapists); Cimbal was his adviser. The term 'psychoanalysis' was be replaced by the term 'developmental psychology' (*Entwicklungspsychologie*).[60] Contrary to what Boehm had said on his own behalf, it was not his cunning or his efforts at persuasion that prevented a ban on psychoanalysis and the activities of the Berlin Institute and DPG. This explanation was nothing but a decoy – the tree that hid the forest. Boehm consistently argued that he was only obeying Freud and that he enjoyed the full support of Ernest Jones and Anna Freud. What went by the wayside in his protestations was the position of the Nazi regime vis-à-vis psychoanalysis. Basically, Freud knew that if the Nazis had wanted to ban psychoanalysis, nothing – no resignations, no protective or anticipatory measures – would have sufficed to prevent them from doing so. Anna Freud realised this in the summer of 1934. She reported to Jones that the Nazi government 'never made an attack on analysis or restricted its activity in any way. The twenty-five members who left did so because they were Jews, not because they were analysts'.[61]

The conclusion to be drawn at this point is that Boehm's efforts in the summer of 1933 – when he managed to navigate his way through the administrative labyrinth by attempting to persuade bureaucrats and National Socialist physicians of the usefulness of psychoanalysis – were essentially a smokescreen. Indeed, the files that he had assembled relating to the political harmlessness of psychoanalysis could never have landed on the right desk if it had not been possible to offer German psychotherapists a place in the new state. On the other hand, this attempt at rapprochement had to be received favourably by those analysts who agreed to align themselves with a kind of psychotherapy that would serve the new regime. This is an essential factor: the point on which these German analysts gave way essentially relates to what Freud himself so greatly feared – the reduction of psychoanalysis to the rank of just another treatment technique. Without this underhand desire to gain social recognition at any cost, German analysts could not have claimed to be useful to the regime. However, the orientation towards the medicalisation of psychoanalysis was already under way before the Nazis came to power. Jones himself favoured it.

Sometimes the stupidity of the Nazi administration was of considerable assistance. Boehm precisely recorded the successive steps he took in his discussions with the Union of the Struggle for German Culture and the Police

Prefecture during the period from 1933 to 1934. All these steps, he explained, had had a single goal. It was a question of not giving the government an excuse to ban psychoanalysis. In some circumstances, the crass ignorance of the administration's doctors proved to be a real asset. To continue its teaching activities, the Berlin Institute needed special permission. To this end, a request had to be made to the Prefecture of Police. A doctor from the Charlottenburg Police Prefecture duly came to inspect the premises of the institute at the beginning of 1934. On this occasion, he asked the maid who received him what kind of instruments were used to treat the institution's patients. The maid said there were no instruments. To complete his written report, the doctor telephoned Boehm the next day and asked for further details. Who worked at the institute and what was their nationality? Who among them was of Aryan origin?

Throughout the series of steps he took at that time, Boehm applied his strategy of taking preventive measures. Despite Freud's opposition to this policy, in the spring of 1933, Boehm instilled fear in his colleagues by trying to speed things up. By dint of insisting – in association with Müller-Braunschweig – he finally obtained the resignation of the Jewish members of the steering committee of the DPG during the general assembly that was held in November 1933. Under cover of his obedience to Freud, he passed on this strategy of fear as the only one capable of preventing the prohibition of psychoanalysis. The ban on psychoanalysis was the red flag that Boehm wielded in order to intimidate his colleagues. There was really no question of a ban, however, since Matthias Göring's policy was clearly oriented towards aligning psychoanalysis with state-sanctioned psychotherapy. Boehm and his colleague also had to prove that there was no conflict of interest between the new direction and that of the IPA. Following the meeting between Boehm, Müller-Braunschweig and Jones in The Hague on 1 October 1933, Johan van Ophuijsen, who was present, reported that the situation in Germany was not as favourable as Boehm claimed.

> The German Psychoanalytic Society is unable to meet all of the written and unwritten requirements for membership in the IPA. One could even ask whether, in its current form, the DPG can still be authorised to be a member of the IPA. But this is a state of emergency,[62]

he wrote in a circular issued by the office of the president of the IPA. Did Jones not heed this warning? Van Ophuijsen's remark suggests that the criterion of urgency was likely to sweep away all considerations of ethics.

Historians have shown that despite authoritarian rule and administrative control at all levels, there was still room for individual and institutional initiatives in Hitler's Germany.[63] The opportunism of two German psychoanalysts was a decisive factor in the misuse of the discipline during the Brownshirt years. The Aryanisation of the board of directors of the DPG and the Berlin Institute served their interests. This is in line with Arendt's conclusions, which highlighted the mediocrity and banality of the zealous servants of the National Socialist state. As early as 1935, Jones was praised for the way he managed the affairs of the IPA, but he was also criticised for the way he handled the departure of the Berlin Institute's Jewish members. The fiction of their spontaneous resignation, as presented by Edward Glover at the Marienbad congress of 1936, remained influential, however.

The collaboration between the two nonentities turned into intense rivalry at the end of the war. Even before the German surrender in May 1945, Schultz-Hencke and Kemper, aided by several others, conceived the idea of creating a new institute for treatment and training. This attempt to avoid charges that they had collaborated with the Nazi regime clearly exposes the path taken by Boehm, who had worked side by side with the German psychotherapeutic schools to accept non-physicians. Müller-Braunschweig undertook to reorganise the DPG and fell out with Schultz-Hencke when he announced that he wanted to establish a training course that would be solely psychoanalytic. At the IPA congress in Zurich in 1949, Müller-Braunschweig requested that the new DPG be admitted to the IPA. Müller-Braunschweig cleverly turned the ensuing discussions towards the subject of the orthodoxy of Schultz-Hencke's neo-analysis.

The suggestion that the new DPG be recognised by the IPA was accepted despite the fact that some of its members had trained at the Göring Institute. At the same time, the IPA duly imposed the condition that Schultz-Hencke should be expelled; following the latter's failure to comply, a small group around Müller-Braunschweig decided to found a new association that would offer a solely analytic training. The possibility of creating a new society – under the name of the German Psychoanalytic Association (DPV) – was agreed by the IPA in September 1950. As a result, there were two opposing currents of psychoanalysis in postwar Germany. The psychotherapeutic current followed the evolution that had begun before 1933 and developed under the Nazis. The other current, under the direction of Müller-Braunschweig, claimed to have its roots in psychoanalysis. Both currents, without mentioning the fact of their collaboration with the Nazis, blamed each other for having collaborated.

The ethical position of the IPA's leadership during the National Socialist era always raises many questions among the new generations of psychoanalysts. Particularly since the 1980s, much research has been undertaken in Germany in order to exhume the history of the psychoanalytic movement in the Third Reich, especially with regard to the way in which the movement's reconstruction was undertaken during the postwar years. The IPA's official recognition of the DPV was announced at the international congress of 1951. For his part, Boehm wanted to gain time by trying to extend the DPG's provisional admission for two years. In Amsterdam, Anna Freud stated that it would not be impossible to admit the new DPG to IPA membership if the

DPG could prove its worth during that period: 'I see no reason why this society, if it proves its worth as Dr. Boehm supposes, should not renew its candidacy for membership.'[64]

The involvement of analysts with the institute linked to the Nazi regime was much discussed in Germany, as can be seen from the following proposals – dating from the end of the 1980s – relating to their collective culpability:

> All generations of German psychoanalysts carry the weight of history in a manner that goes beyond the customary consequences – in effect, although psychoanalysis may be independent of its founder, and inasmuch as it is a science, without any religious or racial tie, an analyst is, for all that, necessarily born of a Jewish genealogy and acquires his professional identity through his identification with the work of Freud.[65]

But the responsibility of the executive committees of the IPA is very much in question in relation to the organisation's decision to assist those analysts who had worked at the Göring Institute to establish themselves overseas after the war. In 1949, while regretting that Werner Kemper, the former director of the Göring Institute's polyclinic, had not stayed in Germany in order to rebuild the DPG, Jones helped him to settle in Brazil. Kemper, who had been named to that post following the arrest of John F. Rittmeister, became a teaching analyst in Rio de Janeiro.[66]

Others, concentrating on the question of the Jewish origins of psychoanalysis, emphasise the disturbing and truly symptomatic dimension of these events. Does analysis make people virtuous?

> They were psychoanalysts, and one would have hoped that something in the very nature of being psychoanalysts would have prevented them from collaborating with an anti-humanist ideology and becoming strangers to the values of responsibility and self-awareness. But it came to nothing, and that leaves us with questions that will disturb us for as long as we are capable of thinking.[67]

As Lacan pointed out, once subjected to psychoanalysis, the dimwit always becomes a crook.

Notes

1 Lore Reich Rubin, 'Anna Freud and the expulsion of Wilhelm Reich from the International Psychoanalytic Association', presentation at Goethe-Institute Boston, 15 March 1997, *International Forum of Psychoanalysis*, vol. 12 (2003), 109–117.

2 Ernest Jones to Anna Freud, letter of 2 May 1933; available at the Archives of the London Institute of Psychoanalysis.

3 *Ibid.*, 'Though we should do all we could to disavow it.'
4 Richard Sterba, *Reminiscences, op. cit.*
5 'Rapport du président Ernest Jones sur la situation des émigrants d'Allemagne au XIIIe Congrès psychanalytique international, du 26 au 31 août 1934, à Lucerne', in Karen Brecht, *Ici, la vie continue*, p. 231.
6 Extract from Carl Müller-Braunschweigs's 'Memorandum on the organisation of the theoretical course', in Karen Brecht, *Ici, la vie continue, op. cit.*, p. 264.
7 This accusation has been levelled at Geoffrey Cocks.
8 Eli Zaretsky, *Secrets of the Soul: A Social and Cultural History of Psychoanalysis* (New York: Vintage, 2005).
9 Mail from Dr Leonard Bruno to the author, 1 February 2010.
10 Freud to Jones, letter 606 F, 7 April 1933, in R. Andrew Paskauskas, *Complete Correspondence of Sigmund Freud and Ernest Jones, op. cit.*, p. 715.
11 Jacques Lacan, 'Science and Truth', *Écrits*, p. 743.
12 Eitingon to Freud, letter 773 E, 2 November 1933, in Michael Schröter, *Correspondance, op. cit.*, p. 804.
13 Letter from Freud to Haim Koffler, 26 February 1930. Cited in Jacquy Chemouni, *La psychanalyse française captive du politique* (Paris: Beauchesne, 2010), pp. 80–81.
14 Freud to Ferenczi, letter 1244 F, 2 April 1933, in Falzeder and Brabant, *The Correspondence of Sigmund Freud and Sándor Ferenczi, Volume 3, op. cit.*, p. 449.
15 Freud to Eitingon, letter 774 F, 1 March 1934, in Michael Schröter, *Correspondance, op. cit.*, p. 809.
16 Mark Edmundson, *The Death of Sigmund Freud: Fascism, Psychoanalysis and the Rise of Fundamentalism* (London: Bloomsbury, 2007).
17 Freud to Eitingon, letter 755 F, 21 March 1933, in Michael Schröter, *Correspondance, op. cit.*, p. 785.
18 Freud to Eitingon, letter 755 F, 21 March 1933, in Michael Schröter, *Correspondance, op. cit.*, p. 785.
19 Regine Lockot, 'Mésusage, disqualification et division au lieu d'expiation: Étapes de la DPG dans le contexte du Congrès de Zurich de 1949', *Topique*, vol. 57 (1995), 247.
20 Eitingon to Freud, letter 756 E, 24 March 1933, in Michael Schröter, *Correspondance, op. cit.*, p. 787.
21 Karen Brecht, *Ici, la vie continue, op. cit.*, p. 95.
22 Saul Friedländer, *Nazi Germany and the Jews, Volume 1, op. cit.*
23 Freud to Eitingon, letter 759 F, 17 April 1933, in Michael Schröter, *Correspondance, op. cit.*, p. 789.
24 Siegfried Bernfeld, 'La discussion communiste sur la psychanalyse et la réfutation de l'hypothèse de l'instinct de mort par Reich' (1932), *Partisans*, no. 66–67 (July/October, 1972), 8–20.
25 Freud to Eitingon, letter 690 F, 9 January 1933, in Michael Schröter, *Correspondance, op. cit.*, p. 725.
26 Sigmund Freud, 'The Question of a *Weltanschauung*' (1932), *Standard Edition*, vol. 22, p. 181.
27 Freud to Eitingon, letter 746 F, 20 November 1932, in Michael Schröter, *Correspondance, op. cit.*, p. 774.
28 Ernest Jones, *Sigmund Freud*, vol. 3, *op. cit.*, p. 198.
29 Fanny Colonomos and Elisabeth Marsault, *Comme des jongleurs insensibles: Les psychanalystes allemands et la montée du nazisme* (Paris: Frénésie, 1988), p. 103.
30 *Ibid.*, p. 104.
31 Extract from a speech delivered at the Sportpalast in Berlin on 30 September 1942. Cited in Eberhard Jäckel, *Hitler idéologue, op. cit.*, pp. 86–87.

32 *Ibid.*
33 Freud to Ferenczi, letter 1244 F, 2 April 1933, in Falzeder and Brabant, *The Correspondence of Sigmund Freud and Sándor Ferenczi, Volume 3*, op. cit., p. 449.
34 Fanny Colonomos and Elisabeth Marsault, *Comme des jongleurs insensibles, op. cit.*, p. 103.
35 Sigmund Freud, 'Why War?' (1933), *Standard Edition*, vol. 22, p. 208.
36 Sigmund Freud, 'The Dissection of the Psychical Personality' (1932), *Standard Edition*, vol. 22, p. 67.
37 Fanny Colonomos and Elisabeth Marsault, *Comme des jongleurs insensibles, op. cit.*, p. 8.
38 Ian Kershaw, *Hitler* (London: Longman, 1991), p. 50.
39 Freud to Jones, letter 606 F, 7 April 1933, in R. Andrew Paskauskas, *Complete Correspondence of Sigmund Freud and Ernest Jones, op. cit.*, p. 716.
40 Freud to Eitingon, letter 759 F, 17 April 1933, in Michael Schröter, *Correspondance, op. cit.*, p. 789.
41 Eitingon to Freud, letter 761 E, 27 April 1933, in Michael Schröter, *Correspondance, op. cit.*, p. 793.
42 Freud to Eitingon, letter 764 F, 13 July 1933, in Michael Schröter, *Correspondance, op. cit.*, note 5, p. 797.
43 Carl Müller-Braunschweig, 'Psychoanalysis and *Weltanschauung*' (1933), cited in Karen Brecht, *Ici, la vie continue, op. cit.*, pp. 245–246.
44 Felix Boehm, 'Report on Events from 1933 to the Amsterdam Congress in August 1951', Archives of the London Institute of Psychoanalysis.
45 Ernest Jones to Anna Freud, letter of 2 October 1933, Archives of the London Institute of Psychoanalysis.
46 Richard Sterba, *Réminiscences, op. cit.*, p. 141.
47 The catalogue of the Ernest Jones Rehabilitation Fund can be accessed via the website of the Institute of Psychoanalysis, British Psychoanalytical Society.
48 Brenda Maddox, *Freud's Wizard: Ernest Jones and the Transformation of Psychoanalysis* (London: John Murray, 2006), p. 225.
49 Matthias Göring, 'Schlussansprache: Anlässlich des allgemeinen ärztlichen Kongress für Psychotherapie, Bad Nauheim, 1934', cited in Karen Brecht, *Ici, la vie continue, op. cit.*, p. 138.
50 Freud to Jones, letter 616, 23 August 1933, in R. Andrew Paskauskas, *Complete Correspondence of Sigmund Freud and Ernest Jones, op. cit.*, p. 829.
51 'It was easy to get on excellent terms with Göring, who is a very sympathetic personality,' Jones wrote to Anna Freud on 20 July 1936. He added that he had no reason to defy Göring other than with regard to the question of teaching. Cited in Regine Lockot, 'Mésusage', *op. cit.*
52 Hannah Arendt, 'The Image of Hell' (1946), in *Essays in Understanding, 1930–1954: Formation, Exile, and Totalitarianism* (New York: Schocken Books, 2005), p. 197.
53 Eitingon to Freud, letter 756 E, 24 March 1933, in Michael Schröter, *Correspondance, op. cit.*, p.786.
54 Eitingon to Freud, letter 760 E, 21 April 1933, in Michael Schröter, *Correspondance, op. cit.*, p. 792.
55 Felix Boehm, 'Anthropophagy: Its Forms and Motifs' (1935), *The International Journal of Psychoanalysis*, no. 16 (1935), 9–21.
56 Edith Ludowyk Gyömröi (née Glück; b. Budapest 1896, d. London 1987) underwent a free analysis with Fenichel in Berlin in 1923. A Jew closely associated with the Communists, she had to insist on being admitted to the Berlin Institute as a student. A member of the Kinderseminar, she emigrated to Prague in 1933 and

stayed in touch with Edith Jacobson, Annie Reich, Barbara Lantos and Kate Friedländer via the bulletins circulated by Fenichel.

57 Edith Ludowyk Gyömröi, 'Memories of the German Psychoanalytical Association', Sigmund Freud Archives, Library of Congress, Washington, DC.
58 Felix Boehm to Edith Ludowyk Gyömröi, letter of 25 April 1933, Archives of the London Institute of Psychoanalysis.
59 Matthias Göring to Walter Cimbal, letter of 6 August 1933, in Karen Brecht, *Ici, la vie continue, op. cit.*, p. 243.
60 Regine Lockot, 'À propos des changements', *op. cit.*, pp. 23–34.
61 Anna Freud to Ernest Jones, letter of 18 August 1934, cited in Zaretsky, *Secrets of the Soul, op. cit.*, p. 226.
62 Karen Brecht, *Ici, la vie continue, op. cit.*, p. 96.
63 Geoffrey Cocks, 'Continuity and Development of Psychoanalysis and Psychotherapy in Germany Since 1939', *International Review of Psychoanalysis*, no. 1 (1988), 51–70.
64 Karen Brecht, *Ici, la vie continue, op. cit.*, p. 200.
65 Helmut Thoma and Horst Kachele, *Psychoanalytic Practice* (Berlin, Heidelberg and New York: Springer Verlag, 1987). Cited by Friedrich W. Eickhoff in 'The unconscious feeling of borrowed culpability and the palimpsest structure of the symptom', consulted online on 25 December 2009 at http://inconscientetsociete.free.n14.php.
66 Héléna Besserman Vianna, *Politique de la psychanalyse face à la didactique et à la torture* (Paris: L'Harmattan, 1997), pp. 167–211.
67 Anna M. Antonovsky, 'Des analystes aryens dans l'Allemagne nazie: les questions de l'adaptation, de désymbolisation et de trahison', *Revue Française de Psychanalyse*, 72.4 (2008), 1067.

Chapter 7

Conclusion

Standards and training of the psychoanalyst

The Weimar Republic offered suitable conditions for the establishment of the first psychoanalytic institution. It was a continuation of a movement initiated during the war, when psychoanalysis was applied to the therapy of traumatic neuroses. The first psychoanalysts on the frontline of war neuroses were psychiatrists, and it was from among them that the founders of the Berlin Psychoanalytic Polyclinic were recruited. After the war, the treatment of the superego and its connection to the death drive became a necessity for Freud's students. In Germany, this desire was transformed, from the beginning of the republic, into a desire to participate in the reconstruction of the nation by making psychoanalysis accessible to all. A few years earlier, Freud had already reflected on the possibility of limiting the duration of analyses. At the time of his speech to the Budapest congress, the matter was still being studied because this particular manoeuvre was envisaged as a means of countering transferential inertia. However, Freud definitively refuted this solution in a major article on the limits of psychoanalysis, which he wrote towards the end of his life.[1] In the meantime, the Berlin Polyclinic experiment had led to the conclusion that it was all but impossible to arbitrarily alter the temporal parameter of an analysis.

With regard to the creation and functioning of the Berlin Institute, one of the most important questions is that of Freud's desire. Was he influenced by those among his colleagues who wanted to take action when the postwar economic crisis provoked fears of a shortage of private clients? Did he simply look on from afar, effectively allowing things to develop as they did, and offer words of advice as and when they were asked for? We have Lacan to thank for showing that it was Freud's desire to ensure the survival of his work that led him to set up a certain type of organisation based on identification and fidelity to himself so as to ensure the future of psychoanalysis. Freud supported the creation of a centre in Berlin in order to stem the flow of the Americanisation and medicalisation of psychoanalysis. His correspondence with Abraham, Ferenczi and Eitingon between 1918 and 1925 does not

DOI: 10.4324/9781003215684-10

suggest a lack of involvement with Berlin. His connection to Eitingon makes it unlikely that anything could have been done without his support and consent. In view of the overlapping historical, biographical and political elements, it is therefore questionable whether Freud allowed himself to be influenced for more than a decade against his will, to let things happen without his involvement in the founding and running of an apparatus that seemed essential to the future of the European psychoanalytic movement in the postwar years.

In the wake of the stench of scandal that had surrounded the beginnings of psychoanalytic practice, there came the moment for the analysts to set something up and make themselves socially useful. For reasons internal to the IPA, which had been moving toward centralisation since 1910, it was also necessary to train new generations of analysts in accordance with guidelines that were sufficiently explicit to be exportable. The two main requirements (to ensure that analysts had themselves undergone analysis and to provide candidates with a theoretical and clinical base in the form of a course of study) were met by encouraging analysts to invent modalities as well as a location adapted to this formation. A second institute, based on the original Berlin model, was created in Vienna. In the 1920s, therefore, the Berliners were at the centre of the international psychoanalytic movement, and the three-stage course was presented as the ultimate in psychoanalytic training. They preferred to recruit candidates who were doctors, contrary to the recommendations of Freud, who had to put all the weight of his authority in the balance in order to preserve a place for the formation of lay analysts. Of course, Freud paid particular attention to psychiatrists who approached him to undertake an analysis, the idea being that by practising psychoanalysis in their turn, they could use their influence at the heart of the medical profession. In reality, what Freud strongly objected to was not anybody in particular – it was the makeover of psychoanalysis into psychotherapy.

In spite of its dual social and didactic orientation – but also because of it – the original Berlin project bore within itself the seeds of a contradiction. In the long term, there was bound to be a conflict between the desire to make psychoanalysis accessible to all and the psychoanalysts' desire for recognition, which led them to standardise their training by taking inspiration from the university and medical models. Was it actually necessary to insert oneself into society by donning the therapist's costume? The peculiarity of German history during the 1930s is certainly a unique, but nonetheless instructive, example of the drift that led a small number of psychoanalysts to join an institute of psychotherapists who were not put off by the idea of the preservation both of the German race and of the nation's 'health capital'. In such a context, how could psychoanalysis have developed without being absorbed by the ideals and keywords of a discourse foreign to its own? From this point of view, the case of Siegfried Bernfeld is highly disturbing. He arrived in Berlin in 1926 to undertake an analysis with Hanns Sachs. Long afterward, in November 1952, a few months before his death, Bernfeld gave a lecture at the

San Francisco Institute on the subject of didactic psychoanalysis. On this occasion, he spoke about his past experience and was signally unsparing concerning the grievances he held against those former colleagues who had organised and standardised analytical training at the Berlin Institute. This critique came from within, as it were, and therein lies one of its most salient features, delivered as it was by a distinguished IPA didactician. Which was why it caused a scandal. Bernfeld's 'San Francisco Earthquake', as some called it, was only published ten years later, in the *Psychoanalytic Quarterly*, accompanied by a careful introduction explaining that had the author wanted to publish it in his lifetime, he would certainly have censored the lecture's autobiographical passages. This, though, seems unlikely, if one takes into account the general tone of the lecture, in which Bernfeld interpreted, on the basis of two distinct factors, the prevalence given to the medical professions at the Berlin Institute. First, he pointed out that the doyens of the analytical movement were completely overwhelmed by the runaway success of psychoanalysis among the younger generation in the aftermath of the war. With the exception of the few clinicians who adhered to socialist ideals, most of the elders of the Berlin analytical movement reacted with anxiety to the phenomenon of the penetration of Freudian ideas into culture. They were afraid that psychoanalysis would get away from them, that they would lose control of the profession and that it would fall into the hands of the new generations of psychologists, educators and social workers who were enthusiastically discovering the new and subversive ideas of psychoanalysis, resonating as they did with the spirit of cultural and political renewal that was one of the essential characteristics of the Weimar Republic.

These second-generation analysts developed a singular form of xenophobia that led them to prefer the isolation that had accompanied them from the beginning to the upsurge of general interest that so disturbed them. Apart from a few socialist doctors, the medical profession in Germany was, by and large, fiercely opposed to the new republic, Bernfeld recalled. The craze for the young discipline notwithstanding, the psychoanalysts of the time were not considered representatives of a respectable profession, even though many doctors were now interested in psychoanalysis, especially young psychiatrists attracted by psychotherapy. As Bernfeld recalled:

> But, strange to say, the psychoanalysts themselves desired respectability. They wished to set themselves up as part of the medical profession, and in order to achieve this aim they felt they had to have clinics, professional schools, and professional societies.[2]

This is a decisive testimony as to how psychoanalysts hoped to become part of Berlin high society. Unbeknownst to those who were working for the opening up of psychoanalysis, this desire for respectability produced certain effects. It is this desire for social recognition and prestige, and not purely the configuration of German society in the 1920s, that explains the gap that was observed very early on between the project to make psychoanalysis accessible to all and the overrepresentation of patients and pupils from the middle and upper classes at the polyclinic. The indigent, the poor, and the destitute turned to the polyclinic increasingly infrequently even though it was readily available to them.

When Wilhelm Reich set up his project to crisscross the Viennese suburbs in a bus to dispense contraceptive advice, he attracted many workers. As a militant activist for the proletarian cause, Reich naturally did not hesitate to visit the slums where his patients lived, realising that analytical treatment was probably less urgent an issue than the need for social welfare. 'What can psychoanalysis do against real misery?' he asked. Admittedly, it should not be forgotten that, for Bernfeld, the accusation of having sacrificed social commitment for respectability certainly related to his own nostalgia for a bygone era, and his critique was essentially directed at psychoanalysts who refused to become politically involved. The fact that he had responded, at Freud's request, to the article that Reich wrote in 1932 did not imply that he had forgotten his own time as a militant in the Austrian youth movement. Nor does it mean that no precarious, excluded, or poor people consulted the Berlin Polyclinic after 1922. Bernfeld was simply highlighting a strong tendency that had been noted, without further comment, by the management of the Berlin Polyclinic in its first report on its activities. The founders of the Berlin Institute mainly recruited candidates with a medical degree while accepting, by way of compromise, a handful of students who were not doctors. In this way, the tutors selected people whose profiles were already much like their own. It would appear that this trend became more pronounced over time, since there was at first a measure of tolerance for students who were not physicians. Thus the initial wish, formulated by Karl Abraham, that one of the preconditions for the practice of psychoanalysis at the polyclinic was sufficient training in neuropsychiatry was not fulfilled. Likewise, the first Berlin didactician, Hanns Sachs, was not a doctor. It was not until Max Eitingon dealt with this mess by taking matters into his own hands at the Bad Homburg congress in 1925 that the problem was solved. He set up the International Training Commission in order to standardise analytical training within psychoanalytical associations by means of procedures for evaluating candidates and appointing analysts as instructors, tutors, and supervisors. Things were different in Vienna, however. From the beginning to the end of his practice, Freud was careful not to let institutional and administrative considerations interfere with didactic analyses. It is thanks to Bernfeld, in fact, that we have an anecdote relating to Freud's perspective on standardised analytic training. In 1922, Bernfeld had wanted to establish himself as an analyst in Vienna. He had heard about the training institute that had opened in Germany and was planning to travel to Berlin to undertake a didactic analysis. When he told Freud about his plans, Freud promptly told him that his idea was utterly absurd and that he should simply throw himself into psychoanalysis and see how things went. Whenever a problem with a patient arose, said Freud, there would always be time to react.

Freud's words, reported by Bernfeld thirty years later, are absolutely explicit: 'Nonsense. Go right ahead. You certainly will have difficulties. When you get into trouble, we will see what we can do about it.'[3] Freud was interested in the personality of his young colleague. He confided that, of all his students, Bernfeld had one of the finest minds he had encountered. Freud also appreciated Bernfeld's rhetorical skills, knew of his activism in the Austrian youth movement before World War I, and was aware that Bernfeld was a committed Zionist. He was putting his trust in someone who had already proven himself. Bernfeld was also a student of philosophy, not a doctor. However, one sign of the attraction that the institution created by Abraham, Simmel and Eitingon held for the analytical world in the 1920s was the fact that Freud's advice did not prevent Bernfeld from going to Berlin.

The regulation of didactic analysis

In 1923, the Berlin Institute decided to standardise and unify the organisation of psychoanalysis for didactic purposes. The students, mostly doctors, who wished to complete their analytical training in the German capital now had to submit to a series of draconian measures:

1. The institute's teaching commission could admit or reject a candidate irrevocably after three preliminary interviews.
2. A personal analysis of at least six months' duration was mandatory.
3. The candidate's training analyst would be appointed by the committee.
4. The committee, on the advice of the training analyst, could decide whether the candidate's analysis was sufficiently advanced to permit his participation in subsequent training stages.
5. The committee would arrange for supervision with an analyst other than the candidate's training analyst.
6. The supervising analyst had the right to withdraw the patient from the candidate in the event of incompetence.
7. Finally, the candidate would have to undertake, in writing, to await the favourable opinion of the institute's board before calling himself or herself an analyst.

How might one explain this change? Bernfeld's interpretation of the event could shed light on the timing and origin of the regulations. In the immediate aftermath of the announcement of Freud's illness in 1923, many of his associates panicked. The generation of students who had followed Freud since his beginnings, who had accompanied him across the desert and endured a good deal of mockery, who had defended him against his detractors, who had been his earliest companions in adversity were literally stunned by the unbearable news: they truly believed that Freud's demise was imminent. When they learned, in the spring of 1924, that a less gloomy prognosis suggested that Freud's life could be prolonged, an unconscious sense of guilt linked to the wish for the death of the founding father emerged. It was precisely at this point that the Berlin analysts took action and decreed that a firm and urgent response was needed to preserve psychoanalysis from any attempt at deviation. Hence the presence of a predominantly melancholic and ambivalent mixture of devotion to the father and, at the same time, a desire to distance oneself from him – entirely characteristic of the style of the Berlin Institute – that influenced the way in which psychoanalysis was transmitted there. The result was the peculiar conception that the spread of psychoanalytical ideas in society was a threat that had to be countered immediately. Authoritarian directives and strict regulations were put in place to protect psychoanalysis from the danger of its bastardisation. Every effort had to be made to ensure that the analytic discipline would continue to be a scientific method in the hands of an elite.

In light of these details, one can perhaps articulate the Berliners' somewhat paradoxical conduct more logically. On the one hand, they had the courage and the boldness to inscribe psychoanalysis in the city by making it accessible to all. This project was contemporaneous with the invention of new, democratic spaces outside the German universities. On the other hand, shortly after its creation, the Berlin Institute received fewer and fewer patients of working-class origin while, at the same time, it established guidelines for training and standards for practice. This regulation came at the expense of innovation and invention. The taste for rules, the imposition of standards, and the strict observance of guidelines supplanted originality and the initial desire to make psychoanalysis accessible to everyone. It makes sense, however, to isolate this series of events from those that were unfolding on the societal level. Could psychoanalysts remove themselves from contemporary political discourse and events, from the state of the civilisation in which they were acting? Could they absent themselves from the complex and tormented political situation of their time, when aspirations for change were facing obscurantist outbursts against a backdrop of economic crisis all the way up until the electoral disaster of March 1932, which was going to allow the country's conservative leaders to rally to the Nazi Party?

The fact remains that the Berliners didn't support the social openness they advocated. The reason for this should be clarified. In 1920, the spread of psychoanalysis to all strata of society took a spectacular leap forward. In Weimar Germany, psychoanalysis became the thing that everyone was talking about, a phenomenon mentioned by Freud in one of his *New Introductory Lectures.* Because of this diffusion of psychoanalysis into society at large, psychoanalysts feared that they would be dispossessed of the Freudian invention that they had so zealously defended. The practice of wild analysis seemed to them to be a threat that had to be fought at all costs. The training of analysts had to respond to the urgent need to contain the risk of dispossession. Psychoanalysis had thus penetrated contemporary discourse: the posture of psychoanalysts could no longer be the same as it had been in the heroic times of the struggle for survival. Psychoanalysts reacted to success by establishing supposedly protective rules. But there was also a gap between the position defended by Freud with regard to lay analysis and the institutionalisation of psychoanalysis as it was first realised in Germany. Bernfeld's interpretation refers to *Totem and Taboo*:

> We believed that the father was dead and even secretly desired his death. Therefore, we are guilty of having wished for the death of our great man. We must now unite to enact and respect principles that will organise our community and govern the reproduction of the analytic species. We will act as if the father is dead, even if he is not.

From the moment that the analytical discourse lined up behind the banners of universality and standardisation, all things original, all things new, and the previously unheard of things crucial to the expansion of the application of psychoanalysis became, in less than ten years, a rigid device framed by a hierarchical organisation where only the most docile stood a chance of being selected as candidates. The establishment of the regulation on didactic psychoanalysis constituted a real turning point in the history of psychoanalysis insofar as it led to the differentiation of didactic analysis from analysis with a therapeutic aim. Berlin served as a field of experimentation for the break, within the associations affiliated to the IPA, between pure psychoanalysis and psychoanalysis applied to therapy. The Berlin Institute, which was the first establishment to put the ideas of the Budapest congress of 1918 into practice, was also the place from which the standardisation of training – which Balint, Bernfeld and, above all, Lacan would criticise – was developed. Eitingon's 'Prussian' institution favoured the organisation of the profession by means of a training that gave access to it rather than by favouring the object that was constitutive of its experience.

Lacan's refusal of standards

The break with the standard established by the superego that linked psychoanalysts to the cult of the dead father was the crux of Jacques Lacan's separation from the IPA. In 1953, when he resigned from the Psychoanalytical Society of Paris (SPP) and joined the group formed around Daniel Lagache in opposition to that of Sacha Nacht, there was a plan afoot to re-establish an institute of psychoanalysis. Before the war, there had been an institute (created in 1934) with financial support from Marie Bonaparte and designed on the model of the Berlin Institute. Nacht, who was opposed to the training of non-medical candidates in the new institute, was very much aligned with those who rejected Freud's position on lay psychoanalysis. In opposition to this bastion of medical power, Lacan and his colleagues founded the French Society of Psychoanalysis (SFP). But Lacan also refused to conform to the standards of practice imposed by the IPA, particularly the rule mandating a fixed duration of sessions. His practice of variable sessions, which he explained for the first time in December 1951 in front of the members of the SFP, was interpreted as an act of insubordination toward the IPA. On this subject, it should be noted that much has been said about Lacan's refusal to obey the rules without further questioning the way in which those rules had been invented and what their aims were. The tendency of analysts to want to become as respectable as doctors and their wish to imitate the university curriculum encouraged the establishment of training regulations. The orthodoxy of the technique was also a reaction formation linked to the demise of Sigmund Freud. It was, finally, a turning point related to the evolution of the theory that privileged the autonomy of the ego and identification with the analyst at the expense of deciphering the formations and the sexual reality of the unconscious.

At the beginning of *Seminar I*, devoted to Freud's papers on technique, Lacan resoundingly declared: 'The fun is over!' His return to Freud was marked by the reading of the great Freudian texts, which at that point people were only reading through the prism of American ego psychology. Lacan restored the function of speech and language to its central place in the analytic experience. Commenting with particular care on the doctrine of resistances, he pointed out the effects on the makeover of speech (its reduction to something of secondary importance) that this doctrine led to. What happens, in fact, when the patient's words count for less than his presentation and gestures? If the psychoanalyst fails to understand that the function of the patient's speech is the only medium at his disposal and that all speech calls for an answer, he goes astray in interpreting the subject's behaviour in order to find in it what the subject does not say. In order to do this, the analyst must address the person concerned, which ultimately leads them to speak. But at the moment that speech is recovered, it becomes suspect because there, where there had been nothing but the analyst's silence, there should have been interpretation. Ultimately, the makeover of speech occurs when the analyst seeks to provoke the confession of his patient. Or when, immersed in his own thoughts, he tries to grasp what it is that is animating the counter-transference. According to Lacan, the depreciation of the function of speech gives rise to empty speech. In this imaginary relationship, the patient can speak for a long time in vain to the analyst without reaching the point where he can assume his desire.

Even though speech is only language, language is an order and it is constituted by laws. This is why Lacan recommends that the analyst should know the fundamental distinction between the signifier as the synchronic structure of the material of language – each element taking there its difference from the others through its use – and the signified defined as the diachronic set of concretely pronounced discourses. The study of the interpretation of dreams, wordplay and its relation to the unconscious, and jokes reveals the impact of the signifier in the unconscious.

The questioning of truth by the Freudian discovery implies that psychoanalysis is not a means of achieving happiness and success. Its misuse consists in transforming it into a technique at the service of contemporary narcissism. Lacan refused to allow psychoanalysis to deny itself. On the ethical, clinical and political levels, whatever the theoretical and temporal distance that separates them, Freud and Lacan come together. They incarnate, each in their own way and with the same creative power, the desire of the analyst.

Notes

1 Sigmund Freud, 'Analysis Terminable and Interminable' (1937), *Standard Edition*, vol. 23, pp. 216–253.
2 Siegfried Bernfeld, 'On Psychoanalytic Training', *Psychoanalytic Quarterly*, No. 31 (1962), 466.
3 *Ibid.*, 463.

Bibliography

All references to the writings of Sigmund Freud are, unless otherwise indicated, to the following edition: Sigmund Freud, *The Standard Edition of the Complete Psychological Works of Sigmund Freud*, trans. James Strachey, Alix Strachey and Alan Tyson (London: Vintage, 2001).

Books

Franz Alexander and Hugo Staub, *The Criminal, the Judge and the Public: A Psychological Analysis* (London: George Allen & Unwin, 1931).

Lou Andreas-Salomé and Anna Freud, *À l'ombre du père: Correspondance, 1919–1937* (Paris: Fayard, 2006).

Bertolt Brecht, *Fear and Misery of the Third Reich* (London: Bloomsbury, 2006).

Karen Brecht, Volker Friedrich, Ludger Hermanns, Isidor J. Kaminer, and Dierk H. Juelich (eds.), *Ici, la vie continue d'une manière fort surprenante…, Contribution à l'Histoire de la Psychanalyse en Allemagne*, text established by Alain Mijolla and Vera Renz (Paris: International Psychoanalytic Association, 1987). Originally published as: *Hier geht das Leben auf eine sehr merkwürdige Weise weiter…, Zur Geschichte der Psychoanalyse in Deutschland* (Hamburg, 1985).

Jacquy Chemouni, *La psychanalyse française captive du politique* (Paris: Beauchesne, 2010).

Geoffrey Cocks, *Psychotherapy in the Third Reich: The Göring Institute* (Oxford: Oxford University Press, 1985).

Fanny Colonomos (ed.), *On forme des psychanalystes: Rapport original sur les dix ans de l'Institut Psychanalytique de Berlin, 1920–1930* (Paris: Denoël, 1985).

Fanny Colonomos and Elisabeth Marsault, *Comme des jongleurs insensibles: Les psychanalystes allemands et la montée du nazisme* (Paris: Frénésie, 1988).

Elizabeth Ann Danto, *Freud's Free Clinics: Psychoanalysis and Social Justice, 1918–1938* (New York: Columbia University Press, 2005).

Mark Edmundson, *The Death of Sigmund Freud* (London: Bloomsbury, 2007).

Kurt R. Eissler, *Freud as an Expert Witness: The Discussion of War Neuroses Between Freud and Wagner-Jauregg* (Madison, CT: International Universities Press, 1986).

Henri-Frédéric Ellenberger, *À la découverte de l'inconscient* (Villeurbane: Simep, 1974).

Ernst Falzeder (ed.), *The Complete Correspondence of Sigmund Freud and Karl Abraham, 1907–1925* (London and New York: Karnac, 2002).

Ernst Falzeder and Eva Brabant (eds.), *The Correspondence of Sigmund Freud and Sándor Ferenczi, Volume 3, 1920–1933*, trans. Peter T. Hoffer (Cambridge, MA: Harvard University Press, 2001).
Hanna Fenichel and David Rapaport (eds.), *The Collected Papers of Otto Fenichel: First Series* (London: Routledge & Kegan Paul, 1954).
Hanna Fenichel and David Rapaport (eds.), *The Collected Papers of Otto Fenichel: Second Series* (London: Routledge & Kegan Paul, 1954).
Otto Fenichel, *The Psychoanalytic Theory of Neurosis* (Abingdon: Routledge, 1996).
Sándor Ferenczi, *Psychanalyse 3, Oeuvres completes, 1919–1926* (Paris: Payot, 1982).
Sándor Ferenczi, *Psychanalyse 4, Oeuvres completes, 1927–1933* (Paris: Payot, 1982).
Saul Friedländer, *Nazi Germany and the Jews, Volume 1: The Years of Persecution, 1933–1939* (New York: HarperCollins, 1997).
Erich Fromm, *Sigmund Freud's Mission* (London: George Allen & Unwin, 1959).
Peter Gay, *Weimar Culture: The Outsider as Insider* (London: Martin Secker & Warburg, 1969).
Phyllis Grosskurth, *Melanie Klein: Her World and Her Work* (London: Hodder & Stoughton, 1986).
Russell Jacoby, *The Repression of Psychoanalysis: Otto Fenichel and the Political Freudians* (Chicago: University of Chicago Press, 1986).
Eberhard Jäckel, *Hitler idéologue* (Paris: Gallimard, 1995).
Ernest Jones (ed.), *Psychoanalysis and the War Neuroses*, vol. 2 (London: International Psychoanalytical Press, 1921).
Ernest Jones, *Sigmund Freud: Life and Work, The Young Freud, 1856–1900*, vol. 1 (London: The Hogarth Press, 1956).
Ernest Jones, *Sigmund Freud: Life and Work, Years of Maturity, 1901–1919*, vol. 2 (London: The Hogarth Press, 1955).
Ernest Jones, *Sigmund Freud: Life and Work, The Last Phase, 1919–1939*, vol. 3 (London: The Hogarth Press, 1957).
Ian Kershaw, *Hitler* (London: Longman, 1991).
Werner Kindt (ed.), *Dokumentation der Jugendbewegung: Grundschriften der deutschen Jugendbewegung*, vol. 1 (Düsseldorf and Cologne: Eugen Diederichs Verlag, 1963).
Jacques Lacan, *Écrits: The First Complete Edition in English*, trans. Bruce Fink (New York and London: Norton, 2006).
Jacques Lacan, *The Seminar of Jacques Lacan, Book I: Freud's Papers on Technique (1953–1954)*, trans. John Forrester (New York and London: Norton, 1991).
Jacques Lacan, *The Seminar of Jacques Lacan, Book X: Anxiety*, trans. A. R. Price (Cambridge: Polity, 2014).
Jacques Lacan, *The Seminar of Jacques Lacan, Book XI: The Four Fundamental Concepts of Psychoanalysis*, trans. Alan Sheridan (London: Penguin, 1978).
Jacques Lacan, *The Seminar of Jacques Lacan, Book XVII: The Other Side of Psychoanalysis*, trans. Russell Grigg (New York and London: Norton, 2007).
Jacques Lacan, *Talking to Brick Walls: A Series of Presentations in the Chapel at Sainte-Anne Hospital* (Cambridge: Polity, 2017).
Walter Laqueur, *Weimar: A Cultural History, 1918–1933* (London: Weidenfeld and Nicolson, 1974).
Gustave Le Bon, *The Crowd* (New York: Dover Books, 2003).
Brenda Maddox, *Freud's Wizard: Ernest Jones and the Transformation of Psychoanalysis* (London: John Murray, 2006).

Perry Meisel and Walter Kendrick (eds.), *Bloomsbury/Freud: The Letters of James and Alix Strachey, 1924–1925* (London: Chatto & Windus, 1986).
Stéphane Michaud (ed.), *Correspondances de Freud* (Paris: Presse de la Sorbonne Nouvelle, 2007).
Jacques-Alain Miller (ed.), *Le Transfert négatif* (Paris: Seuil, 2005).
R. Andrew Paskauskas (ed.), *The Complete Correspondence of Sigmund Freud and Ernest Jones, 1908–1939* (Cambridge, MA: The Belknap Press of Harvard University Press, 1993).
Ernst Pfeiffer (ed.), *Sigmund Freud and Lou Andreas-Salomé: Letters*, trans. William Robson Scott and Elaine Robson Scott (London: The Hogarth Press, 1972).
Jacqueline Poulain-Colombier and Philippe Christophe (eds.), *Le Patient de la psychanalyse* (Paris: L'Harmattan, 2007).
Wilhelm Reich, *Character Analysis*, trans. Theodore P. Wolfe (New York: Noonday Press, 1963).
Wilhelm Reich, *The Function of the Orgasm*, trans. Vincent R. Carfagno (London: Souvenir Press, 1983).
Wilhelm Reich, *The Invasion of Compulsory Sex-Morality* (New York: Farrar, Straus and Giroux, 1971).
Wilhelm Reich, *The Mass Psychology of Fascism*, trans. Vincent R. Carfagno (Harmondsworth: Penguin Books, 1975).
Wilhelm Reich, *Reich Speaks of Freud* (Harmondsworth: Penguin Books, 1975).
Max Schur, *Freud: Living and Dying* (New York: International Universities Press, 1972).
Moustapha Safouan, *Jacques Lacan and the Question of Psychoanalytic Training*, trans. Jacqueline Rose (London: Palgrave Macmillan, 2000).
Michael Schröter (ed.), *Sigmund Freud et Max Eitingon, Correspondance: 1906–1939* (Paris: Fayard, 2009).
Ernst Simmel, *Kriegs-Neurosen und psychisches Trauma* (Munich and Leipzig: Otto Nemnich, 1918).
Richard Sterba, *Reminiscences of a Viennese Psychoanalyst* (Detroit, MI: Wayne State University Press, 1983).
Helmut Thoma and Horst Kachele, *Psychoanalytic Practice* (Berlin, Heidelberg and New York: Springer-Verlag, 1987).
Héléna Besserman Vianna, *Politique de la psychanalyse face à la didactique et à la torture* (Paris: L'Harmattan, 1997).
Eli Zaretsky, *Secrets of the Soul: A Social and Cultural History of Psychoanalysis* (New York: Vintage, 2005).
Stefan Zweig, *The World of Yesterday: Memoirs of a European*, trans. Anthea Bell (London: Pushkin Press, 2011).

Articles and essays

Karl Abraham, 'Character-Formation on the Genital Level of Libido-Development' (1926), *International Journal of Psychoanalysis*, vol. 7 (1926).
Karl Abraham, 'Contribution to the Symposium on Psychoanalysis and the War Neurosis Held at the Fifth International Psychoanalytical Congress in Budapest' (1918), *The International Psychoanalytical Library*, vol. 2 (1921).
Karl Abraham, 'The Influence of Oral Erotism on Character-Formation' (1925), *International Journal of Psychoanalysis*, vol. 6 (1925).

Franz Alexander, 'Le cursus théorique' (1930), in Fanny Colonomos (ed.), *On forme des psychanalystes: Rapport original sur les dix ans de l'Institut psychanalytique de Berlin, 1920–1930* (Paris: Denoël, 1985).

Anna M. Antonovsky, 'Des analystes aryens dans l'Allemagne nazie: les questions de l'adaptation, de désymbolisation et de trahison', *Revue Française de Psychanalyse*, 72. 4 (2008).

Hannah Arendt, 'The Image of Hell' (1946), in Hannah Arendt, *Essays in Understanding, 1930–1954: Formation, Exile, and Totalitarianism* (New York: Schocken, 2005).

Hannah Arendt, 'What is Authority?' (1954), in Hannah Arendt, *The Portable Hannah Arendt* (New York: Penguin, 2000).

Siegfried Bernfeld, 'La discussion communiste sur la psychanalyse et la réfutation de l'hypothèse de l'instinct de mort par Reich' (1932), *Partisans*, no. 66–67 (July/October, 1972).

Siegfried Bernfeld, 'On Psychoanalytic Training', *Psychoanalytic Quarterly*, no. 31 (1962).

Felix Boehm, 'Anthropophagy: Its Forms and Motifs' (1935), *The International Journal of Psychoanalysis*, no. 16 (1935).

Felix Boehm, 'Report on the Events from 1933 to the Amsterdam Congress in 1951', *Archives of the London Institute of Psychoanalysis.*

Geoffrey Cocks, 'Continuity and Development of Psychoanalysis and Psychotherapy in Germany Since 1939', *International Review of Psychoanalysis*, no. 1 (1988).

Max Eitingon, 'Allocution prononcée le 30 Septembre 1928 lors de l'inauguration des nouveaux locaux de l'Institut', in Fanny Colonomos (ed.), *On forme des psychanalystes: Rapport original sur les dix ans de l'Institut psychanalytique de Berlin, 1920–1930* (Paris: Denoël, 1985).

Max Eitingon, 'Max Eitingon: des premiers temps de la psychanalyse (Document I)', in Michael Schröter (ed.), *Sigmund Freud et Max Eitingon: Correspondance, 1906–1939* (Paris: Fayard, 2009).

Max Eitingon, 'Report on the Berlin Psychoanalytical Polyclinic (March 1920–June 1922)', *Bulletin of the International Psychoanalytical Association*, no. 4 (1923).

Otto Fenichel, 'Concerning the Theory of Psychoanalytic Technique', in *Collected Papers: First Series* (London: Routledge & Kegan Paul, 1954).

Otto Fenichel, 'Rapport statistique sur l'activité thérapeutique entre 1920 et 1930' (1930), in Fanny Colonomos (ed.), *On forme des psychanalystes: Rapport original sur les dix ans de l'Institut Psychanalytique de Berlin, 1920–1930* (Paris: Denoël, 1985).

Sándor Ferenczi, 'Élasticité de la technique psychanalytique' (1928), in Sándor Ferenczi, *Psychanalyse 4, Oeuvres completes, 1927–1933* (Paris: Payot, 1982).

Sándor Ferenczi, 'Technical Difficulties in an Analysis of Hysteria' (1919), in Sándor Ferenczi, *Further Contributions to the Theory and Technique of Psychanalysis*, trans. Jane Isabel Suttie (London: Karnac, 1980).

Sándor Ferenczi, 'Psychanalyses des névroses de guerre' (1919), in Sándor Ferenczi, *Psychanalyse 3, Oeuvres completes, 1919–1926* (Paris: Payot, 1982). See also: Sándor Ferenczi, '*Psychoanalysis of War Neurosis*', delivered at the Symposium on Psychoanalysis and the War Neuroses, held at the Fifth International Psychoanalytical Congress, Budapest, September 1918. Published in a collection with Karl Abraham, Ernst Simmel, Ernest Jones and Sigmund Freud, *The International Psychoanalytical Library*, vol. 2 (1921).

Sándor Ferenczi, 'Psychanalyse et politique sociale' (1922), in Sándor Ferenczi, *Psychanalyse 3, Oeuvres completes, 1919–1926* (Paris: Payot, 1982).
Sigmund Freud, 'Character and Anal Erotism' (1908), *Standard Edition*, vol. 9 (London: Vintage, 2001).
Sigmund Freud, 'Civilization and Its Discontents' (1930), *Standard Edition*, vol. 21 (London: Vintage, 2001).
Sigmund Freud, 'The Disposition to Obsessional Neurosis' (1913), *Standard Edition*, vol. 12 (London: Vintage, 2001).
Sigmund Freud, 'The Dissection of the Psychical Personality' (1933), *Standard Edition*, vol. 22 (London: Vintage, 2001).
Sigmund Freud, 'Dr. Anton von Freund' (1920), *Standard Edition*, vol. 18 (London: Vintage, 2001).
Sigmund Freud, 'The Dynamics of Transference' (1912), *Standard Edition*, vol. 12 (London: Vintage, 2001).
Sigmund Freud, 'Fixation to Traumas – The Unconscious' (1917), *Standard Edition*, vol. 16 (London: Vintage, 2001).
Sigmund Freud, 'Freud à propos de Max et Mirra Eitingon (1937), avec commentaires (Document XIII)', in Michael Schröter (ed.), *Sigmund Freud et Max Eitingon, Correspondance: 1906–1939* (Paris: Fayard, 2009).
Sigmund Freud, 'The Future Prospects of Psychoanalytic Therapy' (1910), *Standard Edition*, vol. 11 (London: Vintage, 2001).
Sigmund Freud, 'Group Psychology and the Analysis of the Ego' (1921), *Standard Edition*, vol. 18 (London: Vintage, 2001).
Sigmund Freud, 'Lines of Advance in Psychoanalytic Therapy' (1919) *Standard Edition*, vol. 17 (London: Vintage, 2001).
Sigmund Freud, 'Memorandum on the Electrical Treatment of War Neurotics' (1920), published as an appendix to 'Introduction to Psychoanalysis and the War Neuroses', *Standard Edition*, vol. 17 (London: Vintage, 2001).
Sigmund Freud, 'Moses and Monotheism: Three Essays' (1939), *Standard Edition*, vol. 23 (London: Vintage, 2001).
Sigmund Freud, 'On Beginning the Treatment (Further Recommendations on the Technique of Psychoanalysis)' (1913), *Standard Edition*, vol. 12 (London: Vintage, 2001).
Sigmund Freud, 'On the Teaching of Psychoanalysis in Universities' (1918), *Standard Edition*, vol. 17 (London: Vintage, 2001).
Sigmund Freud, 'Postscript' (1927) to 'The Question of Lay Analysis' (1926), *Standard Edition*, vol. 20 (London: Vintage, 2001).
Sigmund Freud, 'Preface to Max Eitingon's Report on the Berlin Psychoanalytic Polyclinic (March 1920 to June 1922)' (1923), *Standard Edition*, vol. 19 (London: Vintage, 2001).
Sigmund Freud, 'Preface to Ten Years of the Berlin Psychoanalytic Institute' (1930), *Standard Edition*, vol. 21 (London: Vintage, 2001).
Sigmund Freud, 'The Question of Lay Analysis' (1926), *Standard Edition*, vol. 20 (London: Vintage, 2001).
Sigmund Freud, 'The Question of a Weltanschauung' (1933), *Standard Edition*, vol. 22 (London: Vintage, 2001).
Sigmund Freud, 'Recommendations to Physicians Practising Psychoanalysis' (1912), *Standard Edition*, vol. 12 (London: Vintage, 2001).

Sigmund Freud, 'Remembering, Repeating, and Working-Through (Further Recommendations on the Technique of Psychoanalysis, II)' (1914), *Standard Edition*, vol. 12 (London: Vintage, 2001).

Sigmund Freud, 'Some Character-Types met with in Psychoanalytic Work' (1916), *Standard Edition*, vol. 14 (London: Vintage, 2001).

Sigmund Freud, 'Why War?' (1933), *Standard Edition*, vol. 22 (London: Vintage, 2001).

Sigmund Freud, '"Wild" Psychoanalysis' (1910), *Standard Edition*, vol. 11 (London: Vintage, 2001).

Matthias Göring, 'Schlussansprache: Anlässlich des allgemeinen ärztlichen Kongress für Psychotherapie, in Bad Nauheim' (1934), in Karen Brecht, Volker Friedrich, Ludger Hermanns, Isidor J. Kaminer, and Dierk H. Juelich (eds.), *Ici, la vie continue d'une manière fort surprenante…, Contribution à l'Histoire de la Psychanalyse en Allemagne*, text established by Alain Mijolla and Vera Renz (Paris: International Psychoanalytic Association, 1987).

Edith Ludowyk Gyömröi, 'Memories of the German Psychoanalytical Association', *Sigmund Freud Archives* (Washington, DC: Library of Congress).

Karen Horney, 'De l'organisation' (1930), in Fanny Colonomos (ed.), *On forme des psychanalystes: Rapport original sur les dix ans de l'Institut Psychanalytique de Berlin, 1920–1930* (Paris: Denoël, 1985).

Maurice-Moshe Krajzman, 'Max Eitingon, 1881–1943: Construire l'entreprise psychanalytique', *Ornicar?*, no. 48 (1989).

Jacques Lacan, 'British Psychiatry and the War' (1947), *Psychoanalytical Notebooks of the London Society of the New Lacanian School*, no. 33 (2019).

Jacques Lacan, *De la psychose paranoïaque dans ses rapports avec la personnalité* (Paris: Seuil, 1980).

Jacques Lacan, 'Le séminaire de Jacques Lacan' (1975), *Ornicar?*, no. 4 (1975).

Jacques Lacan, 'Science and Truth', in Jacques Lacan, *Écrits: The First Complete Edition in English* (New York and London: Norton, 2006)

Jacques Lacan, 'The Tokyo Discourse', trans. Dany Nobus, *Journal for Lacanian Studies*, vol. 3, no. 1 (London and New York: Karnac, 2005).

Jacques Lacan, 'Variations on the Standard Treatment', in Jacques Lacan, *Écrits: The First Complete Edition in English* (New York and London: Norton, 2006).

Hans Lampl, 'La consultation à la policlinque', in Fanny Colonomos (ed.), *On forme des psychanalystes: Rapport original sur les dix ans de l'Institut psychanalytique de Berlin, 1920–1930* (Paris: Denoël, 1985).

Regine Lockot, 'À propos des changements de nom de l'Association psychanalytique de Berlin', *La Revue lacanienne*, no. 1 (2008).

Olivier Mannoni, 'Freud et Eitingon, les rouages de la machinerie psychanalytique', in Stéphane Michaud (ed.), *Correspondances de Freud* (Paris: Presse de la Sorbonne Nouvelle, 2007).

Carl Müller-Braunschweig, 'Psychanalyse et Weltanschauung' (1933), in Karen Brecht, Volker Friedrich, Ludger Hermanns, Isidor J. Kaminer, and Dierk H. Juelich (eds.), *Ici, la vie continue d'une manière fort surprenante…, Contribution à l'Histoire de la Psychanalyse en Allemagne*, text established by Alain Mijolla and Vera Renz (Paris: International Psychoanalytic Association, 1987).

Gustave Peiser, 'Introduction', in *Berlin entre les deux guerres: une symbiose judéo-allemande? Actes du colloque tenu à l'université Stendhal à Grenoble* (Paris: L'Harmattan, 2000).

Sandór Radó, 'Le cursus pratique', in Fanny Colonomos (ed.), *On forme des psychanalystes: Rapport original sur les dix ans de l'Institut psychanalytique de Berlin, 1920–1930* (Paris: Denoël, 1985).
Klaus Dieter Rath, 'À propos de l'exercice de la psychanalyse en Allemagne', *Journal français de Psychiatrie*, no. 12 (Paris: Érès, 2001).
Wilhelm Reich, 'On the Optimal Conditions for the Analytic Reduction of the Present-Day Material to the Infantile', in Wilhelm Reich, *Character Analysis* (New York: Noonday Press, 1963).
Wilhelm Reich, 'Preface to First Edition' (1933), in Wilhelm Reich, *Character Analysis* (New York: Noonday Press, 1963).
Wilhelm Reich, 'Some Problems of Psychoanalytic Technique' (1933), in Wilhelm Reich, *Character Analysis* (New York: Noonday Press, 1963).
Wilhelm Reich, 'The death instinct', in Wilhelm Reich, *Reich Speaks of Freud* (Harmondsworth: Penguin Books, 1975).
Joseph Roth, 'The Steam Baths at Night', in Joseph Roth, *What I Saw: Reports from Berlin, 1920–1933* (London: Granta, 2011).
Hanns Sachs, 'L'analyse didactique' (1930), in Fanny Colonomos (ed.), *On forme des psychanalystes: Rapport original sur les dix ans de l'Institut psychanalytique de Berlin, 1920–1930* (Paris: Denoël, 1985).
Hanns Sachs, 'The Prospects of Psychoanalysis' (1939), *International Journal of Psychoanalysis*, vol. 20.
Michael Schröter, 'Le Timonier: Max Eitingon et son role dans l'histoire de la psychanalyse', in Michael Schröter (ed.), *Sigmund Freud et Max Eitingon, Correspondance: 1906–1939* (Paris: Fayard, 2009).
Ernst Simmel, 'Sur l'histoire et la signification sociale de l'Institut psychanalytique de Berlin' (1930), in Fanny Colonomos (ed.), *On forme des psychanalystes: Rapport original sur les dix ans de l'Institut psychanalytique de Berlin, 1920–1930* (Paris: Denoël, 1985).
Ernst Simmel, 'L'hôpital psychanalytique et le mouvement psychanalytique' (1937), in Jacqueline Poulain-Colombier and Philippe Christophe (eds.), *Le Patient de la psychanalyse* (Paris: L'Harmattan, 2007).
Laura Sokolowsky, 'La désinsertion de l'Homme aux loups', *La Cause freudienne*, no. 71 (June 2009).
Martin Staemmler, 'Le judaïsme dans la médecine' (1933), in *Ici, la vie continue d'une manière fort surprenante…: Contribution à l'Histoire de la Psychanalyse en Allemagne*, text established by Alain Mijolla and Vera Renz (Paris: International Psychoanalytic Association, 1987).
Richard Sterba, 'Un cas de psychothérapie brève par Sigmund Freud' (1951), in Jacqueline Poulain-Colombier and Philippe Christophe (eds.), *Le Patient de la Psychanalyse* (Paris: L'Harmattan, 2007).
Gregory Zilboorg, 'En Amérique' (1930), in Fanny Colonomos (ed.), *On forme des psychanalystes: Rapport original sur les dix ans de l'Institut Psychanalytique de Berlin, 1920–1930* (Paris: Denoël, 1985).

Index